Textbook of

HUMAN NEUROANATOMY

(Fundamental and Clinical)

Eighth Edition

Textbook of

HUMAN NEUROANATOMY

(Fundamental and Clinical)

Eighth Edition

Inderbir Singh

MS., Ph.D., F. A. M. S.
52, Sector 1, Rohtak 124001
Haryana, India

Jaypee Brothers Medical Publishers (P) Ltd

St Louis (USA) • Panama City (Panama) • New Delhi • Ahmedabad • Bengaluru
Chennai • Hyderabad • Kochi • Kolkata • Lucknow • Mumbai • Nagpur

Published by

Jitendar P Vij

Jaypee Brothers Medical Publishers (P) Ltd

Corporate Office

4838/24 Ansari Road, Daryaganj, **New Delhi** - 110002, India, Phone: +91-11-43574357, Fax: +91-11-43574314

Registered Office

B-3 EMCA House, 23/23B Ansari Road, Daryaganj, **New Delhi** - 110 002, India

Phones: +91-11-23272143, +91-11-23272703, +91-11-23282021, +91-11-23245672, Rel: +91-11-32558559

Fax: +91-11-23276490, +91-11-23245683   e-mail: jaypee@jaypeebrothers.com, Website: www.jaypeebrothers.com

Branches

❑   2/B, Akruti Society, Jodhpur Gam Road Satellite
     Ahmedabad 380 015, Phones: +91-79-26926233   Rel: +91-79-32988717   Fax: +91-79-26927094
     e-mail: ahmedabad@jaypeebrothers.com

❑   202 Batavia Chambers, 8 Kumara Krupa Road, Kumara Park East
     Bengaluru 560 001, Phones: +91-80-22285971, +91-80-22382956, 91-80-22372664 Rel: +91-80-32714073
     Fax: +91-80-22281761,   e-mail: bangalore@jaypeebrothers.com

❑   282 IIIrd Floor, Khaleel Shirazi Estate, Fountain Plaza, Pantheon Road
     Chennai 600 008, Phones: +91-44-28193265, +91-44-28194897 Rel: +91-44-32972089 Fax: +91-44-28193231
     e-mail: chennai@jaypeebrothers.com

❑   4-2-1067/1-3, 1st Floor, Balaji Building, Ramkote Cross Road
     Hyderabad 500 095, Phones: +91-40-66610020, +91-40-24758498 Rel:+91-40-32940929 Fax:+91-40-24758499
     e-mail: hyderabad@jaypeebrothers.com

❑   No. 41/3098, B & B1, Kuruvi Building, St. Vincent Road
     Kochi 682 018, Kerala, Phones: +91-484-4036109, +91-484-2395739, +91-484-2395740
     e-mail: kochi@jaypeebrothers.com

❑   1-A Indian Mirror Street, Wellington Square
     Kolkata 700 013, Phones: +91-33-22651926, +91-33-22276404, +91-33-22276415 Fax: +91-33-22656075,
      e-mail: kolkata@jaypeebrothers.com

❑   Lekhraj Market III, B-2, Sector-4, Faizabad Road, Indira Nagar
     Lucknow 226 016   Phones: +91-522-3040553, +91-522-3040554, e-mail: lucknow@jaypeebrothers.com

❑   106 Amit Industrial Estate, 61 Dr SS Rao Road, Near MGM Hospital, Parel
     Mumbai 400 012, Phones: +91-22-24124863, +91-22-24104532 Rel: +91-22-32926896 Fax: +91-22-24160828
     e-mail: mumbai@jaypeebrothers.com

❑   "KAMALPUSHPA" 38, Reshimbag, Opp. Mohota Science College, Umred Road
     Nagpur 440 009 (MS), Phone: Rel: +91-712-3245220, Fax: +91-712-2704275,
     e-mail: nagpur@jaypeebrothers.com

North America Office
1745, Pheasant Run Drive, Maryland Heights (Missouri), MO 63043, USA Ph: 001-636-6279734
e-mail: jaypee@jaypeebrothers.com, anjulav@jaypeebrothers.com

Central America Office
Jaypee-Highlights Medical Publishers Inc. City of Knowledge, Bld. 237, Clayton, Panama City, Panama
Ph: 507-317-0160

Textbook of Human Neuroanatomy

© 2009, INDERBIR SINGH

This book has been published in good faith that the material provided by author is original. Every effort is made to ensure accuracy of material, but the publisher, printer and author will not be held responsible for any inadvertent error(s). In case of any dispute, all legal matters are to be settled under Delhi jurisdiction only.

First Edition   :   1997
Seventh Edition :   2006
Reprint   :   2008
Eighth Edition   :   2009

ISBN   978-81-8448-703-9

Layout design and composing by the author

Printed at   Ajanta Offset & Packagings Ltd., New Delhi

Preface to the Eighth Edition

I have great pleasure in presenting the **eighth edition** of TEXTBOOK OF HUMAN NEUROANATOMY.

As in previous editions, the main effort has been to present a complicated subject in as simple a manner as possible. The major problem that faces the author of any student textbook is to decide just how much to include out of the limitless volume of information available. Some facts are such that no student can afford to be without them. However, these essentials are often wrapped up in a huge mass of detail which often serves only to obscure the important principles relevant to future clinical studies. It is for this reason that, in this edition, essential matter is clearly demarcated from more advanced detail. Clinical matter is similarly demarcated.

In this edition the book has been given a **strong clinical orientation** which will appeal specially to advanced students.

I am much obliged to Shri Jitendar P. Vij, CMD of Jaypee Brothers for being always extremely helpful and accommodating. His hard work and his pleasant nature make him a delight to work with.

I continue to be obliged to Prof. S.C. Srivastava, and to Dr. R.K. Yadav for very kindly providing a number of photographs.

As always, I am deeply indebted to readers who have sent words of encouragement and suggestions for improvement. I am grateful to all students who have read this book, because without them the book would have no reason to exist.

Rohtak
April 2009   INDERBIR SINGH

Author's address: 52 Sector 1, Rohtak, Haryana, 124001
e-mail: eyebee29@rediffmail.com

Contents

IMPORTANT NOTE

Basic matter that is essential for first professional M.B.B.S students is printed on a white background.

BASIC

Advanced matter is printed on a pink background. This should be read by students who are satisfied about their knowledge of basic matter.

ADVANCED

Sections on CLINICAL matter are printed on a blue background.

CLINICAL

Sections on matter pertaining to development are given on a yellow background.

DEVELOPMENT

1 : Introduction to Neuroanatomy

What is Neuroanatomy?

The human body consists of numerous tissues and organs that are diverse in structure and function. Yet they function together, and in harmony, for the well being of the body as a whole. It is obvious that there has to be some kind of influence that monitors and controls the working of different parts of the body. Although there are other mechanisms that help in such control (e.g. hormones) the overwhelming role in directing the activities of the body rests with the nervous system. Neuroanatomy is the study of the structural aspects of the nervous system. It cannot be emphasised too strongly that the study of structure is meaningless unless correlated with function. Division of a study of the nervous system into neuroanatomy and neurophysiology is only a matter of convenience.

Divisions of the Nervous System

The nervous system may be divided into (a) the *central nervous system*, made up of the brain and spinal cord, and (b) the *peripheral nervous system*, consisting of the peripheral nerves and the ganglia associated with them.

The brain consists of (a) the *cerebrum*, made up of two large cerebral hemispheres, (b) the *cerebellum*, (c) the *midbrain*, (d) the *pons*, and (e) the *medulla oblongata*. The midbrain, pons and medulla together form the *brainstem*. The medulla is continuous, below, with the spinal cord.

Peripheral nerves attached to the brain are called *cranial nerves*; and those attached to the spinal cord are called *spinal nerves*.

The peripheral nerves include those that supply skin, muscles and joints of the body wall and limbs, and those that supply visceral structures e.g., heart, lungs, stomach etc. Each of these sets of peripheral nerves is intimately associated with the brain and spinal cord. The nerves supplying the body wall and limbs are often called *cerebrospinal nerves*. The nerves supplying the viscera, along with the parts of the brain and spinal cord related to them, constitute the *autonomic nervous system*. The autonomic nervous system is subdivided into two major parts: the *sympathetic* and the *parasympathetic* nervous systems.

How neuroanatomy is studied

The study of neuroanatomy begins with the study of those features of the brain and spinal cord (and of the nerves attached to them) that can be seen with the naked eye. This is the study of gross anatomy. It includes the study of the surface features of the brain and spinal cord; and the courses, relations and distribution of peripheral nerves. Some details of the internal structure of the brain and spinal cord can be made out with the naked eye. However, the study of internal structure depends mainly on microscopic examination. Again some details of structure can be made out using ordinary histological methods, but the greater part of the information about the nervous system has been obtained using specialised methods. In recent years such studies have increasingly involved the use of histochemical methods and the study of tissues under the high magnifications possible only with an electron microscope (ultrastructure).

Tissues constituting the nervous system

The nervous system is made up, predominantly, of tissue that has the special property of being able to conduct impulses rapidly from one part of the body to another. The specialised cells that constitute the functional units of the nervous system are called *neurons*. Within the brain and spinal cord neurons are supported by a special kind of connective tissue that is called *neuroglia*. Nervous tissue, composed of neurons and neuroglia, is richly supplied with blood. It has been taught that lymph vessels are not present, but the view has recently been challenged.

The nervous system of man is made up of innumerable neurons. The total number of neurons in the human brain is estimated at more than 10^{12}. The neurons are linked together in a highly intricate manner. It is through these connections that the body is made aware of changes in the environment, or of those within itself; and appropriate responses to such changes are produced e.g., in the form of movement or in the modified working of some organ of the body. The mechanisms for some of these relatively simple functions have come to be known as a result of a vast amount of work done by numerous workers for over a century. There is no doubt that higher functions of the brain, like those of memory and intelligence, are also to be explained on the basis of connections between neurons, but as yet little is known about the mechanisms involved. Neurons are, therefore, to be regarded not merely as simple conductors, but as cells that are specialised for the reception, integration, interpretation and transmission of information.

Nerve cells can convert information obtained from the environment into codes that can be transmitted along their axons. By such coding the same neuron can transmit different kinds of information.

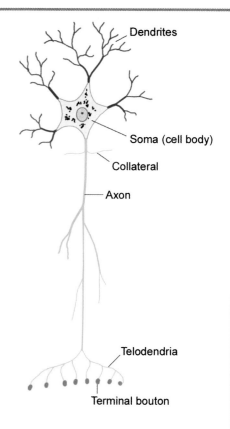

Fig. 1.1. Diagram showing the main parts of a typical neuron.

How the Nervous system can be affected by disease

Some knowledge of anatomy is an essential prerequisite for the practice of any clinical discipline, but no where is this more true than in the diagnosis of neurological disorders. The localisation of the areas of the nervous system involved in disease calls for a fairly thorough knowledge of the location of various masses of grey matter, and of the courses of various tracts. The purpose of this chapter is to provide some illustrations of how a knowledge of neuroanatomy can be of help in neurological diagnosis; and to introduce some terms that are commonly used in clinical practice.

In recent years, considerable advances in neurological diagnosis have become possible by the use of sophisticated imaging techniques like computed tomography (CT), and magnetic resonance imaging (MRI). In interpreting these images a thorough knowledge of the gross anatomy of the head, neck and brain (or of other regions concerned) is invaluable.

Damage to nervous tissue can occur in various ways. Any part of the brain or spinal cord may be damaged by direct injury (*trauma*). Apart from other obvious causes such injury may occur during child birth. If nervous tissue is deprived of blood even for a short period irreversible damage may result. Localised damage of this kind may occur if one of the arteries supplying the brain is blocked. This may occur by clotting of blood within the vessel (*thrombosis*). Such an event is more likely in older individuals in whom the arteries have undergone a degenerative change known as *arteriosclerosis.* A vessel can also be blocked by some extraneous material (e.g., clot, fat, air) reaching it from some other part of the body through the circulation. Such matter is called an *embolus.* Sometimes an artery may rupture, the blood leaking into brain tissue (*haemorrhage*) causing considerable damage. A haemorrhage in the brain is often fatal. Bleeding may be caused by rupture of small abnormal dilatations of arteries (*aneurysms*). Aneurysms may be congenital, or may be produced due to weakening of the arterial wall in the region.

Another cause of brain damage is the presence of any abnormal mass within the cranial cavity. As the cranial cavity cannot expand such a mass inevitably presses on brain tissue. Such a *space occupying lesion* may be a tumour, a collection of pus, a collection of blood (in the epidural space) etc. Apart from producing general signs of increased intracranial tension, local effects are produced depending on the area involved.

Increased intracranial tension, specially when it is rapid in progression, can lead to further brain damage in a number of ways. Swelling of the brain (*cerebral oedema*) following trauma, or infection, can itself act like a space occupying lesion. Brain tissue is pressed against the wall of the cranial cavity leading to damage. Part of the brain may herniate through a wound in the skull.

As pressure on a region of brain tissue increases it can lead to occlusion of blood vessels and infarctions. When intracranial pressure increases to the level of arterial pressure blood flow ceases and brain death ensues.

Nervous tissue may be affected by infections, both acute and chronic. An infection in the brain is referred to as *encephalitis*; and that in the spinal cord is called *myelitis.* Defects in neural tissue may also be caused by *maldevelopment* (congenital anomalies), by *degeneration* in old age, and by various *metabolic disorders.* Finally, alterations in nervous function may occur in the absence of recognisable structural changes. These are called *functional disorders.*

From the above it will be obvious that in some cases a neurological disorder will be of acute onset (as in trauma, vascular accidents, or acute infections). In such cases the patient may at first show signs indicative of widespread functional deficit quite out of proportion to the actual area involved. Deep unconsciousness (*coma*) is often present. In course of time, however, considerable recovery may take place, leaving residual defects dependent upon the area involved. In slowly developing diseases on the other hand, considerable structural damage may occur before symptoms become obvious. In the descriptions that follow we will deal only with signs and symptoms referable to the actual area of lesion.

CLINICAL

Neuron Structure

Elementary Structure of a Typical Neuron

Neurons vary considerably in size, shape and other features. However, most of them have some major features in common and these are described below (Figs. 1.1 to 1.4).

A neuron consists of a *cell body* that gives off a number of *processes*. The cell body is also called the soma or *perikaryon*. Like a typical cell it consists of a mass of cytoplasm surrounded by a cell membrane. The cytoplasm contains a large central nucleus (usually with a prominent nucleolus), numerous mitochondria, lysosomes and a Golgi complex (Fig. 1.2). In the past it has often been stated that centrioles are not present in neurons, but studies with the electron microscope (usually abbreviated to EM) have shown that centrioles are present. In addition to these features, the cytoplasm of a neuron has some distinctive characteristics not seen in other cells. The cytoplasm shows the presence of a granular material that stains intensely with basic dyes; this material is the *Nissl substance* (also called Nissl bodies or granules) (Fig. 1.3). When examined with the EM, these bodies are seen to be composed of rough surfaced endoplasmic reticulum (Fig 1.2). The presence of abundant granular endoplasmic reticulum is an indication of the high level of protein synthesis in neurons. The proteins are needed for maintenance and repair, and for production of neurotransmitters and enzymes.

Another distinctive feature of neurons is the presence of a network of fibrils permeating the cytoplasm (Fig. 1.4). These *neurofibrils* are seen, with the EM, to consist of microfilaments and microtubules. (The centrioles present in neurons may be concerned with the production and maintenance of microtubules).

BASIC

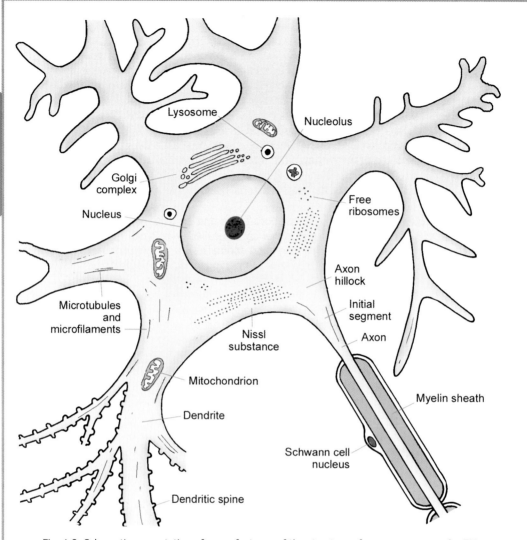

Fig. 1.2. Schematic presentation of some features of the structure of a neuron as seen by EM.

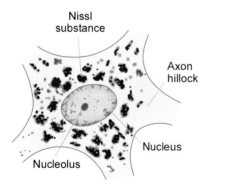

Fig. 1.3. Neuron stained to show Nissl substance. Note that the Nissl substance is not present in the axon (a) and in the region of the axon hillock (ah)

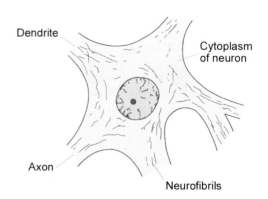

Fig. 1.4. Neuron stained to show neurofibrils. Note that the fibrils extend into both axons and dendrites.

Some neurons contain pigment granules (e.g., neuromelanin in neurons of the substantia nigra). Ageing neurons contain a pigment lipofuscin (made up of residual bodies derived from lysosomes).

The processes arising from the cell body of a neuron are called **neurites**. These are of two kinds. Most neurons give off a number of short branching processes called **dendrites** and one longer process called an **axon**.

The dendrites are characterised by the fact that they terminate near the cell body. They are irregular in thickness, and Nissl granules extend into them. They bear numerous small spines that are of variable shape.

The axon may extend for a considerable distance away from the cell body. The longest axons may be as much as a metre long. Each axon has a uniform diameter, and is devoid of Nissl substance.

In addition to these differences in structure, there is a fundamental functional difference between dendrites and axons. In a dendrite, the nerve impulse **travels towards the cell body** whereas in an axon the impulse travels **away from the cell body**.

We have seen above that the axon is free of Nissl granules. The Nissl-free zone extends for a short distance into the cell body: this part of the cell body is called the **axon hillock**. The part of the axon just beyond the axon hillock is called the **initial segment** (Fig. 1.2).

During its formation each axon comes to be associated with certain cells that provide a sheath for it. The cells providing this sheath for axons lying outside the central nervous system are called **Schwann cells**. Axons lying within the central nervous system are provided a similar covering by a kind of neuroglial cell called an **oligodendrocyte**. The nature of this sheath is best understood by considering the mode of its formation (Fig. 1.5). An axon lying near a Schwann cell (1) invaginates into the cytoplasm of the Schwann cell (2,3). In this process the axon comes to be suspended by a fold of the cell membrane of the Schwann cell: this fold is called the **mesaxon** (3). In some situations the mesaxon becomes greatly elongated and comes to be spirally wound around the axon, which is thus surrounded by several layers of cell membrane (4,5). Lipids are deposited between adjacent layers of the membrane. These layers of the mesaxon, along with the lipids, form the **myelin sheath**. Outside the myelin sheath a thin layer of Schwann cell cytoplasm persists to form an additional sheath which is called the **neurilemma** (also called the neurilemmal sheath or Schwann cell sheath). Axons having

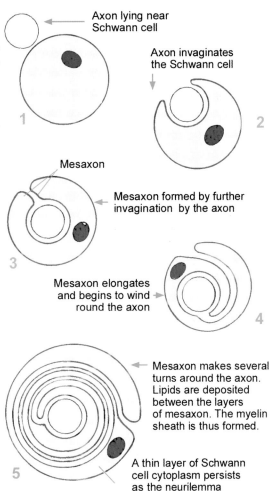

Fig. 1.5. Stages in the formation of the myelin sheath by a Schwann cell. The axon which first lies near the Schwann cell (1), invaginates into its cytoplasm (2,3), and comes to be suspended by a mesaxon. The mesaxon elongates and comes to be spirally wound around the axon (4,5). Lipids are deposited between the layers of the masaxon.

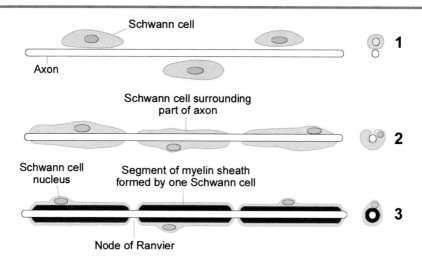

Fig. 1.6. Scheme to show that each Schwann cell forms a short segment of the myelin sheath. The small figures at the extreme right are transverse sections through the nerve fibre, at the corresponding stages.

a myelin sheath are called **myelinated axons**. The presence of a myelin sheath increases the velocity of conduction (for a nerve fibre of the same diameter). It also reduces the energy expended in the process of conduction.

An axon is related to a large number of Schwann cells over its length (Fig. 1.6). Each Schwann cell provides the myelin sheath for a short segment of the axon. At the junction of any two such segments there is a short gap in the myelin sheath. These gaps are called the **nodes of Ranvier**.

There are some axons that are devoid of myelin sheaths. These **unmyelinated axons** invaginate into the cytoplasm of Schwann cells, but the mesaxon does not spiral around them (Fig. 1.7). Another difference is that several such axons may invaginate into the cytoplasm of a single Schwann cell.

An axon may give off a variable number of branches (Fig. 1.1). Some branches, that arise near the cell body and lie at right angles to the axon are called **collaterals**. At its termination the axon breaks up into a number of fine branches called **telodendria** that may end in small swellings (**terminal boutons** or **bouton terminaux**). An axon (or its branches) can terminate in two ways. Within the central nervous system, it always terminates by coming in intimate relationship with another neuron, the junction between the two neurons being called a synapse (page 10). Outside the central nervous system, the axon may end in relation to an effector organ (e.g., muscle or gland), or may end by synapsing with neurons in a peripheral ganglion.

Axons (and some dendrites that resemble axons in structure: see below) constitute what are commonly called **nerve fibres**.

Grey and White Matter

Sections through the spinal cord or through any part of the brain show certain regions that appear whitish, and others that have a darker greyish colour. These constitute the **white and grey matter**

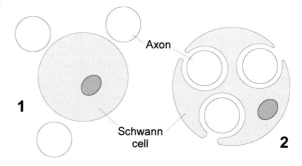

Fig. 1.7. Relationship of unmyelinated axons to a Schwann cell.

respectively. Microscopic examination shows that the cell bodies of neurons are located only in grey matter that also contains dendrites and axons starting from or ending on the cell bodies. Most of the fibres within the grey matter are unmyelinated. On the other hand the white matter consists predominantly of myelinated fibres. It is the reflection of light by myelin that gives this region its whitish appearance. Neuroglia and blood vessels are present in both grey and white matter.

The arrangement of the grey and white matter differs at different situations in the brain and spinal cord. In the spinal cord and brainstem the white matter is on the outside whereas the grey matter forms one or more masses embedded within the white matter (Fig. 2.1). In the cerebrum and cerebellum there is an extensive, but thin, layer of grey matter on the surface. This layer is called the **cortex**. Deep to the cortex there is white matter, but within the latter several isolated masses of grey matter are present (Fig. 8.9). Such isolated masses of grey matter present anywhere in the central nervous system are referred to as **nuclei**. As grey matter is made of cell bodies of neurons (and the processes arising from or terminating on them) nuclei can be defined as groups of cell bodies of neurons. Aggregations of the cell bodies of neurons may also be found outside the central nervous system. Such aggregations are referred to as **ganglia**. Some neurons are located in **nerve plexuses** present in close relationship to some viscera. These are, therefore, referred to as **ganglionated plexuses**.

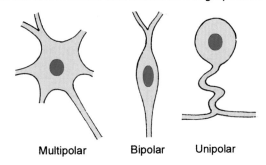

Multipolar   Bipolar   Unipolar

Fig. 1.8. Multipolar, bipolar and unipolar neurons.

The axons arising in one mass of grey matter terminate very frequently by synapsing with neurons in other masses of grey matter. The axons connecting two (or more) masses of grey matter are frequently numerous enough to form recognisable bundles. Such aggregations of fibres are called **tracts**. Larger collections of fibres are also referred to as **funiculi, fasciculi** or **lemnisci**. (A lemniscus is a ribbon like band). Large bundles of fibres connecting the cerebral or cerebellar hemispheres to the brainstem are called **peduncles**.

Aggregations of processes of neurons outside the central nervous system constitute **peripheral nerves**.

Neuropil

Many regions of the brain and spinal cord are occupied by a complex meshwork of axon terminals, dendrites and processes of neuroglial cells. This meshwork is called the neuropil.

Variability in Neuron Structure

Variation in the shape of neuronal cell bodies

Neurons vary considerably in the size and shape of their cell bodies (somata) and in the length and manner of branching of their processes. The cell body varies in diameter from about 5 µm, in the smallest neurons, to as much as 120 µm in the largest ones. The shape of the cell body is dependent on the number of processes arising from it. The most common type of neuron gives off several processes and the cell body is, therefore, **multipolar** (Fig. 1.8). Some neurons have only one axon and one dendrite and are **bipolar**.

Another type of neuron has a single process (which is highly convoluted). After a very short course this process divides into two. One of the divisions represents the axon; the other is functionally a dendrite, but its structure is indistinguishable from that of an axon. This neuron is described as **unipolar**, but from a functional point of view it is to be regarded as bipolar. (To avoid confusion on this account this kind of neuron has been referred to, in the past, as a *pseudounipolar* neuron but this term has now been discarded). Depending on the shapes of their cell bodies some neurons are referred to as *stellate* (star shaped) or *pyramidal*.

In addition to the variations in size and shape, the cell bodies of neurons may show striking variations in the appearance of the Nissl substance. In some neurons, the Nissl substance is very prominent and is in the form of large clumps. In some others, the granules are fine and uniformly distributed in the cytoplasm, while yet other neurons show gradations between these extremes. These differences are correlated with function.

Variations in axons

The length of the axon arising from the cell body of a neuron is also subject to considerable variability. Some neurons have long axons, and connect remote regions. These are called *Golgi type I* neurons. In other neurons axons are short and end near the cell body. They are called *Golgi type II* neurons or *microneurons*: these are often inhibitory in function. Very rarely, a neuron may not have a true axon.

As stated earlier, axons also differ in the nature of the sheaths covering them, some of them being myelinated and others unmyelinated. Axons also show considerable variation in the diameter of their cross sections.

Variations in dendrites

Dendrites arising from a neuronal cell body vary considerably in number, and in the extent and manner of branching. They also differ in the distribution of spines on them. These characteristics are of functional importance. The *area* occupied by the dendrites of a neuron is referred to as its *dendritic field*. Different kinds of neurons have differing dendritic fields (See page 9).

Neurons also show considerable variation in the number and nature of synapses established by them.

FURTHER DETAILS ABOUT NEURONS

Axon hillock and initial segment:

The axon hillock and the initial segment of the axon are of special functional significance. This is the region where action potentials are generated (spike generation) resulting in conduction along the axon. The initial segment is unmyelinated. It often receives axo-axonal synapses that are inhibitory. The plasma membrane here is rich in voltage sensitive channels.

Axoplasmic flow:

The cytoplasm of neurons is in constant motion. Movement of various materials occurs through axons. This *axoplasmic flow* takes place both away from and towards the cell body. The flow away from the cell body is greater. Some materials travel slowly (0.1 to 2 mm a day) constituting a *slow transport*. In contrast other materials (mainly in the form of vesicles) travel 100 to 400 mm a day constituting a *rapid transport*.

Slow transport is unidirectional, away from the cell body. It is responsible for flow of axoplasm (containing various proteins) down the axon. Rapid transport is bi-directional and carries vesicular material and mitochondria. Microtubules play an important role in this form of transport. Retrograde axoplasmic flow may carry neurotropic viruses (see below) along the axon into the neuronal cell body.

Axoplasmic transport of tracer substances introduced experimentally can help to trace neuronal connections.

Role of axoplasmic transport in spread of disease

Some infections that affect the nervous system travel along nerves.

(a) Rabies is a disease (often fatal) caused by a bite of a rabid dog (and some other animals including monkeys). The saliva of an infected animal contains the rabies virus. The virus travels from the site of the bite to the central nervous system, along nerves, by reverse axoplasmic flow and causes infection there. As this means of transport is slow there is a delay of a few days between the bite and appearance of symptoms. The duration of this delay depends on the length of the nerve fibres concerned. A bite on the face produces symptoms much faster than one on the foot.

(b) The virus of poliomyelitis is also transported (from the gastrointestinal tract) to the nervous system through reverse axoplasmic flow.

(c) In contrast tetanus travels from the site of infection to the brain through spaces in the endoneurium of nerve fibres.

CLINICAL

Some features of dendrites

(a) Dendrites can be distinguished immuno-cytochemically from axons because of the presence in them of microtubule associated protein MAP-2 not present in axons.

(b) Dendritic spines vary in size and shape. Some spines contain aggregations of smooth endoplasmic reticulum (in the form of flattened cisternae with associated dense material). The complex is referred to as the ***spine apparatus***.

(c) Actin filaments are present in dendritic spines.

(d) Some variations in the dendritic field are as follows. The field may be ***spherical*** (as in stellate cells), ***hemispherical, disc-like, conical*** or ***flat***. In some neurons (e.g., pyramidal), the neuron may have two separate dendritic fields. Apart from shape there is considerable variability in *extent* of the dendritic field. Some neurons (e.g., Golgi neurons of the cerebellum) have dendritic fields covering a very wide area. More than eighty per cent of the neuronal surface area (excluding the axon) may be situated on the dendritic tree. The frequency of branching of dendrites is correlated with the number of synapses on them. In some neurons the dendritic spines may number several thousand. Finally, it may be emphasised that the dendritic tree is not a 'fixed' entity, but may undergo continuous remodelling. This affords a basis for modification of neuronal behaviour.

ADVANCED

Sex chromatin in neurons

Each cell of a human male has 44+X+Y chromosomes; and each cell of a female has 44+X+X chromosomes. Of the two X-chromosomes in a female only one is functionally active. The other (inactive) X-chromosome forms a mass of dark staining hetero-chromatin that can be identified in suitable preparations and can be useful in determining whether a particular tissue belongs to a male or a female. Because of this association with sex this mass of hetero-chromatin is called the ***sex chromatin***. It is also called a ***Barr body*** after the name of the scientist who discovered it. In most cells the sex chromatin lies just under the nuclear membrane (Fig. 1.9). In some cells the sex chromatin occupies a different position from that described above. In neurons it forms a rounded mass lying very close to the nucleolus and is, therefore, called a ***nucleolar satellite***. In neutrophil leucocytes it may appear as an isolated round mass attached to the rest of the nucleus by a narrow band, thus resembling the appearance of a ***drumstick***.

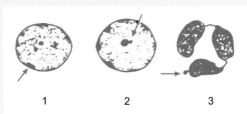

1 2 3

Fig. 1.9. Sex chromatin. 1 – Typical position deep to nuclear membrane. 2 – As a nucleolar satellite in a neuron. 3 – As a drumstick in a neutrophil leucocyte.

The Synapse

We have seen that synapses are sites of junction between neurons. Synapses may be of various types depending upon the parts of the neurons that come in contact. In the most common type of synapse, an axon terminal establishes contact with the dendrite of a receiving neuron to form an **axodendritic synapse**. Synapses on dendrites may be located on spines or on the smooth areas between spines. The axon terminal may synapse with the cell body (**axosomatic synapse**) or, less commonly, with the axon of the receiving neuron (**axoaxonal synapse**). An axoaxonal synapse may be located either on the initial segment (of the receiving axon) or just proximal to an axon terminal.

In some parts of the brain (e.g., the thalamus) we see some synapses in which the presynaptic element is a dendrite instead of an axon. Such synapses may be **dendro-axonic** or **dendro-dendritic**. In yet others the soma of a neuron may synapse with the soma of another neuron (**somato-somatic** synapse), or with a dendrite (**somato-dendritic** synapse).

The axon may terminate in a single bulb-like end called a **bouton** (or **synaptic bag**). Alternatively, the terminal part of the axon may bear a number of such enlargements each of which synapses with the receiving neuron. We have seen that dendrites bear numerous spines. Axon terminals may synapse either with the spines or with smooth portions of the dendrite between the spines. Occasionally, an axon terminal may end by synapsing with the terminal bouton of another axon forming what is called a **serial synapse**. In certain situations several neurons may take part in forming complex synapses. Such areas, encapsulated by neuroglial cells, form **synaptic glomeruli**. Such glomeruli are found in the cerebellum, the olfactory bulb, the lateral geniculate body and in some other situations.

At some sites several synapses may be present around a short length of a dendrite and may be enclosed within a glial capsule. Such a complex is called a **synaptic cartridge**.

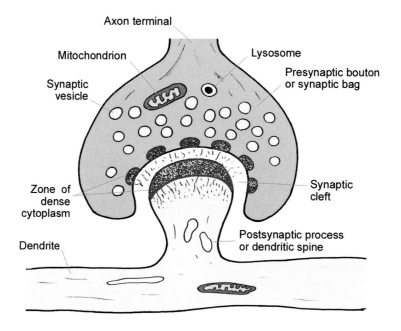

Fig. 1.10. Scheme showing the structure of a typical synapse
as seen by EM.

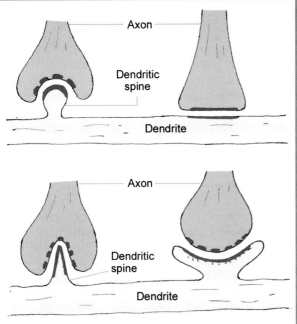

Fig. 1.11. Some variations in the orientation of axodendritic synapses

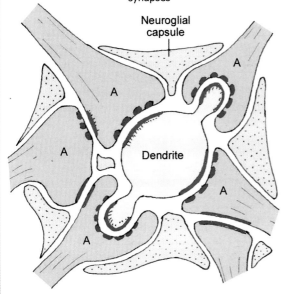

Fig. 1.12. Diagram to show a synaptic glomerulus.

A synapse transmits an impulse only in one direction. The two elements taking part in a synapse can, therefore, be spoken of as *presynaptic* and *postsynaptic* (Fig. 1.10). In an axo-dendritic synapse, the terminal enlargement of the axon may be referred to as the *presynaptic bouton* or *synaptic bag*. The region of the dendrite receiving the axon terminal is the *postsynaptic process*. The two are separated by a space called the *synaptic cleft*. Delicate fibres or granular material may be seen within the cleft. On either side of the cleft there is a region of dense cytoplasm. On the presynaptic side this dense cytoplasm is broken up into several bits. On the postsynaptic side the dense cytoplasm is continuous and is associated with a meshwork of filaments called the *synaptic web*.

The thickened areas of membrane on the presynaptic and postsynaptic sides constitute the *active zone* of a synapse. Neuro-transmission takes place through this region. Some variations in the structure of the active zone are described below.

Within the presynaptic bouton numerous synaptic vesicles can be seen. Mitochondria and lysosomes may also be present. The presynaptic bouton contains numerous microtubules (that extend into it from the axon). The tubules end near the presynaptic membrane. Synaptic vesicles are attached to the microtubules by short stalks. The postsynaptic process may also show membranous structures of various shapes, microtubules, filaments and endoplasmic reticulum.

Various proteins and enzymes are present in relation to presynaptic and postsynaptic regions. Some of them (F-actin, spectrin) form a filamentous network that immobilises vesicles until they are to be released.

Neurotransmitters

The transmission of impulses through synapses involves the release of chemical substances called *neurotransmitters* that are present within synaptic vesicles. When a nerve impulse reaches a terminal bouton neurotransmitter is released into the synaptic cleft. Under the influence of the neurotransmitter the postsynaptic surface becomes depolarised resulting in a nerve impulse in the postsynaptic neuron. In the case of inhibitory synapses, the presence of the neurotransmitter causes hyperpolarisation of the postsynaptic membrane. The neurotransmitter released into the synaptic cleft acts only for a very short duration. It is either destroyed (by enzymes) or is withdrawn into the terminal bouton.

When an action potential reaches the presynaptic terminal, voltage sensitive calcium channels are opened up so that there is an influx of calcium ions leading to a series of chemical changes. As a result of these changes synaptic vesicles pour the neurotransmitter stored in them into the synaptic cleft. The neurotransmitter reaches and binds onto receptor molecules present in the postsynaptic membrane. This alters permeability of the postsynaptic membrane to ions of calcium, sodium, potassium or chloride leading to depolarisation (or hyperpolarisation at inhibitory synapses). The best known (or classical) neurotransmitters responsible for fast but short-lived action of the kind described above are acetylcholine, noradrenaline and adrenaline. For long, all nerve terminals were regarded as either *cholinergic* or *adrenergic*, until it was recognised that these were not the only neurotransmitters present. Other fast neurotransmitters whose presence is now well established are dopamine and histamine.

It is also recognised that apart from the neurotransmitters mentioned above numerous other chemical substances are associated with synapses. Some of these, which probably act as neurotransmitters, are serotonin, gama-aminobutyric acid (GABA), glutamate, aspartate and glycine.

It is now known that at some synapses the effect of a neurotransmitter may last for seconds or even minutes. Repeated synaptic activity can have long lasting effects on the receptor neuron including structural changes such as the formation of new synapses, alterations in the dendritic tree, or growth of axons. Such effects produced under the influence of chemical substances are described as *neuromediation*, the chemical substances concerned being called *neuromediators*. This term includes *neurohormones*, synthesised in neurons and poured into the blood stream through terminals resembling synapses in structure. Similar chemical substances are also poured into the cerebrospinal fluid or into intercellular spaces to influence other neurons in a diffuse manner.

Lastly, some chemical substances associated with synapses do not influence synaptic transmission directly, but influence the effects of transmitters or of neuromediators. Such chemical substances are referred to as *neuromodulators*. Several peptides found in the nervous system probably act as neuromodulators. These include substance P, vasoactive intestinal polypeptide (VIP), somatostatin, cholecystokinin and many others.

The following factors can influence synaptic transmission (and thereby the speed of responses).

(a) Drugs like caffeine produce their stimulatory effect by stimulating synaptic transmission.

(b) Synaptic transmission may decrease in old age because calcium ion channels become fewer. In the case of the heart this may impair the stimulating effect of exercise on heart rate and cardiac output.

(c) Synaptic transmission is disturbed in some diseases like myasthenia gravis.

(d) It is also affected in poisoning by organophosphates. In this condition the action of acetylcholine esterase is inhibited and acetyl choline accumulates. This can lead to spasm of respiratory muscles and death.

Classification of Synapses

Synapses may be of various types depending on the neuronal elements taking part. They may also be classified on the basis of their ultrastructure, and on the basis of the neurotransmitters released by them. From a physiological standpoint a synapse may be excitatory or inhibitory.Synapses in different situations can vary considerably in overall shape (Fig. 1.11); in the size, shape and nature of synaptic vesicles and in the configuration of the presynaptic and postsynaptic areas of dense cytoplasm.

Fig. 1.13. Classification of synapses on the basis of ultrastructure and neurotransmitters present		
Asymmetric / symmetric	Shape of vesicles	Neurotransmitter associated
Asymmetric	Small spherical	Acetyl choline Glutamine Serotonin Some other amines
	Dense cored	Noradrenaline Adrenaline Dopamine
Symmetric	Pleomorphic	GABA Glycine

Two main types of synapses are recognised on the basis of their ultrastructure.

Asymmetric or Type I synapses: In these synapses the subsynaptic zone of dense cytoplasm is thicker on the presynaptic side. The synaptic cleft is about 30 nm. Such synapses are excitatory.

Symmetric or Type II synapses: In these synapses the subsynaptic zones of dense cytoplasm are thin and of similar thickness on both sides. The synaptic cleft measures about 20 nm.

Various synapses intermediate in structure between these two main types are also encountered.

The vesicles to be seen within synapses can also be of various types. Some vesicles are clear while others have dense cores. They may be pleomorphic (i.e., a mixture of various shapes). The appearance of vesicles can often be correlated with the neurotransmitter present. On the basis of these characters some sub-varieties of Type 1 and Type II synapses that have been recognised are given in Fig. 1.13.

Through its ramifications an axon usually establishes synapses with several different neurons; but in some situations it synapses with one neuron only. Some axons bear boutons that do not come into direct contact with other neurons. Such boutons may represent areas where neurotransmitters are released into surrounding areas, and can have widespread rather than localised effect.

At some sites specialised regions may be seen in relation to synapses. They are mentioned here as they are given specific names.

In some synapses in the retina and internal ear vesicles are arranged around a rod-like element placed at right angles to the cell membrane. This configuration is called a **synaptic ribbon**. Within some dendritic spines collections of flattened cisternae (endoplasmic reticulum) with associated dense material are seen. These are given the name **spine apparatus**.

Electrical Synapses

Synapses involving the release of neurotransmitters are referred to as **chemical synapses**. At some sites one cell may excite another without the release of a transmitter. At such sites adjacent cells have direct channels of communication through which ions can pass from one cell to another altering their electrical status. Such synapses are called **electrical synapses**.

At the site of an electrical synapse plasma membranes (of the two elements taking part) are closely applied, the gap between them being about 4 nm. Proteins called *connexins* project into this gap from the membrane on either side of the synapse. The proteins are so arranged that small open channels are created between the two synaptic elements.

Electrical synapses are common in lower vertebrates and invertebrates. They have been demonstrated at some sites in the brains of mammals (e.g., in the inferior olive and cerebellum).

Junctions between receptors and neurons, or between neurons and effectors, share some of the features of typical synapses and may also be regarded as synapses. Junctions between cardiac myocytes, and between smooth muscle cells, are regarded as electrical synapses.

Influence of neural activity on synapses

It has been shown that neural activity acts as a stimulus for development of new synapses and for increase in their size, specially in early postnatal life. Some experiments show that even in later life (in some situations) brief synaptic activity can have an influence on the subsequent activity of the synapse. This is specially true in areas like the hippocampus and may be associated with memory.

Peripheral Nerves

Peripheral nerves are collections of nerve fibres. These are of two functional types.

(a) Some nerve fibres carry impulses from the spinal cord or brain to peripheral structures like muscle or gland: they are called *efferent* or *motor* fibres. Efferent fibres are axons of neurons (the cell bodies of which are) located in the grey matter of the spinal cord or of the brainstem.

(b) Other nerve fibres carry impulses from peripheral organs to the brain or spinal cord: these are called *afferent* fibres. Many (but not all) afferent fibres are concerned in the transmission of sensations like touch, pain etc.: they are, therefore, also called *sensory* fibres. Afferent nerve fibres are processes of neurons that are located (as a rule) in sensory ganglia.

In the case of spinal nerves these ganglia are located on the dorsal nerve roots. In the case of cranial nerves they are located on ganglia situated on the nerve concerned (usually near its attachment to the brain). The neurons in these ganglia are usually of the unipolar type (page 8). Each unipolar neuron gives off a peripheral process which passes into the peripheral nerve forming an afferent nerve fibre. It also gives off a central process that enters the brain or spinal cord.

From what has been said above it will be clear that the afferent nerve fibres in peripheral nerves are functionally dendrites. However, their histological structure is exactly the same as that of axons.

Basic Structure of Peripheral Nerve Fibres

Each nerve fibre has a central core formed by the axon. This core is called the *axis cylinder*. The plasma membrane surrounding the axis cylinder is the *axolemma*. The axis cylinder is surrounded by a myelin sheath (page 5). This sheath is in the form of short segments that are separated at short intervals called the *nodes of Ranvier* (Fig. 1.6). The part of the nerve fibre between two consecutive nodes is the *internode*.

Each segment of the myelin sheath is formed by one Schwann cell. Outside the myelin sheath there is a thin layer of Schwann cell cytoplasm. This layer of cytoplasm is called the *neurilemma*. The method of formation of these sheaths has been described on page 5.

Each nerve fibre is surrounded by *endoneurium* (Fig. 1.14). This is a layer of connective tissue The endoneurium holds adjoining nerve fibres together and facilitates their aggregation to form bundles or *fasciculi*. Apart from collagen fibres the endoneurium contains fibroblasts, Schwann cells, endothelial cells and macrophages.

Each fasciculus is surrounded by the *perineurium,* which is a thicker layer of connective tissue. The perineurium is made up of layers of flattened cells separated by layers of collagen fibres. The perineurium probably controls diffusion of substances in and out of axons.

A very thin nerve may consist of a single fasciculus, but usually a nerve is made up of several fasciculi. The fasciculi are held together by the *epineurium*. This is a fairly dense layer of connective tissue that surrounds the entire nerve.

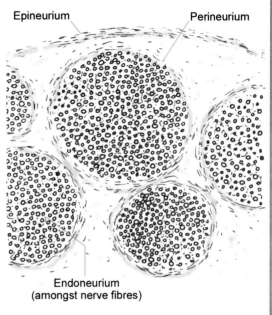

Fig. 1.14. Diagram showing the connective tissue supporting nerve fibres of a peripheral nerve

The epineurium contains fat that cushions nerve fibres. Loss of this fat in bedridden patients can lead to pressure on nerve fibres and paralysis.

Blood vessels to a nerve travel through the connective tissue that surrounds it. Severe reduction in blood supply can lead to *ischaemic neuritis* and pain.

Fig. 1.15. Classification of fibres in peripheral nerves.

Type	Subtype	EFFERENT	AFFERENT
A	Alpha (α)	To extrafusal muscle fibres	From encapsulated receptors in skin, joints, gut Primary sensory fibres from muscle spindles (Group I) Secondary sensory fibres from muscle spindles (Group II)
	Delta (δ)	Some collaterals of Aα fibres to intrafusal muscle fibres	From thermoreceptors and nociceptors
	Gamma (γ)	To intrafusal muscle fibres	
B		Preganglionic autonomic	From skin, viscera From free n. endings in connective tissue of muscle (Group III)
C		Postganglionic autonomic	Interoceptive fibres From thermoreceptors and nociceptors (Group IV)

Classification of Fibres in Peripheral Nerves according to Diameter and Velocity of Conduction

In a transverse section across a peripheral nerve it is seen that the nerve fibres vary considerably in diameter. Fibres of larger diameter are myelinated while those of smallest diameters are unmyelinated. It is well established that by and large fibres of larger diameter conduct impulses more rapidly than those of smaller diameter. Various schemes for classification of nerve fibres on the basis of their diameter and their conduction velocity have been proposed. The best known classification is as follows.

Type A

The fastest conducting fibres are called Type A fibres. Their conduction velocity is 30 to 120 m/sec; and their diameter varies from 1 to 2 μm. They are myelinated.

Type A fibres are further divided (in descending order of diameter and conduction velocity) into three subtypes: alpha (Aα), delta (Aδ) and gamma (Aγ). Type A fibres perform both motor and sensory functions as follows:

Motor Type A fibres
1. Aα fibres supply extrafusal fibres in skeletal muscle.
2. Aγ fibres supply intrafusal fibres in muscle spindles.
3. Aδ fibres are collaterals of Aα fibres (to extrafusal fibres) that innervate some intrafusal fibres.

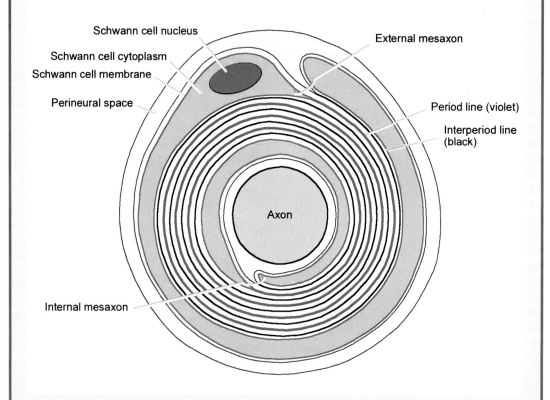

Fig. 1.16. Scheme to explain the significance of period and intraperiod lines seen in the myelin sheath at high EM magnifications.

Sensory Type A fibres

1. Aα sensory fibres carry impulses from encapsulated receptors in skin, joints and muscle. They include primary sensory afferents from muscle spindles (also called Group I fibres); and secondary afferents from spindles (also called Group II fibres). Some of them carry impulses from the gut.

2. Aδ sensory fibres are afferents from thermo-receptors and nociceptors (pain receptors).

Type B

Type B fibres have a conduction velocity of 4 to 30 m/sec; and their diameter is less than 3 µm. They are myelinated. They are either preganglionic autonomic efferent fibres (motor), or afferent fibres from skin and viscera, and from free nerve endings in connective tissue of muscle (also called Group III fibres).

Type C

In contrast to type A and type B fibres, type C fibres are unmyelinated. They have a conduction velocity of 0.5 to 4 m/sec; and their diameter is 0.5 to 4 µm. These are postganglionic autonomic fibres, and some sensory fibres conveying pain. (These include nociceptive fibres from connective tissue of muscle: Group IV fibres. Note that the terms Group I to IV all refer to afferents from muscle tissue). Some fibres from thermoreceptors and from viscera also fall in this category.

Unmyelinated axons are numerous in dorsal nerve roots and in cutaneous nerves. Many unmyelinated axons are also present in nerves to muscles and in ventral nerve roots. Most autonomic nerve fibres are unmyelinated although myelinated fibres are also present in preganglionic nerves.

The classification of nerve fibres is summarised in Fig. 1.15.

FURTHER DETAILS REGARDING STRUCTURE OF PERIPHERAL NERVES

Further Consideration of the Structure of the Myelin Sheath.

From Fig. 1.16 it will be seen that each layer of plasma membrane helping to form the myelin sheath has an internal or cytoplasmic surface that comes in contact with the internal surface of the next layer; and an external surface that meets the external surface of the next layer. When the myelin sheath is examined with the higher magnifications of the electron microscope it shows alternate thick and thin lines. The thick lines (called **period lines** or **major dense lines**) represent the fused cytoplasmic surfaces of two adjacent layers of the plasma membrane, whereas the thin lines (called **intraperiod lines** or **minor dense lines**) represent the fused external surfaces of two adjacent membranes. Some other terms of interest are shown in Fig. 1.16.

Incisures of Schmidt Lanterman

With the light microscope oblique clefts can often be seen in the myelin sheath (Fig. 1.17). These clefts are called the **Schmidt Lanterman clefts**. Many workers have considered these clefts to be artefacts. However, EM studies show the clefts to be areas where adjoining layers of Schwann cell plasma membrane (forming the myelin sheath) have failed to fuse (Fig. 1.18) leaving (i) a layer of Schwann cell cytoplasm that passes spirally around the axon in the position of the period line; and (ii) a spiral space through which the perineural space communicates with the periaxonal space in the position of the intraperiod line. This space provides a path for passage of substances into the myelin sheath and axon, from the space around the nerve fibre. The clefts enlarge greatly when a nerve fibre undergoes Wallerian degeneration.

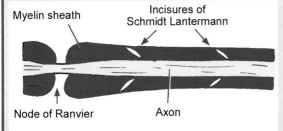

Myelin sheath — Incisures of Schmidt Lantermann

Node of Ranvier — Axon

Fig. 1.17. Diagram to show the incisures of Schmidt Lanterman. Also see Fig. 1.1

Nodes of Ranvier

We have seen that the myelin sheath is in the form of segments separated at ***nodes of Ranvier***. We have also noted that the part of the nerve fibre between two such nodes is called the internode. The length of the internode is greater in thicker fibres and shorter in thinner ones. It varies from 150 to 1500 µm.

The nerve fibres within a nerve frequently branch. When they do so the bifurcation always lies at a node.

The nodes of Ranvier have great physiological importance. When an impulse travels down a nerve fibre it does not proceed uniformly along the length of the axis cylinder, but jumps from one node to the next. This is called ***saltatory conduction***.

(In unmyelinated neurons the impulse travels along the axolemma. Such

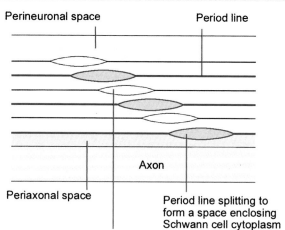

Fig. 1.18. Simplified scheme to show how the incisures of Schmidt Lanterman are formed.

conduction is much slower than saltatory conduction and consumes more energy).

EM studies reveal several interesting details about the nodes of Ranvier (Fig. 1.19). Immediately next to a node the myelin sheath shows an expansion called the ***paranodal bulb***. There are longitudinal furrows on the surface of the paranodal bulb. These furrows are filled in by Schwann cell cytoplasm containing many mitochondria. Finger-like processes of this cytoplasm extend towards the naked part of the axon and come in contact with it. These processes interdigitate with those from neighbouring Schwann cells. In the intervals between these processes the axon is covered by a ***gap substance*** that plays a role in regulating the flow of the nerve impulse by influencing the passage of ions into, and out of, the axon.

At a node of Ranvier the axon itself is much thinner than in the internode. The part of the axon passing through the paranodal bulb shows infoldings of its axolemma (cell membrane) that correspond to the grooves on the surface of the paranodal bulb (Fig. 1.20).

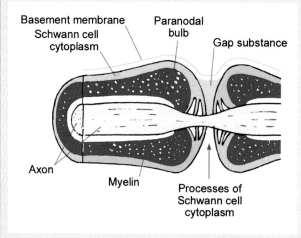

Fig. 1.19. Some details of a node of Ranvier.

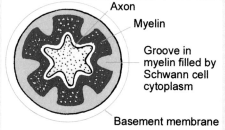

Fig. 1.20. Transverse section across paranodal bulb. Note the fluted appearance of the myelin and of the axon

Chemical composition of myelin

Myelin contains protein, lipids and water. The main lipids present include cholesterol, phospholipids, and glycosphingolipids. Other lipids are present in smaller amounts.

Myelination can be seriously impaired, and there can be abnormal collections of lipids, in disorders of lipid metabolism. Various proteins have been identified in myelin sheaths and abnormality in them can be the basis of some neuropathies.

Some facts about myelination

1. It has been observed that myelin sheaths are present only around axons having a diameter more than 1.5 μm in peripheral nerves, and over 1 μm within the central nervous system. However, many axons of these or greater diameter may remain unmyelinated.

2. In general, the larger the axon diameter, the thicker the myelin sheath, and the greater the internodal distance.

3. All Schwann cells associated with a particular axon are believed to be present in relation to it before myelination begins, there being no division of Schwann cells thereafter. Axon diameter and internodal length are also probably determined before myelination begins. However, these dimensions increase with growth.

4. In peripheral nerves Schwann cells accompany nerve fibres as the latter grow towards their destinations. In contrast, in the CNS the axons extend to their destination before oligodendrocytes become associated with them.

5. Myelination does not occur simultaneously in all axons. A myelinated tract becomes fully functional only after its fibres have acquired myelin sheaths. Nerve fibres are not fully myelinated at birth. Myelination is rapid during the first year of life and becomes much slower thereafter. This is to be correlated with the gradual ability of an infant to perform more complicated actions.

6. At their exit from the CNS axons in peripheral nerves pass through a central-peripheral transition region where Schwann cells come into relationship with glial cells. This junction normally lies at a node of Ranvier that is called the PNS-CNS compound node (PNS = Peripheral nervous system; CNS = Central nervous system).

Blood Nerve Barrier

Peripheral nerve fibres are separated from circulating blood by a blood-nerve barrier. Capillaries in nerves are non-fenestrated and their endothelial cells are united by tight junctions. There is a continuous basal lamina around the capillary. The blood-nerve barrier is reinforced by cell layers present in the perineurium.

Functional relationship between axons and Schwann cells

Schwann cells are not to be regarded merely as a passive covering for axons. A close functional relationship exists between the two as follows.

1. Signals traveling along axons probably influence the differentiation of Schwann cells. Such signals seem to determine proliferation and survival of Schwann cells and also determine whether or not they will form myelin.

2. In contrast, signals arising in Schwann cells can influence the growth of axons and their diameter. Schwann cells are essential for repair of damaged peripheral nerves.

In the preceding sections we have considered some aspects of the arrangement of neurons. Further consideration of the arrangement of neurons within the nervous system requires some knowledge of the structure of the spinal cord, and of its relationship to spinal nerves. These topics will be discussed in the next chapter. We will resume consideration of the arrangement of neurons in Chapter 3.

Degeneration and Regeneration of Neurons

Prolonged pressure on a nerve can cause temporary loss of function. This can occur in unconsciousness or even in deep sleep, and in bedridden patients. Pressure on the radial nerve can cause the condition known as *Saturday night palsy*. Pressure on blood vessels supplying a nerve can lead to a painful condition called *ischaemic neuritis*.

When the axon of a neuron is crushed or cut across a series of degenerative changes are seen in the axon distal to the injury, in the axon proximal to the injury, and in the cell body.

The changes in the part of the axon distal to the injury are referred to as *anterograde degeneration* or *Wallerian degeneration*. They take place in the entire length of this part of the axon. A few hours after injury the axon becomes swollen and irregular in shape, and in a few days it breaks up into small fragments (Fig. 1.21). The neurofibrils within it break down into granules. The myelin sheath breaks up into small segments. It also undergoes chemical changes that enable degenerating myelin to be stained selectively. The region is invaded by numerous macrophages that remove degenerating axons, myelin and cellular debris. These macrophages probably secrete substances that cause proliferation of Schwann cells and also produce nerve growth factors. The Schwann cells increase in size and produce a large series of membranes that help to form numerous tubes. We shall see later that these tubes play a vital role in regeneration of nerve fibres.

Degenerative changes in the neuron proximal to the injury are referred to as *retrograde degeneration*. These changes take place in the cell body and in the axon proximal to injury.

The cell body of the injured neuron undergoes a series of changes that constitute the phenomenon of *chromatolysis* (Fig. 1.22). The cell body enlarges tending to become spherical. The nucleus moves from the centre to the periphery. The Nissl substance becomes much less prominent and appears to dissolve away: hence the term chromatolysis. Ultrastructural and histochemical alterations occur in the cell body. The severity of the reaction shown by the cell body is variable. In some cases chromatolysis ends in cell death, followed by degeneration of all its processes. The reaction is more severe when the injury to the axon is near the cell body. If the cell survives, the changes described above are reversed after a period of time.

It is sometimes observed that changes resulting from axonal injury are not confined to the injured neuron, but extend to other neurons with which the injured neuron synapses. This phenomenon is referred to as *transneuronal degeneration*. The degeneration can extend through several synapses (as demonstrated in the visual pathway).

Changes in the proximal part of the axon are confined to a short segment near the site of injury (Fig. 1.21). If the injury is sharp and clean the effects extend only up to one or two nodes of Ranvier proximal to the injury. If the injury is severe a longer segment of the axon may be affected. The changes in the affected part are exactly the same as described for the distal part of the axon. They are soon followed by active growth at the tip of the surviving part of the axon. This causes the terminal part of the axon to swell up (Fig. 1.21 F). It then gives off a number of fine branches. These branches grow into the connective tissue at the site of injury in an effort to reach the distal cut end of the nerve (Fig. 1.21 G.H). We have seen that the Schwann cells of the distal part of the nerve proliferate to form a series of tubes. When one of the regenerating axonal branches succeeds in reaching such a tube, it enters it and then grows rapidly within it. The tube serves as a guide to the growing fibre. Axonal branches that fail to reach one of the tubes degenerate. It often happens that more than one axonal branch enters the same tube. In that case the largest branch survives and the others degenerate. The axon terminal growing through the Schwann cell tube ultimately reaches, and establishes contact with, an appropriate peripheral end organ. Failure to do so results in degeneration of the newly formed axon. The new axon formed in this way is at first very thin and devoid of a myelin sheath (Fig. 1.21 I). However, there is progressive increase in its thickness and a myelin sheath is formed around it (Fig. 1.21 J).

From the above account it will be clear that chances of regeneration of a cut nerve are considerably increased if the two cut ends are near each other, and if scar tissue does not intervene between them.

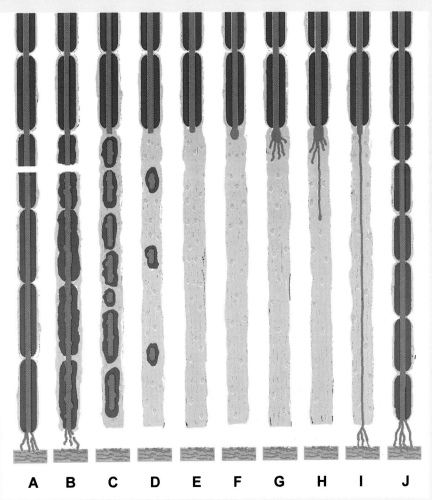

Fig. 1.21. Stages in the degeneration of a nerve fibre after injury (A to E) and its subsequent regeneration (F to J). For explanation see text.

Normal neuron

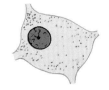

Neuron showing chromatolysis

Fig. 1.22. Diagram illustrating the changes seen in the cell body of a neuron during chromatolysis.

It has been observed that tubes formed by Schwann cells begin to disappear if they are not invaded by axons for a long time.

Axons in the CNS do not regenerate as in peripheral nerves. However, it has been seen that if a peripheral nerve is implanted into the CNS, axons tend to grow into the nerve. This may provide a method by which regeneration of tracts could be achieved within the CNS. It appears probable that implanted peripheral nerves provide the necessary environment for regeneration of axons (which the CNS is itself unable to provide).

Chances of regeneration of a damaged nerve are better under the following conditions.

(a) The nerve is crushed but there is no separation of the two ends. The endoneural sheath should be intact.

(b) Separation of cut ends should be minimal. Scar tissue should not intervene between the two ends.

(c) Infection should not be present.

If the gap between the two cut ends is great the growing axonal buds get mixed up with connective tissue to form a mass called a *neuroma*.

Sometimes during regeneration of a mixed nerve axons may establish contact with the wrong end organs. For example, fibres that should reach a gland may reach the skin. When this happens in the auriculotemporal nerve it gives rise to *Frey's syndrome*. Instead of salivation there is increased perspiration, increased blood flow and pain over skin.

For effects of damage to individual nerves see the author's Textbook of Anatomy.

Apart from injury, neurons may be affected by degeneration. Loss, by degeneration, of myelin sheaths can give rise to several conditions the most important of which is *multiple sclerosis*. The condition is confined to the central nervous system, and peripheral nerves are spared. Symptoms include weakness and various sensory disturbances. Multiple sclerosis is believed to be an autoimmune disease.

Neuroglia

In addition to neurons, the nervous system contains several types of supporting cells. These are:

(a) *Neuroglial cells*, found in the parenchyma of the brain and spinal cord.

(b) *Ependymal cells*, lining the ventricular system.

(c) *Schwann cells*, forming sheaths for axons of peripheral nerves. They are also called lemnocytes or peripheral glia.

(d) *Capsular cells* (also called *satellite cells* or *capsular gliocytes*) that surround neurons in peripheral ganglia.

(e) Various types of supporting cells found in relation to motor and sensory terminals of nerve fibres.

Some workers use the term neuroglia for all these categories while others restrict the term only to supporting cells present within the brain and spinal cord. The latter convention is used in the description that follows.

Neuroglial cells may be divided into two major categories.

1. MACROGLIA (or large glial cells)

These are of two types.

(a) *Astrocytes*, which may be subdivided into fibrous and protoplasmic astrocytes.

(b) *Oligodendrocytes*.

2. MICROGLIA (or small glial cells)

Macroglial cells are derived from ectoderm of the neural tube. Microglial cells are, on the other hand, of mesodermal origin.

All neuroglial cells are much smaller in size than neurons. However, they are far more numerous. It is interesting to note that the number of glial cells in the brain and spinal cord is ten to fifty times as much as that of neurons. Neurons and neuroglia are separated by a very narrow extracellular space.

In ordinary histological preparations only the nuclei of neuroglial cells are seen. Their processes can be demonstrated by special techniques.

Astrocytes

These are small star-shaped cells that give off a number of processes (Fig. 1.23). The processes are often flattened into leaf-like laminae that may partly surround neurons and separate them from other neurons. The processes frequently end in expansions in relation to blood vessels or in relation to the surface of the brain. Small swellings called **gliosome**s are present on the processes of astrocytes. These swellings are rich in mitochondria. Fibrous astrocytes are seen mainly in white matter. Their processes are thin and are asymmetrical. Protoplasmic astrocytes are, on the other hand, seen mainly in grey matter. Their processes are thicker than those of fibrous astrocytes and are symmetrical. Intermediate forms between fibrous and protoplasmic astrocytes are also present. Protoplasmic extensions of astrocytes surround nodes of Ranvier, but the significance of this is not understood.

The processes of astrocytes are united to those of other astrocytes through gap junctions. Astrocytes communicate with one another through calcium channels. Such communication is believed to play a role in regulation of synaptic activity, and in metabolism of neurotransmitters and of neuromodulators.

Astrocytes play a role in maintenance of the blood brain barrier. Substances secreted by end feet of astrocytes probably assist in maintaining a membrane, the **glia limitans externa**, which covers the exposed surfaces of the brain. They also help to maintain the basal laminae of blood vessels that they come in contact with.

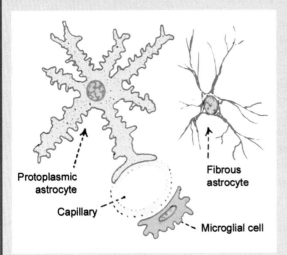

Protoplasmic astrocyte

Fibrous astrocyte

Capillary

Microglial cell

Fig. 1.23. Astrocytes and microglial cells.

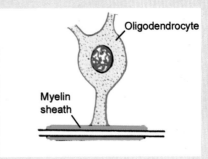

Oligodendrocyte

Myelin sheath

Fig. 1.24. Oligodendrocyte and its relationship to a neuron.

Oligodendrocytes

These cells have rounded or pear-shaped bodies with relatively few processes (olig = scanty). These cells provide myelin sheaths to nerve fibres that lie within the brain and spinal cord. Their relationship to nerve fibres is basically similar to that of Schwann cells to peripheral nerve fibres (page 5). However, in contrast to a Schwann cell that ensheaths only one axon, an oligodendrocyte may enclose several axons. Oligodendrocytes are classified into several types depending on the number of neurons they provide sheaths to. As a rule oligodendrocytes present in relation to large diameter axons provide sheaths to fewer axons than those related to axons of small diameter. The plasma membranes of oligodendrocytes comes into contact with axolemma at nodes of Ranvier.

The composition and structure of myelin sheaths formed by oligodendrocytes show differences from those formed by Schwann cells. The two are different in protein content and can be distinguished by immunocytochemical methods. As damage to neurons within the central nervous system is not followed by regeneration, oligodendrocytes have no role to play in this respect. Also note that in multiple sclerosis myelin formed by oligodendrocytes undergoes degeneration, but that derived from Schwann cells is spared.

Microglia

These are the smallest neuroglial cells. The cell body is flattened. The processes are short. These cells are frequently seen in relation to capillaries. As already stated they differ from other neuroglial elements in being mesodermal in origin. They are probably derived from monocytes that invade the brain during fetal life. They are more numerous in grey matter than in white matter. They become active after damage to nervous tissue by trauma or disease and act as phagocytes.

FUNCTIONS OF NEUROGLIA

The following are the functions of neuroglia.

(a) They provide mechanical support to neurons.

(b) In view of their non-conducting nature they serve as insulators and prevent neuronal impulses from spreading in unwanted directions.

(c) They are believed to help neuronal function by playing an important role in maintaining a suitable metabolic environment for the neurons. They can absorb neurotransmitters from synapses thus terminating their action. It has been held that they play a role in maintaining the blood-brain barrier, but this view is open to question.

(d) As mentioned above, oligodendrocytes provide myelin sheaths to nerve fibres within the central nervous system.

(e) Ependymal cells are concerned in exchanges of material between the brain and the cerebrospinal fluid.

(f) Neuroglial cells are responsible for repair of damaged areas of nervous tissue. They proliferate in such regions (*gliosis*). These cells (specially microglia) may act as macrophages. (Macrophages are cells that can engulf and destroy unwanted material). Large areas of gliosis can be seen by eye and in MRI scans.

Tumours of Nervous Tissue

1. Precursors of neural cells can give rise to *medulloblastomas*. Once mature neurons are formed they lose the power of mitosis and do not give origin to tumours.

Certain tumours called *germinomas* appear near the midline mostly near the third ventricle. They arise from germ cells that also give rise to teratomas.

2. Most tumours of the brain arise from neuroglial cells. *Astrocytomas* are most common. *Oligodendromas* are also frequent.

3. Tumours can also arise from ependyma and from Schwann cells.

A Brief Review of Techniques used in the Study of Neuroanatomy

1. The earliest observations on the brain and peripheral nerves were made on unfixed animal material. Discovery of methods of fixation, and the development of simple microscopes enabled much more detailed studies to be made, but substantial advances became possible only after methods for preparing tissue sections and for staining them became available. The technique of silver impregnation was discovered in the later part of the eighteenth century by workers including Ranvier and Golgi.

2. Early discoveries that paved the way for techniques allowing the tracing of neural pathways included the staining of 'chromatin granules' by Nissl, who also discovered the phenomenon of chromatolysis about a hundred years ago. About the same time Weigert discovered a method for staining normal myelin, and Marchi discovered his method for degenerating myelin.

3. Changes taking place in degenerating neurons were first described by Waller in 1850 (hence the term Wallerian degeneration). After the discovery of Marchi's method for staining degenerating myelin the way was opened for tracing of neural pathways after placing of experimental lesions in animals. However, methods for the demonstration of degenerating axons, and of axon terminals became available only in the middle of the present century (Glees, 1946; Nauta and Gygax, 1951). With the relatively recent development of stereotactic methods it has become possible to create accurate and controlled neural damage even deep within the brain.

4. While the various neuron-tracing methods developed over a century have added considerably to our knowledge of the structure of the nervous system, information thus obtained has been confirmed and greatly amplified by neuro-physiological methods. These involve controlled stimulation at one point with recording of evoked potentials at other sites. Neurophysiological methods have greatly increased in sophistication with the development of stereotaxis, of advanced electronic stimulating and recording devices, and of microelectrodes that can record potential changes even in individual neurons or from individual nerve fibres.

5. More recent advances in the study of neuroanatomy have gone hand in hand with technical developments. The capabilities of light microscopes have increased with the development of refined optics, and with innovations like dark field illumination, use of polarised light, phase contrast, and microscopy with ultraviolet light. One recent advance is the confocal microscope that provides three dimensional views of microscopic structures (without the need for preparation of thin sections and reconstructions).

Histochemistry and Immunological Techniques

6. Histochemical techniques have added greatly to understanding of neurology, specially in association with the results of physiological experiments. In this connection the development of immuno-histochemistry has been of great importance. This technique has made possible precise localisation of various neurotransmitters, neuromediators neuro-modulators and other substances, and has revolutionised concepts about the variety of nerve cells and nerve fibres.

Immuno-histochemical localisation has greatly improved following availability of monoclonal antibodies, and use of molecular genetics for producing antigens of great purity.

Electronmicroscopy

7. A revolutionary explosion of knowledge of the finer details of the structure of neurons, of nerve fibres, and of synapses has taken place with the development of suitable methods for preparation and examination of tissues using the electron microscope. In turn the availability of detailed information has led to the possibility of useful correlations with the results of biochemical and physiological advances. The utility of electronmicroscopy has been greatly increased by combining it with techniques like autoradiography (see below), histochemistry, and immunological methods.

Autoradiography

8. When amino acids or sugars normally present in the body are labelled with radioactive substances and are injected into an animal, they become incorporated at specific sites. These sites can be located in tissue sections by covering a section with a photographic emulsion and allowing the radioactive material to act on it for some days. When the emulsion is developed granules of silver are seen over the sites where the incorporated material is present. This technique is called autoradiography. It has been found that if labelled amino acids or sugars are injected into a part of the brain, these substances are absorbed by neurons and are transported along their axons. These neurons can be revealed by autoradiography. The preparations can be studied both by light microscopy and electronmicroscopy.

Use of marker substances

9. It has been found that if axons are exposed to the enzyme horse radish peroxidase (HRP), the enzyme is taken up into the axons and transported in a retrograde direction to reach the cell bodies concerned. Alternatively if HRP is injected into neuronal cell bodies it is transported down the axons. The presence of enzyme can be seen using appropriate methods. This has provided a new technique

for tracing neuronal pathways. Some fluorochrome dyes act in a manner similar to HRP. Some fluorescent dyes injected into embryonic cells pass into their daughter cells thus enabling the origin of the latter to be traced.

Neuronal implantation

10. It has been shown that embryonic neural tissue implanted into the brain can survive and can be functionally integrated with the host tissue. Such implantation may offer a method for replacing dead or deficient neurons at particular sites (e.g., the corpus striatum). They may also be used to encourage regeneration of axons after injury.

The brief review given above will help the student to realise that our knowledge of neuroanatomy is not static, but is making rapid progress. In reading the chapters that follow the student would do well to keep this in mind; and to be aware that some of the statements they read may well be modified, or discarded, with time.

Early Development of Nervous system

Apart from its blood vessels and some neuroglial elements, the whole of the nervous system is derived from ectoderm. At the time when the nervous system begins to develop the embryo is in the form of a three-layered disc (Figs 1.25, 1.26). In the middle line observe the prochordal plate (cranially) and the primitive streak caudally. The cranial end of the primitive streak is thickened. This thickened cranial end is called the ***primitive knot***. Between the prochordal plate and the primitive knot we see a midline structure the developing ***notochord***. The notochord lies between ectoderm and endoderm.

The part of the ectoderm that is destined to give origin to the brain and spinal cord is situated on the dorsal aspect of the embryonic disc, in the midline, and overlies the developing notochord (Figs. 1.27 A, B). It soon becomes thickened to form the ***neural plate*** (Fig. 1.27 B).

The neural plate becomes depressed along the midline as a result of which the ***neural groove*** is formed (Fig. 1.27 C). This groove becomes progressively deeper. At the same time, the two edges of the neural plate come nearer each other, and eventually fuse, thus converting the neural groove into the ***neural tube*** (Fig. 1.27 D). The neural tube is formed from the ectoderm overlying the notochord and, therefore, extends from the prochordal plate to the primitive knot (Fig. 1.26). The process of formation of the neural tube is referred to as ***neurulation***.

These stages in the formation of the neural tube do not proceed simultaneously all over the length of the neural plate. The middle part is the first to become tubular, so that for some time the neural tube is open cranially and caudally. These openings are called the ***anterior*** and ***posterior neuropores***, respectively. The fusion of the two edges of the neural plate extends cranially, and caudally, and eventually the neuropores disappear leaving a closed tube.

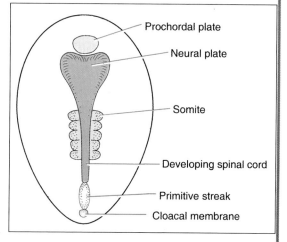

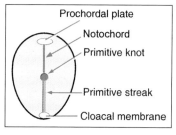

Fig. 1.25. Early embryonic disc before formation of the neural plate.

Fig. 1.26. Embryonic disc showing the neural plate.

Even before the neural tube has completely closed, it is divisible into an enlarged cranial part and a caudal tubular part (Fig. 1.26). The enlarged cranial part forms the brain. The caudal tubular part forms the spinal cord. It is at first short, but gradually gains in length as the embryo grows.

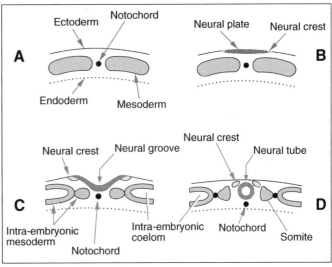

DEVELOPMENT

Fig. 1.27. Formation of neural tube. (A) Embryonic disc before formation of neural plate. (B) Neural plate formed by thickening of ectoderm. (C) Neural plate is converted to a groove. (D) The groove is converted to a tube. Note the neural crest which lies along the edges of the neural plate (B), or neural groove (C). After formation of the neural tube the neural crest lies dorsal to it (D).

Faulty formation of neural tube

1. The whole length of the neural tube remains unclosed. This results in the condition called *posterior rachischisis.*

2. The neural tube remains open in the region of the brain. This results in *anencephaly.* Brain tissue which is exposed brain tissue degenerates.

3. Non-fusion of the neural tube is of necessity associated with non-closure of the cranium (*cranium bifidum*) or of the vertebral canal (*spina bifida*).

4. The brain may be too small (*microcephaly*) or too large (*macrocephaly*).

5. Parts of the nervous system may be absent.

These conditions and other abnormalities are considered further in Chapter 8.

CLINICAL

Formation of neurons and neuroglial cells

The neurons and many neuroglial cells are formed in the neural tube.

The neural tube is at first lined by a single layer of cells, (Fig. 1.28 A). These proliferate to form several layers (Fig. 1.28 B). Nearest the lumen of the tube is the *matrix cell layer* (also called primitive ependymal or germinal layer). The cells of this layer give rise to nerve cells, to neuroglial cells, and also to more germinal cells. Next comes the *mantle layer* in which are seen the developing nerve cells, and neuroglial cells. The outermost layer, termed the *marginal zone*, contains no nerve cells. It consists of a reticulum formed by protoplasmic processes of developing neuroglial cells (*spongioblasts*). It provides a framework into which the processes of nerve cells developing in the mantle layer can grow. (According to recent investigations the wall of the neural tube consists of only one layer of elongated cells. The multilayered appearance is produced by nuclei being placed at different levels as in a pseudostratified epithelium).

The stages in the formation of a nerve cell are as follows:

1. One of the germinal cells passes from the germinal layer to the mantle layer and becomes an *apolar neuroblast* (Fig. 1.29 A).

DEVELOPMENT

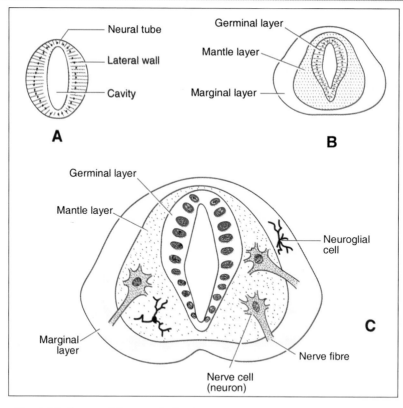

Fig. 1.28. Layers of the neural tube. (The epithelium appears to be multilayered but it is actually pseudostratified.)

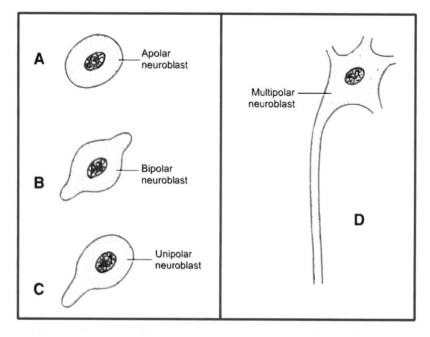

Fig. 1.29. Stages in formation of a typical neuroblast.

2. Two processes develop and convert the apolar neuroblast to a *bipolar neuroblast* (Fig. 1.29 B).

3. One of the processes of the neuroblast disappears, and it can now be called a *unipolar neuroblast* (Fig. 1.29 C).

4. The process of the cell that does not disappear now elongates, and on the side opposite to it numerous smaller processes form. At this stage the cell is called a *multipolar neuroblast* (Fig. 1.29 D).

5. The main process of the multipolar neuroblast now grows into the marginal layer, and becomes the *axon* of the nerve cell (Fig. 1.29 B). The axon can grow to a considerable length. It may either remain within the central nervous system, or may grow out of it as an efferent nerve fibre of a peripheral nerve. At its destination it establishes connections, either with the cell bodies and dendrites of other neurons, or with an effector organ (e.g. muscle).

6. The smaller processes of the neuroblast are the *dendrites*. These ramify and establish connections with other nerve cells.

7. At first the cytoplasm of the nerve cell is homogeneous. Later *Nissl's granules* make their appearance. After their formation, neurons lose the ability to divide.

Neuroglial cells are also formed from germinal cells of the ependymal layer. These cells (*glioblasts*) migrate to the mantle and marginal zones as *medulloblasts* (also called *spongioblasts*), which differentiate either into *astroblasts*, and subsequently into *astrocytes*, or into *oligodendroblasts* and then into *oligodendrocytes*. There is a third type of neuroglial cell called *microglia*. This type does not develop from the cells of the neural tube, but migrates into it along with blood vessels. These cells are believed to be of mesodermal origin.

We have seen above that the ependymal (or neuroepithelial) cells give rise both to neuroblasts and to neuroglia. However, these two cell types are not formed simultaneously. The neuroblasts are formed first. Neuroglial cells are formed after the differentiation of neuroblasts is completed.

The formation of the myelin sheath by Schwann cells and oligodendrocytes has already been explained. Nerve fibres in different parts of the brain, and spinal cord, become myelinated at different stages of development. The process begins during the fourth month of intrauterine life, but is not

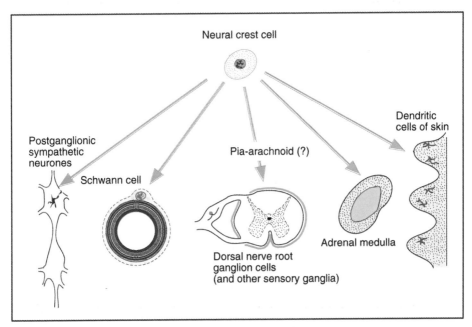

Fig. 1.30. Some derivatives of the neural crest. Many additional derivatives are now believed to exist.

completed until the child is two to three years old. Nerve fibres become fully functional only after they have acquired their myelin sheaths.

The blood vessels of the brain, and their surrounding connective tissue, are not derived from the neural tube. These are mesodermal in origin and invade the developing brain and spinal cord from the surrounding mesoderm.

The development of the *pia mater* and the *arachnoid mater* (*leptomeninges*) is not definitely understood. According to some workers, these are derived from the neural crest. The *dura mater* develops from the mesoderm surrounding the neural tube.

There can be errors in the closure of the neural tube. This leads to congenital anomalies line *anencephaly* and *rachischisis*. These are considered in page 93.

The Neural Crest

At the time when the neural plate is being formed, some cells at the junction between the neural plate and the rest of the ectoderm become specialised (on either side) to form the primordia of the neural crest (Figs. 1.27 B, C). With the separation of the neural tube from the surface ectoderm, the cells of the neural crest appear as groups of cells lying along the dorsolateral sides of the neural tube (Fig. 1.27 D). The neural crest cells soon become free (by losing the property of cell to cell adhesiveness). They migrate to distant places throughout the body. In subsequent development, several important structures are derived from the neural crest. These include some neurons of sensory and autonomic ganglia, Schwann cells, and possibly the pia mater and the arachnoid mater. Many other derivatives of the neural crest are recognised in widespread tissues.

Several diseases and syndromes are associated with the disturbances of the neural crest i.e., Hirschsprung's disease (aganglionic megacolon), aorticopulmonary septal defects of heart, cleft lip, cleft palate, frontonasal dysplasia, neurofibromitosis, tumour of adrenal medulla and albinism etc.

2 : The Spinal Cord : Gross Anatomy and Some Features of Internal Structure

The spinal cord (or spinal medulla) is the most important content of the vertebral canal. The upper end of the spinal cord becomes continuous with the medulla oblongata at the level of the **upper border** of the first cervical vertebra. The lower end of the spinal cord lies at the level of the lower border of the first lumbar vertebra. The level is, however, variable and the cord may terminate one vertebra higher or lower than this level. The level also varies with flexion or extension of the spine.

The lowest part of the spinal cord is conical and is called the **conus medullaris**. The conus is continuous, below, with a fibrous cord called the **filum terminale** (Fig. 2.2).

When seen in transverse section the grey matter of the spinal cord forms an H-shaped mass (Fig. 2.1). In each half of the cord the grey matter is divisible into a larger ventral mass, the **anterior (or ventral) grey column**, and a narrow elongated **posterior (or dorsal) grey column**. In some parts of the spinal cord a small lateral projection of grey matter is seen between the ventral and dorsal grey columns. This the **lateral grey column**. The grey matter of the right and left halves of the spinal cord is connected across the middle line by the **grey commissure** which is traversed by the **central canal.** The lower end of the central canal expands to form the **terminal ventricle** which lies in the conus medullaris. The cavity within the spinal cord continues for a short distance into the filum terminale. The central canal of the spinal cord contains cerebrospinal fluid. The canal is lined by ependyma.

The white matter of the spinal cord is divided into right and left halves, in front by a deep **anterior median fissure**, and behind by the **posterior median septum**. In each half of the cord the white matter medial to the dorsal grey column forms the **posterior funiculus** (or posterior white column).

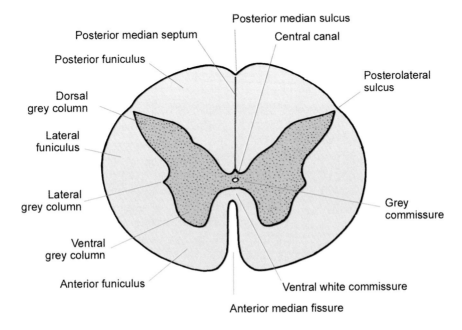

Fig. 2.1. Main features to be seen in a transverse section through the spinal cord.

The white matter medial and ventral to the anterior grey column forms the **anterior funiculus** (or anterior white column), while the white matter lateral to the anterior and posterior grey columns forms the **lateral funiculus**. (The anterior and lateral funiculi are collectively referred to as the **anterolateral funiculus**).

The white matter of the right and left halves of the spinal cord is continuous across the middle line through the **ventral white commissure** which lies anterior to the **grey commissure**. Some myelinated fibres running transversely in the grey commissure, posterior to the central canal are referred to as the **dorsal white commissure**.

Spinal Nerves & Spinal Segments

The spinal cord gives attachment, on either side, to a series of spinal nerves. Each spinal nerve arises by two roots, **anterior (or ventral)** and **posterior (or dorsal)** (Fig. 2.4). Each root is formed by aggregation of a number of rootlets that arise from the cord over a certain length (Fig. 2.5). **The length of the spinal cord giving origin to the rootlets of one spinal nerve constitutes one spinal segment**. However, this definition applies only to the superficial attachment of nerve roots. The neurons associated with one spinal nerve extend well beyond the confines of a spinal segment.

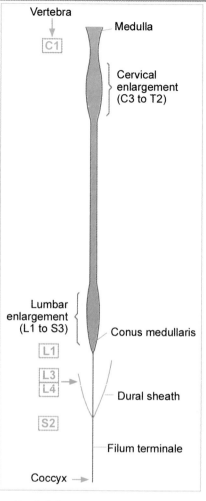

Fig. 2.2. Important vertebral levels in relation to the spinal cord.

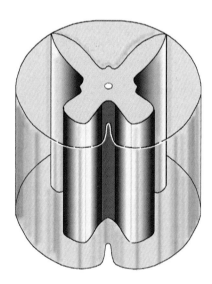

Fig. 2.3. Three dimensional view of grey matter of a segment of the spinal cord, to explain the use of the term column for subdivisions of grey matter.

The spinal cord is made up of thirty one segments: 8 cervical, 12 thoracic, 5 lumbar, 5 sacral and one coccygeal.

Note that in the cervical and coccygeal regions the number of spinal segments, and of spinal nerves, does not correspond to the number of vertebrae.

The rootlets that make up the dorsal nerve roots are attached to the surface of the spinal cord along a vertical groove (called the **postero-lateral sulcus**) opposite the tip of the posterior grey column (Fig. 2.4). The rootlets of the ventral nerve roots are attached to the anterolateral aspect of the cord opposite the anterior grey column. The ventral and dorsal nerve roots join each other to form a spinal nerve. Just proximal to the junction of the two roots the dorsal root is marked by a swelling called the **dorsal nerve root ganglion**, or **spinal ganglion** (Fig. 2.4).

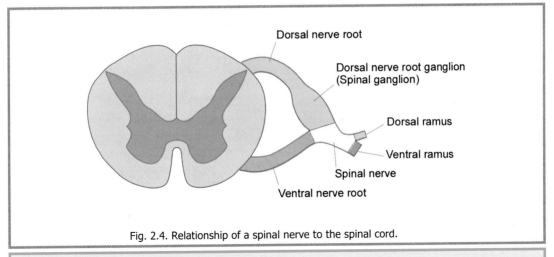

Fig. 2.4. Relationship of a spinal nerve to the spinal cord.

The dorsal nerve root ganglia (and the sensory ganglia of cranial nerves) can be infected with a virus. This leads to the condition called ***herpes zoster***. Vesicles appear on the skin over the area of distribution of the nerve. The condition is highly painful.

DEVELOPMENT

In early fetal life (third month) the spinal cord is as long as the vertebral canal, and each spinal nerve arises from the cord at the level of the corresponding intervertebral foramen. In subsequent development the spinal cord does not grow as much as the vertebral column and its lower end, therefore, gradually ascends to reach the level of the third lumbar vertebra at the time of birth, and to the lower border of the first lumbar vertebra in the adult.

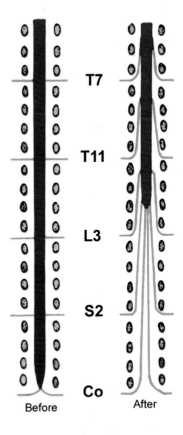

Fig. 2.6. Scheme to show the effect of recession of the spinal cord (during development) on the course of the roots of spinal nerves.

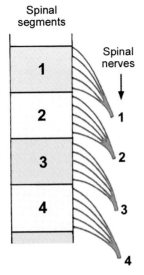

Fig. 2.5. Scheme to illustrate the concept of spinal segments

As a result of this upward migration of the cord the roots of spinal nerves have to follow an oblique downward course to reach the appropriate intervertebral foramen (Fig. 2.6). This also makes the roots longer. The obliquity and length of the roots is most marked in the lower nerves and many of these roots occupy the vertebral canal below the level of the spinal cord. These roots constitute the *cauda equina*.

Another result of the upward recession of the spinal cord is that the spinal segments do not lie opposite the corresponding vertebrae. This fact is clinically important. For estimating the position of a spinal segment in relation to the surface of the body it is important to remember that a vertebral spine is always lower than the corresponding spinal segment. As a rough guide it may be stated that in the cervical region there is a difference of one segment (e.g., the 5th cervical spine overlies the 6th cervical segment); in the upper thoracic region there is a difference of two segments (e.g., the 4th thoracic spine overlies the 6th thoracic segment); and in the lower thoracic region there is a difference of three segments (e.g., the 9th thoracic spine lies opposite the 12th thoracic segment).

The spinal cord is not of uniform thickness. The spinal segments that contribute to the nerves of the upper limbs are enlarged to form the *cervical enlargement* of the cord. Similarly, the segments innervating the lower limbs forms the *lumbar enlargement* (Fig. 2.2).

In addition to spinal nerves the upper five or six cervical segments of the spinal cord give origin to a series of rootlets that emerge on the lateral aspect (midway between the anterior and posterior nerve roots of spinal nerves). These rootlets join to form the spinal root of the accessory nerve. This nerve travels upwards to enter the cranial cavity through the foramen magnum.

The spinal cord is surrounded by the *meninges*. These are the *dura mater*, the *arachnoid mater*, and the *pia mater*. The dura mater is a thick fibrous membrane. The arachnoid mater and pia mater are thin membranes. The space between the dura mater and the wall of the vertebral canal is called the *extradural (or epidural) space*, while the space between the dura and the arachnoid is called the *subdural space*. The arachnoid and pia are separated by the *subarachnoid space* which contains the *cerebrospinal fluid* (CSF) (Fig. 2.7).

The spinal dura mater forms a loose tubular covering for the spinal cord. We have seen that the spinal cord (and overlying pia mater) extends downwards only up to the lower border of the first lumbar vertebra. The dura and arachnoid (along with the subarachnoid space containing CSF), however extend up to the second sacral vertebra.

Between these two levels the subarachnoid space contains the spinal nerve roots forming the cauda equina.

In this region, a needle can be introduced into the subarachnoid space without danger of injury to the spinal cord. This procedure is called *lumbar puncture* (Fig. 2.2). (Further description in Chapter 20).

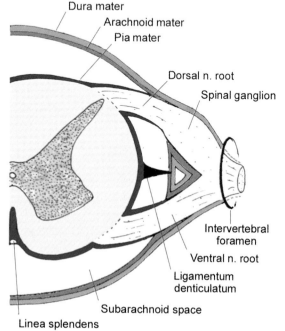

Fig. 2.7. Transverse section through spinal cord to show the formation of meningeal sheaths over the roots of a spinal nerve.

The dorsal and ventral roots of spinal nerves pass through the spinal dura mater separately. Sheaths derived from dura extend over the nerve roots. These dural sheaths reach up to the intervertebral foramina and are attached to the margins of these foramina. The dorsal and ventral nerve roots unite in the intervertebral foramina to form the trunks of spinal nerves. The pia mater and arachnoid mater also extend on to the roots of spinal nerves as sheaths. These sheaths reach up to the site where the nerve roots pass through dura mater (Fig. 2.7).

We have seen that below the level of the conus medullaris the spinal cord is continuous with the filum terminale. The filum terminale is made up mainly of pia mater. Below the level of the second sacral vertebra the filum terminale is surrounded by an extension of dura mater. It ends by gaining attachment to the dorsum of the first segment of the coccyx (Fig. 2.2).

SEGMENTAL INNERVATION:

Any condition that leads to pressure on the spinal cord, or on spinal nerve roots, can give rise to symptoms in the region supplied by nerves. In such cases it is important to be able to localize the particular spinal segments, or roots, involved. For this purpose it is necessary to know which areas of skin, (and which muscles) are innervated through each segment.

DERMATOMES

Areas of skin supplied by individual spinal nerves are called **dermatomes**. To understand the arrangement of dermatomes it is necessary to know some facts about the development of the limbs.

The upper and lower limbs are derived from limb buds. These are, paddle-shaped, outgrowths that arise from the side-wall of the embryo. They are at first directed forward and laterally from the body of the embryo (Fig. 2.8). Each bud has a **preaxial (or cranial) border** and a **postaxial border** (Fig. 2.9). The thumb and great toe are formed on the preaxial border.

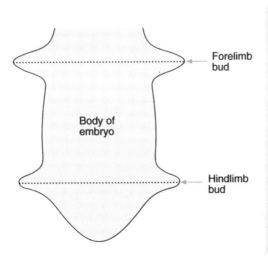

Fig. 2.8. Scheme to show that the longitudinal axis of the limb buds is transverse to the long axis of the embryonic body.

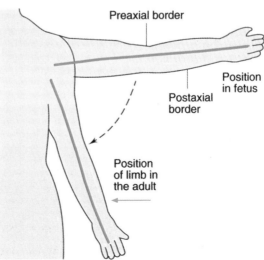

Fig. 2.9. Scheme showing that with the 'adduction' of the embryonic limb, the preaxial border becomes the lateral border.

DEVELOPMENT

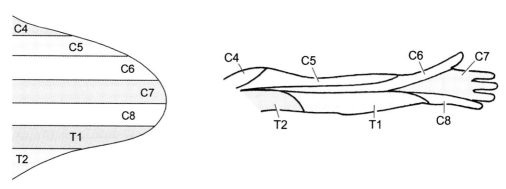

Fig. 2.10. Dermatomes of the upper limb in an embryo.

Fig. 2.11. Dermatomes of the upper limb in an adult.

The forelimb bud is derived from the part of the body wall belonging to segments C4, C5, C6, C7, C8, T1 and T2. It is, therefore, innervated by the corresponding spinal nerves. The hindlimb bud is formed opposite the segments L2, L3, L4, L5, S1 and S2. As the limbs grow skin supplied by these nerves gets "pulled away" into the limbs. This has great effect on the arrangement of dermatomes (Figs. 2.10, 2.11). The dermatomes of the body are shown in Fig. 2.12.

CLINICAL

Now note the following facts about dermatomes These are of clinical significance.

(a) Spinal nerve C1 does not supply any area of skin.

(b) The areas supplied by different spinal nerves overlap in such a way that any given area is supplied by two (or more) nerves. The overlap is less for fibres carrying sensation of touch and more for those carrrying pain and temperature.

(e) Because of overlap maps of dermatomes are only approximate.

(d) Because of what has been said above (about the development of the limbs) the lateral (preaxial) aspect of the upper limb is supplied (in sequence) by segments C4 to C6 and the medial aspect by segments C8 to T2. The segment C7 supplies an intermediate strip.

(e) The layout becomes complex in the lower limb because a twisting of the limb during development.

(f) As a rule, the arrangement of dermatomes is simple over the trunk, as successive horizontal strips of skin are supplied by each spinal nerve of the region. However, the arrangement is unusual over the pectoral region. The skin of the upper part of the pectoral region is supplied by spinal segments C3 and C4 (upto the level of the sternal angle). Below this level we find that in fact the area just below the level of the sternal angle is supplied by segment T2. This is so because nerves C5 to T1 have been pulled away into the upper limb. For the same reason there is no overlap between the areas supplied by C4 and T2.

SEGMENTAL INNERVATION OF MUSCLES

The nerve supply of muscles can also be described on the basis of spinal nerves from which the fibres are derived (or in terms of spinal segments).

(a) It is rare for a muscle to be supplied only by one segment. One example is innervation of intrinsic muscles of the hand.

(b) Most muscles derive innervation from two or more segments.

(c) The segments supplying muscles acting on a joint also supply the joint itself.

(d) Muscles having a common action are usually supplied by the same spinal segments.

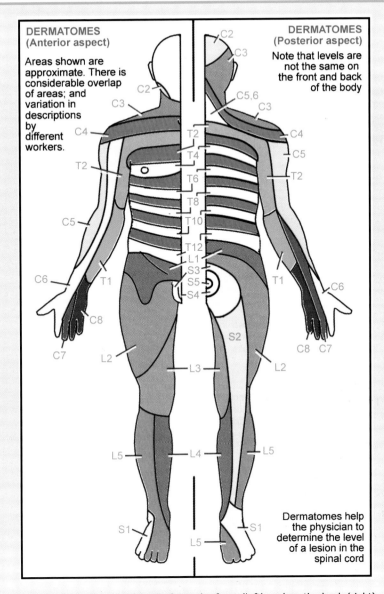

Fig. 2.12. Dermatomes of the body on the front (left) and on the back (right).

The spinal segments supplying a muscle are often given differently in different books. This can be due to individual variations in the subjects studied, or due to different methods of investigation used. It is difficult to remember the segmental supply. A simplified presentation of the segments supplying the muscles of the upper limb is given in Fig. 2.13 and of the lower limb in Fig. 2.14. The integrity of spinal segments can also be tested by examining reflexes mediated by the segment. These are considered in Chapter 5 and are summarised below..

Some Important Spinal Levels

(1) **Knee jerk** or **patellar tendon reflex** (L2, L3, L4); (2) **Ankle jerk** or **Achilles tendon reflex** (L5, S1, S2).

(3) **Biceps tendon reflex** (C5, C6); (4) **Triceps tendon reflex** (C6, C7, C8).

(5) **Supinator jerk** (or radial periosteal reflex) (C7, C8). (6) **Wrist tendon reflex** (C8, T1).

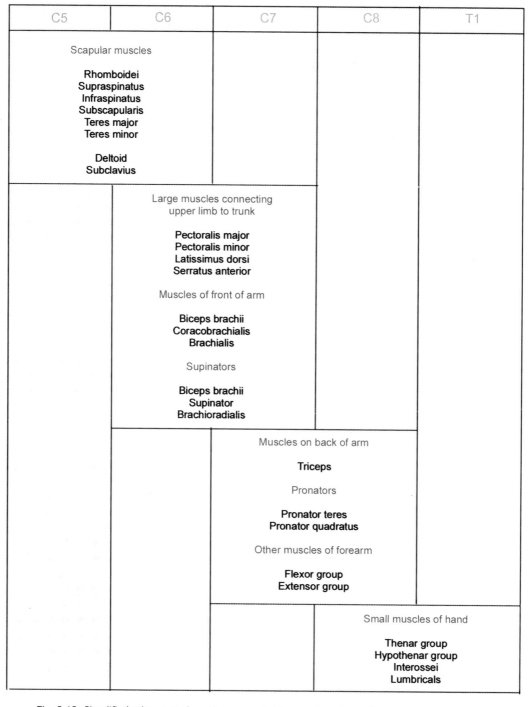

C5	C6	C7	C8	T1

Fig. 2.13. Simplified scheme to show the segmental innervation of muscles of the upper extremity.

(7) *Abdominal reflexes*: upper (T6,7), middle (T8,9) and lower (T10 to T12)
(8) *Cremasteric reflex* (T12 to L2). (9) *Gluteal reflex* (L4 to S1).
(10) *Plantar reflex* (L5 to S2). (11) *Anal reflex* (S4,5, coccygeal).
(12) Movements of the head (C1 to C4).(13) Movements of the diaphragm (C3 to C5).

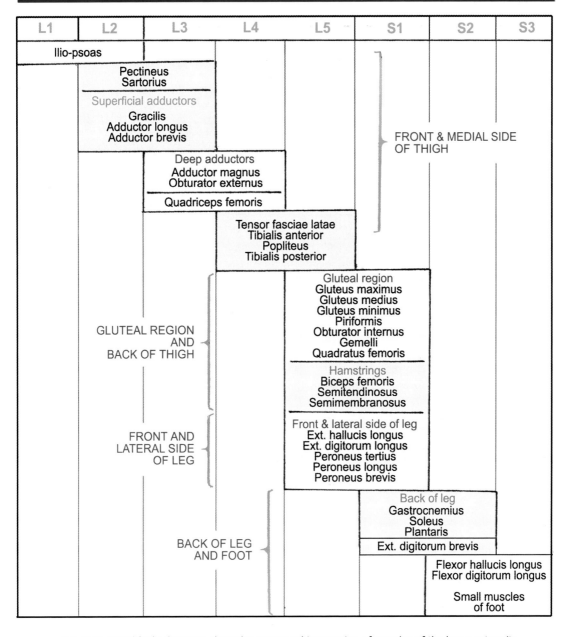

Fig. 2.14. Simplified scheme to show the segmental innervation of muscles of the lower extremity.

Injury above C3 causes paralysis of all respiratory muscles

(14) Movements of the upper extremity (C5 to T1). Injury above this level paralyses all four limbs *(quadriplegia)*.

(15) Movements of the lower extremity (L1 to S2). Injury above this level paralyses both lower limbs *(paraplegia)*.

(16) Filling of the urinary bladder (T12 to L2), and evacuation (S3 to S5).

(17) Erection of the penis (S2 to S4).

(18) Ejaculation (L1 and L2) (smooth muscle), and (S3 and S4) (striated muscle).

CLINICAL

FOR FURTHER DETAILS ABOUT THE SPINAL CORD SEE CHAPTER 5

3 : Basic Neuronal Arrangements

CLASSIFICATION OF NEURONS AND OF NERVE FIBRES IN PERIPHERAL NERVES ACCORDING TO FUNCTION

The nerve fibres that make up any peripheral nerve can be divided into two major types as follows.

(a) Fibres that carry impulses from the CNS to an **effector organ** (e.g., muscle or gland) are called **efferent** or **motor** fibres.

(b) Fibres that carry impulses from peripheral structures (e.g., skin) to the CNS are called **afferent fibres**. Some afferent fibres carry impulses that make us conscious of sensations like touch or pain: such fibres may, therefore, be called **sensory fibres**. Other afferent fibres convey information which is not consciously perceived, but is necessary for reflex control of various activities of the body.

Both afferent and efferent fibres can be further classified on the basis of the tissues supplied by them. The tissues and organs of the body can be broadly divided into two major categories – somatic and visceral. **Somatic structures** are those present in relation to the body wall (or soma). They include the tissues of the limbs (which represent a modified part of the body wall). Thus, the skin, bones, joints and striated muscles of the limbs and body wall are classified as somatic. In contrast, the tissues that make up the internal organs like the heart, lungs or stomach are classified as visceral. These include the lining epithelia of hollow viscera, and smooth muscle.

A distinction between somatic and visceral structures may also be made on embryological considerations.

(1) Structures developing from specialised areas of ectoderm e.g., the retina and membranous labyrinth, are classified as somatic while the epithelium of the tongue (and taste buds) which is of endodermal origin is classified as visceral.

(2) Striated muscle may be derived, embryologically, from three distinct sources. These are:
   (a) the somites developing in the paraxial mesoderm;
   (b) the somatopleuric mesoderm of the body wall; and
   (c) the mesoderm of the branchial arches.

The musculature of the limbs and body wall develops partly from somites and partly **in situ** from the mesoderm of the body wall. The nerves supplying this musculature are classified as somatic. The muscles that move the eyeball, and the muscles of the tongue are also derived from somites and the nerves supplying them are, therefore, also classified as somatic. However, striated muscle that develops in the mesoderm of the branchial arches is classified as visceral. Hence, the muscles of the face, the muscles of mastication, and the muscles of the pharynx and larynx are regarded as visceral.

Keeping in view the distinction between afferent and efferent fibres on one hand, and somatic and visceral structures on the other, we may divide fibres in peripheral nerves into four broad categories. These are:

(a) Somatic efferent,   *(b) Visceral efferent,*
(c) Somatic afferent, and   *(d) Visceral afferent.*

With the exception of somatic efferent fibres each of the categories named above is subdivided into a *general* and a *special* group. We thus have a total of seven *functional components* as follows.

1. *Somatic efferent* (or *somatomotor fibres)* fibres supply striated muscle of the limbs and body wall. They also supply the extrinsic muscles of the eyeballs, and the muscles of the tongue.

2. *General visceral efferent* fibres (also called *visceromotor fibres*) supply smooth muscle and glands. The nerves to glands are called *secretomotor* nerves.

3. *Special visceral efferent* fibres supply striated muscle developing in branchial arch mesoderm. They are frequently called *branchial efferent* or *branchiomotor* fibres. The muscles supplied include those of mastication, and of the face, the pharynx and the larynx.

4. *General somatic afferent* fibres are those that carry:

 (a) *sensations* of touch, pain and temperature from the skin (*exteroceptive impulses*);

 (b) *proprioceptive impulses* arising in muscles, joints and tendons conveying information regarding movement and position of joints.

5. *Special somatic afferent* fibres carry impulses of:

    (a) vision,

    (b) hearing, and

    (c) equilibrium.

6. *General visceral afferent* fibres (also called visceral sensory fibres) carry sensations e.g., pain from viscera (*visceroceptive* sensations).

7. *Special visceral afferent* fibres carry the sensation of taste.

A typical spinal nerve contains fibres of the four general categories. The special categories are present in cranial nerves only.

We will now consider the general disposition of the neurons associated with each functional type of nerve fibre.

Somatic Efferent Neurons

We have already seen that these neurons supply striated muscle. In the spinal cord the cell bodies of these neurons lie in the ventral grey column. They are often referred to as anterior horn cells. The neurons are large and multipolar and their Nissl substance is prominent. They are designated as *alpha neurons* to distinguish them from smaller anterior horn cells called *gamma neurons* (Fig. 3.1).

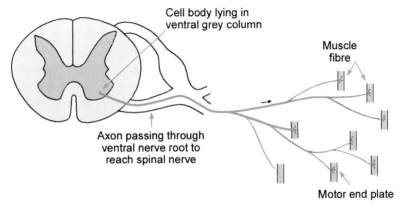

Cell body lying in
ventral grey column

Muscle
fibre

Axon passing through
ventral nerve root to
reach spinal nerve

Motor end plate

Fig. 3.1. Scheme to show the typical arrangement of a somatic efferent neuron.

The axon of a somatic efferent neuron leaves the spinal cord through a ventral nerve root to enter the spinal nerve concerned. During its course through the spinal nerve (and its branches) the axon divides into a variable number of branches each one of which ultimately ends by supplying one muscle fibre. The region of junction between a terminal branch of the axon and the muscle fibre has a special structure and is called the ***motor end plate*** or ***neuromuscular junction.*** Depending on the number of branchings one anterior horn cell supplies a variable number of muscle fibres. One anterior horn cell and the muscle fibres supplied by it constitute one ***motor unit.*** In large muscles, where strength of contraction is more important than precision, a motor unit may contain up to 2000 muscle fibres. On the other hand in muscles where precision is all important (e.g., in muscles of the eyeball) the motor unit may supply as few as six fibres.

The somatic efferent fibres of cranial nerves are axons of neurons, the cell bodies of which lie in somatic efferent nuclei in the brainstem. Their axons pass through the third, fourth and sixth cranial nerves to supply the extrinsic muscles of the eyeballs; and through the twelfth cranial nerve to supply muscles of the tongue.

Special Visceral Efferent Neurons (Branchiomotor Neurons)

These are seen only in relation to cranial nerves. The cell bodies of these neurons are located in the branchial efferent nuclei of the brainstem. Their axons pass through the fifth, seventh, ninth, tenth, and eleventh cranial nerves to supply striated muscle derived from the branchial arches. The relationship of these neurons to striated muscle is the same as that of somatic efferent neurons.

General Visceral Efferent Neurons

These are the neurons that constitute the autonomic nervous system (sympathetic and parasympathetic). They supply smooth muscle or glands. The nerves to glands are called ***secretomotor*** nerves. The pathway for the supply of smooth muscle or gland always consists of two neurons that synapse in a ganglion (Fig. 3.2). The first neuron carries the impulse from the CNS to the ganglion and is, therefore, called the ***preganglionic*** neuron. The second neuron carries the impulse from the ganglion to smooth muscle or gland and is called the ***postganglionic*** neuron.

The cell bodies of preganglionic neurons of the sympathetic nervous system are located in the lateral grey column of the spinal cord in the thoracic and upper two lumbar segments (Fig. 19.3). Their cell bodies are multipolar, but are smaller than those of somatic efferent neurons. The Nissl substance in them is also less prominent. The axons leave the spinal cord through the anterior nerve

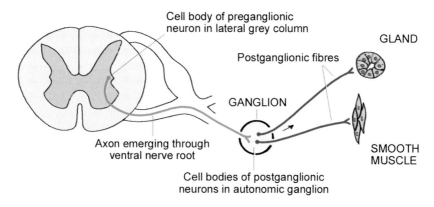

Fig. 3.2. Scheme to show the typical arrangement of a general visceral efferent neuron.

roots of spinal nerves and terminate in a sympathetic ganglion. The cell bodies of postganglionic neurons are located in sympathetic ganglia, and in some cases in peripherally situated ganglia and plexuses. The axons of these postganglionic neurons terminate in relation to smooth muscle in the walls of blood vessels and in viscera. They also supply the arrectores pilorum muscles of the skin, and give a secretomotor supply to sweat glands.

The cell bodies of preganglionic neurons of the parasympathetic nervous system are located in two different situations (Fig. 19.3).

(a) One group is located in the lateral grey column of the spinal cord in the second, third and fourth sacral segments. Their axons end in peripheral ganglia (or plexuses) situated in intimate relationship to pelvic viscera. These ganglia contain the cell bodies of postganglionic neurons. The axons of these neurons are short and end by supplying smooth muscle or glands of the viscera concerned.

(b) The other group of parasympathetic preganglionic neurons is located in the general visceral efferent nuclei of cranial nerves. The axons of these neurons terminate in autonomic ganglia associated with the third, seventh, ninth and tenth cranial nerves. The postganglionic neurons are situated in these ganglia. They supply smooth muscle or glands.

Afferent Neurons

We have seen that afferent nerve fibres can be divided into four categories *viz.,* general somatic afferent, special somatic afferent, general visceral afferent and special visceral afferent. The basic arrangement of the neurons that give origin to all four categories of afferent fibres is similar, and the description that follows applies to all of them.

The cell bodies of neurons that give rise to efferent fibres of peripheral nerves are located within the brain and spinal cord. In contrast, the cell bodies of neurons that give rise to afferent fibres are located outside the CNS. In the case of spinal nerves the cell bodies lie in the spinal ganglia; and in the case of the cranial nerves they lie in sensory ganglia (e.g., the trigeminal ganglion) associated with these nerves. We may illustrate the arrangement with reference to a spinal nerve (Fig. 3.3). The cells of the dorsal nerve root ganglion are of the unipolar variety described on page 7. Each cell gives off a single process that divides into a peripheral process and a central process. The peripheral process extends into the spinal nerve and courses through its branches to reach the tissue or organ supplied. It may branch repeatedly during its course. We have already seen that these peripheral processes are functionally dendrites as they convey impulses towards the cell body, but they are indistinguishable in structure from axons. These processes constitute the sensory fibres of peripheral

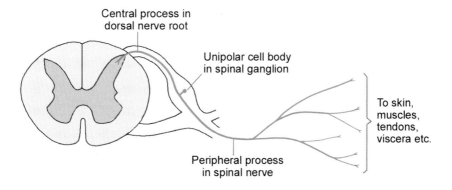

Central process in
dorsal nerve root

Unipolar cell body
in spinal ganglion

To skin,
muscles,
tendons,
viscera etc.

Peripheral process
in spinal nerve

Fig. 3.3. Scheme to show the typical arrangement of an afferent neuron.

nerves. The sensory impulses brought by these processes from various organs of the body are conveyed to the spinal cord by the central processes (representing axons). Within the spinal cord the central processes usually run a short course and terminate by synapsing with cells in the posterior grey column. Some of the central processes are, however, long. They enter the posterior funiculus and run upwards to the medulla as ascending tracts.

The sensory ganglia of the fifth, seventh, ninth and tenth cranial nerves are made up of cells similar to those of the spinal ganglia. Their central processes end by synapsing with cells in the sensory nuclei of these nerves. The sensory ganglia of the eighth nerve (i.e., the cochlear and vestibular ganglia) are peculiar in that their neurons are bipolar, the two processes corresponding to the central and peripheral processes of unipolar neurons.

Arrangement of Neurons within the Central Nervous System

So far we have considered the arrangement of neurons:

(a) having cell bodies that lie within the brain and spinal cord, and sending out efferent processes that leave the CNS to form the motor fibres of peripheral nerves; and

(b) having cell bodies located in ganglia outside the CNS, but sending processes into it.

The bulk of the CNS is, however, made up of neurons that lie entirely within it. As explained earlier, the cell bodies of these neurons are invariably located in masses of grey matter. The axons may be short, ending in close relation to the cell body (***short axon neurons*** or ***Golgi type II neurons***), or may be long (***long axon neurons*** or ***Golgi type I neurons***) and may travel to other masses of grey matter lying at considerable distances from the grey matter of origin. The neurons within the

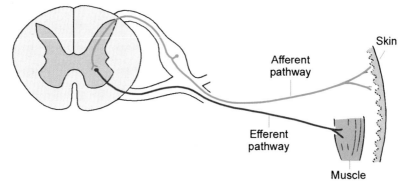

Fig. 3.4. A spinal reflex arc composed of two neurons.

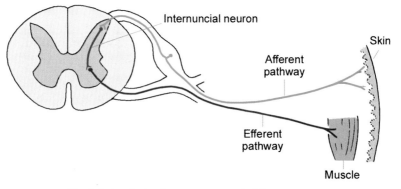

Fig. 3.5. A spinal reflex arc composed of three neurons.

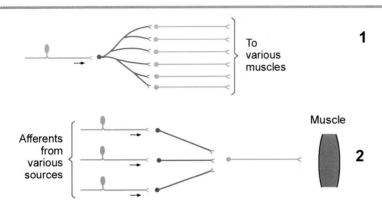

Fig. 3.6. Schemes to illustrate two roles which internuncial neurons may play. The internuncial neurons are shown in red lines.

CNS are interconnected in an extremely intricate manner. The description that follows illustrates some of the basic arrangements encountered.

The simplest pathways are those concerned with reflex activities, such as the contraction of a muscle in response to an external stimulus. For example, if the skin of the sole of a sleeping person is scratched, the leg is reflexly drawn up. Let us see how this happens. The simplest possible arrangement is shown in Fig. 3.4. The stimulus applied to skin gives rise to a nerve impulse which is carried by the peripheral process of a unipolar neuron to the spinal ganglion. From here the impulse passes into the central process which terminates by directly synapsing with an anterior horn cell supplying the muscle which draws the leg up. The complete pathway constitutes a **reflex arc** and in the above example it consists of two neurons – one afferent and the other efferent. As only one synapse is involved the reflex is **monosynaptic**. In actual practice, however, the reflex arc is generally made up of three neurons as shown in Fig. 3.5. The central process of the dorsal nerve root ganglion cell ends by synapsing with a neuron lying in the posterior grey column. This neuron has a short axon that ends by synapsing with an anterior horn cell, thus completing the reflex arc. The third neuron interposed between the afferent and efferent neurons is called an **internuncial neuron,** or simply an **interneuron.** For obvious reasons such a reflex is said to be **polysynaptic**. It is important to know that various tendon reflexes are dependent on monosynaptic reflex arcs.

The purpose served by an interneuron may be basically of three types. Firstly, the axon arising from an interneuron may divide into a number of branches and may synapse with a number of different efferent neurons. As a result an impulse coming along a single afferent neuron may result in an effector response by a large number of efferent neurons. Secondly, afferent impulses brought by a number of afferent neurons may converge on a single efferent neuron through the agency of interneurons. Some of these impulses tend to induce activity in the efferent neuron (i.e., they are **facilitatory)** while others tend to suppress activity (i.e., they are **inhibitory).** Thirdly, through interneurons an afferent neuron may establish contact with efferent neurons in the opposite half of the spinal cord, or in a higher or lower segment of the cord.

Some reflexes are protective e.g., withdrawal of the hand when a hot object is touched. In such a movement involving withdrawal joints of the extremity are flexed. Such reflexes are, therefore, also called **flexor reflexe**s. When a person is standing a series of reflexes are active to prevent him from falling. As these keep the body straight (with the hip and knee joints extended) they are called **extensor reflexes**, or **antigravity reflexes**. Maintenance of posture, through such reflexes) is influenced by the membranous labyrinth, the cerebellum and other centres in the brain. Vision is also important in maintaining correct posture.

Every time a stimulus reaches a neuron it does not mean that it must become active and must produce an impulse. A neuron receives inputs from many neurons (in some cases from hundreds of them). Some of these inputs are facilitatory and others are inhibitory. Activity in the neuron (in the form of initiation of an impulse) depends on the sum total of these inputs. Thus, each neuron may be regarded as a decision-making centre. The greater the number of neurons involved in any pathway, the greater the possibility of such interactions. Viewed in this light it will become clear that interneurons interposed in a pathway increase the number of levels at which 'decisions' can be taken. It will also be appreciated that most of the neurons within the nervous system are, in this sense, interneurons which are involved in numerous highly complex interactions on which the working of the nervous system depends.

From what has been said above it will be seen that some activities occur due to reflex action, and may involve only neurons within the spinal cord. However, most activities of the spinal cord are subjected to influence from higher centres. In the more complicated types of activity several higher centres may be involved and the pathways may be extremely complicated. Afferent impulses reaching these higher centres (e.g., the cerebral cortex) would appear to be somehow stored and this stored information (of which we may or may not be conscious) is used to guide responses to similar stimuli received in future. This accounts for memory and for learning processes.

From the above it will be appreciated that in a study of the nervous system we must first of all have some knowledge of the various masses of grey matter in the CNS and of their interconnections. The functional significance of some of these connections is easily understood, but in many others it is only a matter of conjecture. Some of the connections can be demonstrated anatomically. Evidence of others can be obtained by physiological methods, while a large number of finer connections no doubt remain unknown.

Projection, Association and Commissural Fibres

When a considerable number of fibres pass from a mass of grey matter in one part of the brain to another mass of grey matter in another part of the brain or spinal cord these are referred to as *projection fibres.* Fibres interconnecting different areas of the cerebral cortex or of the cerebellar cortex are called *association fibres*, while fibres connecting identical areas of the two halves of the brain are called *commissural fibres.*

All fibres crossing from one side of the brain or spinal cord to the opposite side are not commissural. When fibres originating in a mass of grey matter in one half of the CNS end in some other mass of grey matter in the opposite half they are referred to as *decussating fibres,* and the sites where such crossings take place are referred to as *decussations.*

4 : Sensory Receptors and Neuromuscular Junctions

We have seen that peripheral nerves contain afferent (or sensory) fibres, and efferent (or motor fibres). In relation to the peripheral endings of afferent nerve fibres there are receptors that respond to various kinds of stimuli.

Most efferent nerve fibres supply muscle, and at the junction of a nerve fibre with muscle we see neuromuscular junctions. In this chapter we will study the structure of various kinds of sensory receptors, and of neuromuscular junctions.

BASIC

Sensory Receptors

Preliminary remarks about receptors and their classification

The peripheral terminations of afferent fibres are responsible for receiving stimuli and are, therefore, referred to as receptors. Receptors can be classified in various ways.

1. From a functional point of view receptors can be classified on the basis of the kind of information they provide. They may be of the following types.

(**a**) *Cutaneous receptors* are concerned with touch, pain, temperature and pressure. These are also called *exteroceptive receptors* or *exteroceptors*.

(**b**) *Proprioceptive receptors* (or *proprioceptors*) provide information about the state of contraction of muscles, and of joint movement and position. This information is necessary for precise control of movement and for maintenance of body posture. By and large these activities occur as a result of reflex action and the information from these receptors may or may not be consciously perceived.

(**c**) *Interoceptive receptors* (or *interoceptors*) are located in thoracic and abdominal viscera and in blood vessels. These include specialised structures like the carotid sinus and the carotid body.

(**d**) The above three categories also include receptors that are stimulated by damaging influences which are perceived as pain, discomfort or irritation. Such receptors are referred to as *nociceptors*.

(**e**) *Special sense receptors* of vision, hearing, smell and taste are present in the appropriate organs. As these receptors (like those from the skin) provide information about factors external to the body they are in a sense exteroceptors.

2. Receptors may also be classified on the basis of the manner in which they are stimulated as follows.

(**a**) *Mechanoreceptors* are stimulated by mechanical deformation. These include receptors for touch, pressure, stretch etc. They also include end organs in the internal ear. After receiving a stimulus some receptors quickly return to the original state and are in a position to record repeated stimulation discretely. Such receptors are termed fast adapting. In contrast, slow adapting receptors record repeated stimuli as if there was one continuous stimulus (e.g., that of position sense at joints).

(**b**) *Chemoreceptors* are stimulated by chemical influences e.g., receptors in taste buds, or in the carotid bodies.

(**c**) *Photoreceptors* are stimulated by light e.g., rods and cones of the retina.

(**d**) *Thermoreceptors* respond to alterations in temperature.

(**e**) *Osmoreceptors* respond to changes in osmotic pressure.

Many receptors are polymodal in that they may respond to more than one kind of stimulus.

3. A third way of classifying receptors is on the basis of their structure. Essentially, most receptors consist of peripheral terminations of sensory nerve fibres that receive the sensory input directly. The somata of the neurons concerned are located in spinal ganglia. As the receptor element is part of a neuron the general term *neuronal receptor* is applied to them.

At some sites the sensory input is received by an epithelial cell which transmits the same to a peripheral nerve fibre. A synapse-like arrangement is seen at the junction of the epithelial cell with the axon terminal. In distinction to neuronal receptors these are termed *epithelial receptors*.

In the olfactory epithelium we have *neuroepithelial receptors*. Here, the receptor cell is a modified neuron that lies within the epithelial lining and directly gives off neuronal processes that travel centrally towards the CNS.

Although the receptor element in a neuronal receptor is a nerve terminal such terminals are often intimately surrounded by epithelial elements as described below.

Depending upon the orientation of these epithelial elements many types of endings have been described, but only the better known of these are given below. In the past, efforts have been made to correlate structural variations with specific sensory modalities. However, it is now realised that one type of sensation may be perceived by more than one variety of receptor. At the same time the same type of ending may subserve different functions in different locations. Finally, it is possible that the same receptor may respond to different kinds of stimuli under different circumstances. In spite of these reservations it appears reasonable to assume that some of the end organs described below are concerned predominantly with particular sensations. It must be remembered, however, that receptors act together and not in isolation and that it is the total pattern of impulses received by the nervous system that determines the nature of the sensations perceived.

For a sensation to be perceived through a receptor three essential steps are involved. Firstly, the receptor terminal has to receive an adequate stimulus. Secondly, the stimulus has to be translated to a change in electrical potential by depolarisation of membrane. Finally, this change in potential has to excite an action potential (in the nerve fibre concerned) that travels to the CNS.

We will now examine the structure of some sensory receptors. These are illustrated in Fig. 4.1.

Exteroceptive Receptors

Free Nerve Endings

When the terminals of sensory nerves do not show any particular specialisation of structure they are called free nerve endings. Such endings are widely distributed in the body. They are found in connective tissue. They are also seen in relation to the epithelial lining of the skin, cornea, alimentary canal, and respiratory system.

Free nerve endings are particularly numerous in relation to hair follicles. They respond mainly to deformation of hair i.e., they are fast adapting mechanoreceptors. The abundance of free nerve endings in relation to hair follicles is to be correlated with the fact that hair increase the sensitivity of skin to touch. Free nerve endings may also be thermoreceptors and nociceptors.

Some free nerve endings present in relation to hair follicles are described as *lanceolate endings*. These terminals are seen running along the hair root, below the opening of the sebaceous duct. The terminations of the nerve fibres are flattened with sharp edges that make direct contact with epithelial cells of the hair root.

Tactile Corpuscles (of Meissner)

These are small oval or cylindrical structures seen in relation to dermal papillae in the hand and foot, and in some other situations. These corpuscles are believed to be responsible for touch. They are slow adapting mechano-receptors.

Each corpuscle is about 80 µm long and 30 µm broad. It consists of an outer capsule and a central core. The capsule is made up of several layers of greatly folded cells and is continuous with the perineurium of nerves supplying the corpuscle. The core contains cells and nerve fibres. Each corpuscle is supplied by several myelinated nerve fibres. Some unmyelinated fibres may also be present.

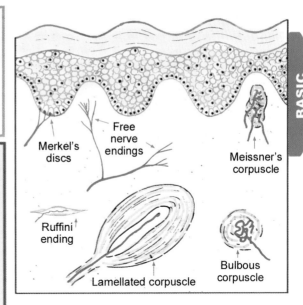

Fig. 4.1. Some sensory receptors present in relation to skin. The receptors are not drawn to scale.

BASIC

Lamellated Corpuscles (of Pacini)

Pacinian corpuscles are circular or oval structures. These are much larger than tactile corpuscles. They may be up to 2 mm in length, and up to 0.5 mm across. They are found in the subcutaneous tissue of the palm and sole, in the digits, and in various other situations. Lamellated corpuscles are believed to be fast adapting mechanoreceptors specially sensitive to vibration. They also respond to pressure.

Each corpuscle has a capsule, an intermediate zone, and a central core. The capsule is arranged in about thirty concentric layers (like the layers of an onion). The intermediate zone is cellular. The core consists of an outer layer of cells from which cytoplasmic lamellae project inwards and interdigitate with each other. In the centre of the core there is generally a single nerve fibre. The terminal part of the fibre is expanded into a bulb. Pacinian corpuscles are supplied by thick myelinated nerve fibres (Type A).

Bulbous Corpuscles (of Krause)

These are spherical structures about 50 µm in diameter. They consist of a capsule within which a nerve fibre terminates in a club-shaped manner. Their significance is controversial. Some authorities regard them to be degenerating or regenerating terminals of nerve fibres rather than as specialised endings.

Tactile Menisci (Merkel cell receptors)

These are small disc-like structures seen in relation to specialised epithelial cells (Merkel cells) present in the stratum spinosum of the epidermis. The discs are expanded ends of nerve fibres. Merkel cells bear spine-like protrusions that interdigitate with surrounding epidermal cells. Tactile menisci are slow adapting mechanoreceptors sensitive to pressure. They are supplied by large myelinated nerve fibres. Apart from surface epithelium of the skin, Merkel cell receptors may be found in relation to the sheaths of hair follicles.

ADVANCED

Ruffini endings

These are spindle-shaped structures present in the dermis of hairy skin. Some are also found in non-hairy skin. Similar receptors are also present in relation to joints, in the gums, and in the glans penis.

Within a fibrocellular sheath there are collagen fibres amongst which there are numerous unmyelinated endings of myelinated nerve fibres. Ruffini endings are slow adapting cutaneous mechanoreceptors responsive to stresses in dermal collagen. They resemble the Golgi tendon organs described below.

Summary of functions of cutaneous receptors

We can summarise the functions of cutaneous receptors as follows.

(**a**) Merkel discs and Ruffini endings are slowly adapting mechanoreceptors.

(**b**) Pacinian corpuscles and some types of free nerve endings act as rapidly adapting mechanoreceptors.

(**c**) Other free nerve endings act as nociceptors and thermoreceptors.

(**d**) Pacinian corpuscles and Ruffini endings lie deep to skin in the dermis or in tissue deep to skin. Their receptive fields are large and sensations mediated through them are not accurately localised. Pacinian corpuscles are useful mainly for appreciation of vibration. Ruffini endings respond to stretching of the dermis.

(**e**) In contrast to Pacinian corpuscles and Ruffini endings, Merkel cell receptors and Meissner's corpuscles have small receptor fields (specially over the fingers) and allow good tactile localisation.

(**f**) Apart from their sensory functions afferent nerve fibres may play a role in inflammation and repair of tissue, probably by releasing peptides (in particular substance P) at their endings. However, these views are not fully established at present.

Proprioceptive Receptors

Golgi Tendon Organs

They are also called the neurotendinous organs of Golgi. These organs are located at the junction of muscle and tendon. Each organ is about 500 μm long and about 100 μm in diameter. It consists of a capsule made up of concentric sheets of cytoplasm (Fig. 4.2). Inside the capsule there are small bundles of tendon fibres. The organ is innervated by one or more myelinated nerve fibres that divide to form several branches (spray-like arrangement). These receptors are stimulated by pull upon the tendon during active contraction of the muscle, and to a lesser degree by passive stretching.

In the past Golgi tendon organs have been considered to be involved in myotactic reflexes that prevent the development of excessive tension in muscle. However, it is now believed that their role is mainly in providing proprioceptive information; and that they are slow adapting receptors.

Similar endings are also present in ligaments of joints. At this site they serve as slow adapting, high threshold, receptors. Impulses from them lead to reflex inhibition of adjacent muscles, preventing excessive stresses on ligaments.

Muscle Spindles

These are spindle-shaped sensory end organs located within striated muscle (Fig.4.2). The spindle is bounded by a fusiform connective tissue capsule (forming an external capsule) within which there are a few muscle fibres of a special kind. These are called *intrafusal fibres* in contrast to *extrafusal fibres* that constitute the main bulk of the muscle. Each spindle contains six to fourteen intrafusal fibres. Each intrafusal fibre is surrounded by an internal capsule of flattened fibroblasts and collagen.

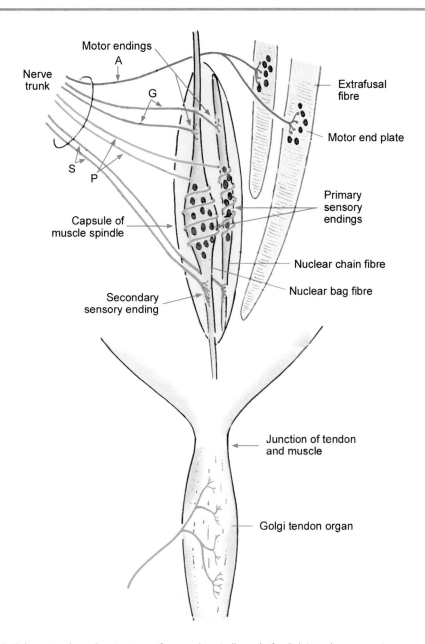

Fig. 4.2. Scheme to show the structure of a muscle spindle and of a Golgi tendon organ. A=axon of alpha neuron supplying extrafusal fibre. G= axons of gamma neurons supplying intrafusal fibres. P, S=afferents from primary and secondary sensory endings respectively.

Intrafusal fibres contain several nuclei that are located near the middle of the fibre. In some fibres this region is dilated into a bag: these are ***nuclear bag fibres***. In other intrafusal fibres the nuclei lie in a single row, there being no dilatation: these are ***nuclear chain fibres***.

Each muscle spindle is innervated by sensory as well as motor nerves. The sensory endings are of two types, primary and secondary. The motor innervation of intrafusal fibres is (mainly) by axons of gamma neurons located in the ventral grey column of the spinal cord (Also see below). The sensory endings respond to stretch. Primary sensory endings are rapidly adapting while secondary endings

BASIC

are slow adapting. However, the precise role of these receptors is complex and varies in different types of fibres.

Spindles provide information to the CNS about the extent and rate of changes in length of muscle. Nuclear bag fibres are stimulated by rapid changes, while nuclear chain fibres react more slowly. Contraction of intrafusal fibres makes the spindle more sensitive to stretch.

ADVANCED

Some further details about muscle spindles are as follows.

1. The nuclear bag fibres are considerably larger than the nuclear chain fibres. They extend beyond the capsule and gain attachment to the endomysium of extrafusal fibres. The nuclear chain fibres, on the other hand, remain within the capsule to which their ends are attached. On the basis of their ultrastructure and physiological properties nuclear bag fibres are divided into two types. Bag1 (or dynamic bag1) fibres respond to rapid changes in muscle length. Bag2 (or static bag2) fibres are less responsive to such changes.

The various types of intrafusal fibres differ from extrafusal fibres, and from each other, in ultrastructure and in some features of histochemistry.

2. The primary sensory fibres wind spirally around the nuclear region of intrafusal fibres and are, therefore, referred to as ***annulospiral endings***. The secondary endings (also called ***flower spray endings***) are seen mostly on nuclear chain fibres and are located away from the nuclear region. Both primary and secondary nerve fibres are derived from large myelinated axons, but are themselves unmyelinated.

3. The motor endings on intrafusal fibres of muscle spindles are of three types.

(**a**) Terminals of gamma-efferents that end on the equator of the nuclear bag, and do not show typical end plates.

(**b**) Gamma-efferents ending some distance away from the equator of the nuclear bag and having typical end plates. These are also called P2 endings.

(**c**) Terminals of delta-efferents (equivalent to beta-efferents of some species), which are collaterals of alpha-fibres supplying extrafusal muscle fibres. These terminals are located near the ends of nuclear bag fibres. They are also called P1 endings.

The motor nerve fibres innervating intrafusal fibres are thin but are myelinated. Those ending over nuclear bags do not show end plates. The P2 endings show typical end plates. P1 endings show en grappe end plates.

Receptors present in relation to joints

Four types of receptors have been demonstrated in relation to joints.

1. ***Type I***. These resemble Ruffini endings. They are innervated by myelinated nerve fibres, and serve as slowly adapting mechanoreceptors. These receptors are responsible for the sense of joint position and movement.

2. ***Type II***. These are similar to Pacinian corpuscles. They are fast adapting mechano-receptors, supplied by myelinated nerve fibres.

3. ***Type III***. These are similar to neurotendinous organs of Golgi. Impulses arising in them are probably responsible for reflex inhibition of muscle contraction, thus preventing excessive movement.

4. ***Type IV.*** These are free nerve endings, probably responsible for pain.

Neuromuscular Junctions

BASIC

We have seen that skeletal muscle fibres are supplied by ramifications of somatic efferent neurons. We have also seen that axonal branches arising from one neuron may innervate a variable number of muscle fibres (that constitute a motor unit).

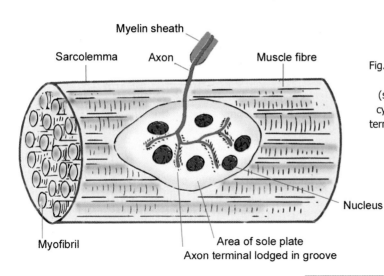

Fig. 4.3. Motor end plate seen in relation to a muscle fibre (surface view). Schwann cell cytoplasm covering the nerve terminal has not been shown for sake of clarity.

A. En plaque endings

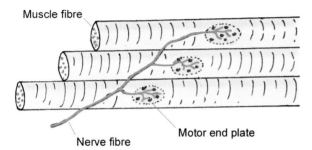

B. En grappe endings

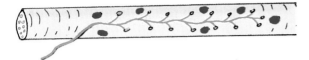

C. Trail endings

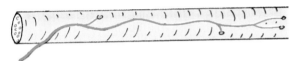

Fig. 4.4. Various types of neuromuscular junctions.

Each skeletal muscle fibre receives its own direct innervation. The site where the nerve ending comes into intimate contact with the muscle fibre is a neuromuscular (or myoneural) junction. Details of these junctions vary in different skeletal muscle fibres as follows.

1. Motor end plates or 'en plaque' endings:

In most neuromuscular junctions the nerve terminal comes in contact with a specialised area near the middle of the muscle fibre. This area is roughly oval or circular, and is referred to as the **sole plate**. The sole plate plus the axon terminal constitute the **motor end plate**. Motor end plates are considered in detail below.

2. 'En Grappe' endings:

On reaching a muscle fibre some axon terminals divide into a number of small ramifications each ending in an expansion applied to the surface of the muscle fibre. These are referred to as 'en grappe' endings.

3. Trail endings:

In some cases the nerve fibre runs for some distance along the length of the muscle fibre giving off several ramifications that come in contact with the latter.

'En grappe' and trail endings are seen mainly in relation to intrafusal muscle fibres (present in muscle spindles)(Fig. 4.4).

BASIC

ADVANCED

BASIC

STRUCTURE OF A TYPICAL MOTOR END PLATE:

In the region of the motor end plate axon terminals are lodged in grooves in the sarcolemma covering the sole plate. Between the axolemma (over the axon) and the sarcolemma (over the muscle fibre) there is a narrow gap (about 40 nm) occupied by various proteins that form a basal lamina. It follows that there is no continuity between axoplasm and sarcoplasm.

Axon terminals are lodged in grooves in the sarcolemma covering the sole plate. In section (Fig. 4.5) this groove is seen as a semicircular depression. This depression is the *primary cleft*. The sarcolemma in the floor of the primary cleft is thrown into numerous small folds resulting in the formation of *secondary* (or subneural) *clefts*.

In the region of the sole plate the sarcoplasm of the muscle fibre is granular. It contains a number of nuclei and is rich in mitochondria, endoplasmic reticulum and Golgi complexes.

Axon terminals are also rich in mitochondria. Each terminal contains vesicles similar to those seen in presynaptic boutons. The vesicles contain the neurotransmitter acetyl choline. Acetyl choline is released when nerve impulses reach the neuromuscular junction. It initiates a wave of depolarisation in the sarcolemma resulting in contraction of the entire muscle fibre. Thereafter the acetyl choline is quickly destroyed by the enzyme acetyl choline esterase. The presence of acetyl choline receptors has been demonstrated in the sarcolemma of the sole plate.

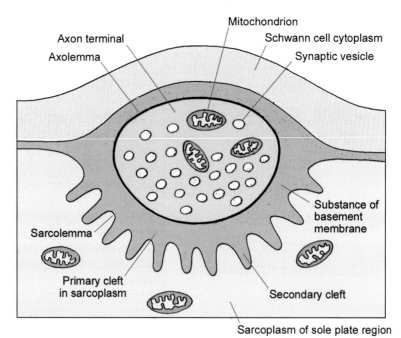

Fig. 4.5. Neuromuscular junction. This figure is a section across one of the axon terminals (and related) structures shown in Fig. 4.3.

ADVANCED

Nerve endings on smooth muscle

Nerve fibres innervating smooth muscle are unmyelinated. They end a short distance away from the myocyte surface. (In other words axolemma and sarcolemma do not come into contact). At most places, the nerve fibres are covered by Schwann cell cytoplasm. However, at places this cytoplasm is retracted exposing a segment of the axon. This segment of the axon shows the presence of vesicles. Neurotransmitter released from the vesicles diffuses to the myocytes.

In sympathetic terminals the vesicles contain catecholamines (usually noradrenaline). Monamine oxidases present in relation to sympathetic endings destroy catecholamines and thus regulate sympathetic activity. At parasympathetic terminals the vesicles in axon terminals are clear. They contain acetyl choline.

Recently it has been shown that some autonomic terminals contain neither noradrenaline nor acetyl choline. These are described as *non-adrenergic non-cholinergic* endings. The neurotransmitter present at these endings is probably a purine (adenosine triphosphate). Such fibres have been demonstrated in the walls of the alimentary and urinary tracts, and also in the CNS. These endings are believed to be predominantly inhibitory.

Other effector endings:

Apart from muscle, effector endings are present in relation to glands (secretomotor endings), to myoepithelial cells, and to adipose tissue.

SOME FACTS ABOUT MUSCLE ACTION

1. We have seen that a muscle fibre requires a stimulus for contraction to occur. Stimuli below a threshold level do not cause contraction. When a stimulus above the threshold strength is applied the muscle contracts to its full extent. This is the ***all or none law***.

2. It is very important to understand that the all or none law applies only to individual muscle fibres and not to the muscle as a whole. The force exerted by a muscle depends on the number of muscle fibres that are in contraction at a particular moment. This allows for a graded strength of muscle action depending upon need. A corollary of this is that large muscles with greater number of fibres can exert more power than smaller muscles. The concept of motor units has been already discussed. Large muscles that are required to act with great strength have larger motor units.

3. If a muscle fibre is stimulated repeatedly it fails to contract after some time. This is ***muscle fatigue***. Fatigue is caused by exhaustion of acetyl choline in the motor end plate, lack of oxygen and nutrients, and accumulation of lactic acid.

4. In a resting muscle some fibres are always in a state of contraction. After some time other fibres take over this function so that fatigue does not occur. This partial contraction gives the muscle its normal state of firmness. This is called ***muscle tone***. If this tone was not present the body would collapse. Muscle tone is controlled by various reflexes dependant on impulses arising in muscle spindles and tendon end organs. These have already been described.

5. When the nerve supply of a muscle is interrupted, tone is lost and the muscle becomes flaccid. Partial loss of tone is called ***hypotonia***. In upper motor neuron lesions the tone is exaggerated (***hypertonia***) and the muscle becomes rigid.

6. The capacity of a muscle to maintain activity over a period of time is called ***endurance***. This depends mainly on availability of glycogen. It is increased by training, as in atheletes. In most persons endurance reaches a maximum by the age of twenty, and declines after the age is fifty.

7. Apart from production of muscle contraction, nerve supply has a trophic effect. This maintains the integrity of the muscle. Denervation of a muscle leads to atrophy.

The functional status of a muscle is also influenced by activity (or the lack of it). If a normal limb is immobilised (e.g. by a plater cast) there is some degree of atrophy and the muscles become weak. Strength can be regained by suitable exercises (physiotherapy). Similarly, mormal muscles can hypertrophy and become stronger by exercise (as in atheletes).

MYASTHENIA GRAVIS

This is a disease marked by great weakness of skeletal muscle. The body produces antibodies against acetyl choline receptors. As a result many of these are destroyed. Transmission at the myoneural junction is much reduced resulting in weakness of muscles. Some improvement is obtained by administration of anti-choline esterase drugs like neostigmine.

Some elementary features of the spinal cord have been considered in Chapter 2. The arrangement of white and grey matter and the division of grey matter into ventral, dorsal and lateral columns has been seen.

We have also noted that the white matter of the spinal cord is divisible into anterior, posterior, and lateral funiculi. These funiculi are made up of fibres running up and down the cord. These constitute the ascending and descending tracts which will be considered in Chapter 9.

The relative amount of grey and white matter, and the shape and size of the grey columns, vary at different levels of the spinal cord (Fig. 5.1). The amount of grey matter to be seen at a particular level can be correlated with the mass of tissue to be supplied. It is, therefore, greatest in the region of the cervical and lumbar enlargements which supply the limbs. The amount of white matter undergoes progressive increase as we proceed up the spinal cord. This is a result of the fact that:

(a) progressively more and more ascending fibres are added as we pass up the cord, and

(b) the number of descending fibres decreases as we go down the cord as some of them terminate in each segment.

In the paragraphs that follow we will consider some details about the grey matter of the spinal cord.

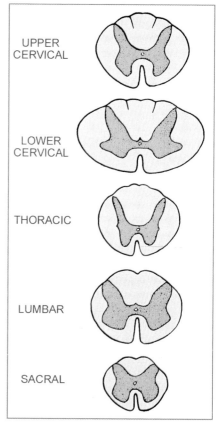

UPPER CERVICAL

LOWER CERVICAL

THORACIC

LUMBAR

SACRAL

Fig. 5.1. Diagrams to show differences in appearance of transverse sections through various levels of the spinal cord.

Grey Matter of the Spinal Cord

Subdivisions of Grey Matter

The grey matter of the spinal cord may be subdivided in more than one manner.

Traditionally, the ventral grey column has been divided into a ventral part, the **head**, and a dorsal part, the **base.** Similarly, the dorsal grey column has been subdivided (from anterior to posterior side) into a **base,** a **neck**, and a **head**. These subdivisions have, however, been found to have little importance.

Nuclei in spinal grey matter

An attempt has been made to recognise discrete collections of neurons (or nuclei) in various regions of the spinal grey matter. These are illustrated in the left half of Fig. 5.2.

The neurons of the ventral grey column (***ventral horn cells***) are arranged in the form of several discrete and elongated groups. We can recognise

(a) a ***medial group*** which may be subdivided into ***dorsomedial*** and ***ventromedial*** parts;

(b) a ***lateral group*** consisting of ***dorsolateral, ventrolateral*** and ***retrodorsolateral*** parts; and

(c) a ***central group*** represented by the ***phrenic*** and ***accessory nuclei*** (in the cervical region) and by the ***lumbosacral nucleus*** (in the lumbosacral region). Some large cells present along the anterior margin of the ventral grey column are called ***spinal border cells.***

Within the ***dorsal grey column*** the following relatively discrete areas may be recognised.

(**a**) The ***substantia gelatinosa*** which lies near the apex.

(**b**) ***Nucleus proprius*** (or ***dorsal funicular*** group).

(**c**) ***Dorsal nucleus*** (also called the ***thoracic nucleus*** or ***Clark's column***) lying on the medial side of the base.

(**d**) A thin layer of cells lying superficial to the substantia gelatinosa and constituting the ***posteromarginal nucleus***, also called the ***marginal zone.***

Between the ventral and dorsal grey columns an ***intermediate zone*** is sometimes described. This contains the ***intermediolateral*** and ***intermediomedial*** nuclei (or columns).

In the right half of Fig. 5.2. the ventral grey column is shown to be subdivided by a line passing forwards and medially. The part of the column lateral to this line (containing the greater part of the lateral group of nuclei) is present only in the region of the cervical and lumbar enlargements of the spinal cord. From this it can be inferred that the lateral group of nuclei innervate the musculature of the limbs. (Some neurons occupying the position of the ventrolateral group are seen in the first and second sacral segments of the spinal cord. They are believed to supply perineal musculature).

The dorsal nucleus is present only in the thoracic and upper lumbar segments. The intermediolateral group of neurons is present (a) from segments T1 to L2, and (b) in segments S2, S3 and S4.

From the examples given above it will be clear that at a given level of the spinal cord only some of the nuclear groups named in the preceding paragraphs are present.

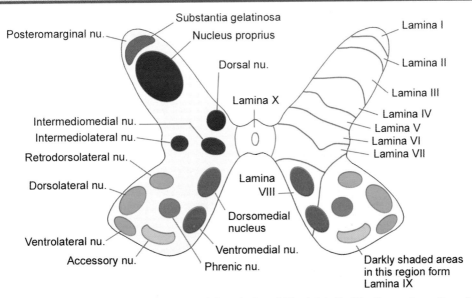

Fig. 5.2. Subdivisions of the grey matter of the spinal cord. The left half of the figure shows the cell groups usually described. The right half shows the newer concept of laminae.

Division of spinal grey matter into laminae

Recent studies have shown that from the point of view of neuronal connections the grey matter of the spinal cord may be divided into ten areas or laminae. These are illustrated in the right half of Fig. 5.2.

Lamina I corresponds to the posteromarginal nucleus (lamina marginalis), *lamina II* to the substantia gelatinosa, and *laminae III* and *IV* to the nucleus proprius. (Laminae I to IV correspond to the head of the dorsal grey column. Some workers include lamina III in the substantia gelatinosa). *Lamina V* corresponds to the neck of the dorsal grey column and *lamina VI* to the base. The lateral part of lamina V corresponds to the formatio reticularis. *Lamina VII* corresponds to the intermediate grey matter and includes the intermediomedial, intermediolateral, and dorsal nuclei. It is believed to be made up predominantly of interneurons. At the level of the cervical and lumbar enlargements this lamina extends into the lateral part of the ventral horn. *Lamina VIII* occupies most of the ventral horn in the thoracic segments, but at the level of the limb enlargements it is confined to the medial part of the ventral horn. *Lamina IX* is made up of the various discrete groups of ventral horn cells already described. *Lamina X* forms the grey matter around the central canal.

From the point of view of function, and of neuronal organisation, it has been proposed that (instead of division into ventral and dorsal grey columns) the spinal grey matter should be divided into a *central core* where the organisation of neurons is diffuse and non-discriminative; and into *dorsal and ventral appendages.* Laminae VII and VIII have been (tentatively) assigned to the central core, laminae I to VI to the dorsal appendage, and lamina IX to the ventral appendage.

Significance of Neurons in Grey Matter of Spinal Cord

The *ventral horn cells* of the spinal cord may be functionally divided into three major categories as follows.

(**a**) The most prominent neurons with large cell bodies and prominent Nissl substance are designated *alpha neurons*. These are somatic efferent neurons (Fig. 3.1). Their axons (*alpha efferents)* leave the spinal cord through the ventral nerve roots of spinal nerves and innervate skeletal muscle. They occupy lamina IX of the ventral grey column.

(**b**) Some smaller neurons designated as *gamma neurons* are also located in lamina IX. They supply intrafusal fibres of muscle spindles (Fig. 4.2). Sensory impulses arising in the spindle travel to the spinal cord and reach the alpha neurons. The gamma neurons thus influence the activity of alpha neurons indirectly through muscle spindles.

(**c**) A considerable number of smaller neurons in the ventral grey column are internuncial neurons. They are most abundant in Lamina VII. Some ramifications of the central processes of cells in the dorsal nerve root ganglia (bringing afferent impulses from the periphery), and axons descending from higher centres, terminate in relation to these internuncial neurons. The axons of internuncial neurons convey these impulses to alpha and gamma neurons.

(**d**) Another variety of neuron that is believed (on physiological grounds) to exist in the ventral grey column is the so called *Renshaw cell*. These cells receive the terminations of collaterals arising from the axons of alpha neurons. The axons of Renshaw cells carry the impulses back to the cell bodies of the same alpha neurons, and thus help to regulate their activity.

The *neurons of the dorsal grey column* may be subdivided as follows.

(**a**) Some of these are internuncial neurons similar to those in the ventral grey column.

(**b**) Many dorsal column neurons receive afferent impulses through the central processes of neurons in dorsal nerve root ganglia. These dorsal column neurons give off axons that enter the white matter of the spinal cord either on the same or opposite side. These axons may behave in one of the following ways.

(1) They may ascend or descend for some segments before terminating in relation to neurons at other levels of the spinal cord. Such axons constitute *intersegmental tracts.*

(2) A considerable number of axons arising from dorsal column neurons run upwards in the spinal cord and constitute *ascending tracts* which terminate in various masses of grey matter in the brain. These tracts form a considerable part of the white matter of the spinal cord.

The *neurons of the intermediolateral group* (lateral grey column) are visceral efferent neurons. They are present at two levels of the spinal cord.

(**a**) One group is present in the thoracic and upper two or three lumbar segments. These are preganglionic neurons of the sympathetic nervous system. Their axons terminate in relation to postganglionic neurons in sympathetic ganglia (and occasionally in some other situations). Axons of these postganglionic neurons are distributed to various organs, and to blood vessels (Figs. 19.1, 19.2).

(**b**) The second group of visceral efferent neurons is found in the second, third and fourth sacral segments of the spinal cord. These are preganglionic neurons of the parasympathetic nervous system. Their axons leave the spinal cord through the ventral nerve roots to reach spinal nerves. They leave the spinal nerves as the *pelvic splanchnic nerves* which are distributed to some viscera in the pelvis and abdomen (Fig. 19.6). They end by synapsing with ganglion cells located in intimate relationship to the viscera concerned. The postganglionic fibres arising in these ganglia are short and supply smooth muscle and glands in these viscera.

The location of the various types of neurons described above in relation to laminae of spinal grey matter is of interest.

Afferent fibres carrying sensations from the skin end predominantly in laminae I to IV. Proprioceptive impulses reach laminae V and VI. These laminae also receive numerous fibres from the cerebral cortex.

Lamina VII gives off fibres that reach the midbrain and cerebellum (through spino-cerebellar, spino-tectal and spino-reticular tracts). It receives fibres from these regions through tectospinal, reticulo-spinal and rubrospinal tracts.

Renshaw cells are located in a forward extension of lamina VII (into the interval between laminae VIII and IX).

Lamina VIII is made up mainly of interneurons that receive fibres from various sources. They give efferents to gamma neurons and thus influence muscle spindles.

Lamina IX contains the alpha and gamma neurons that give off efferent fibres to skeletal muscle. Motor neurons in different parts of the ventral grey column show remarkable differences in the orientation and extent of their dendritic fields. Many of the dendrites of neurons in the ventromedial, central and ventrolateral columns run longitudinally in the form of bundles. These neurons, therefore, come into intimate contact with each other. This arrangement is seen in relation to neurons that supply postural muscles. In contrast, the dendrites of neurons in the dorsolateral column have very little contact with those of neighbouring neurons. This column supplies muscles in distal parts of the limbs and the discrete nature of the neurons may be associated with fine control necessary for movements produced by these muscles.

Spinal Reflexes

We have seen that the nervous system is involved in various types of reflex activity. The basic pathways for such reflexes have been considered on page 44. Many of these reflexes can be demonstrated clinically, and constitute a valuable aid in establishing the integrity of various levels of the nervous system. Some of the reflexes that are used for this purpose are described below.

Myotatic or Stretch Reflexes

Sudden stretching of a muscle (by tapping its tendon) produces reflex contraction of the muscle. The pathway for this reflex involves two neurons only. Stretching of the muscle stimulates proprioceptive nerve endings located in muscle spindles and other receptors. These impulses are carried to the spinal cord by neurons that synapse with motor neurons in the ventral grey columns (Fig. 3.5). Fibres arising from these motor neurons reach the muscle and produce contraction. Stretch reflexes are abolished if any part of the pathway for it (i.e., the reflex arc) is interrupted. Under certain conditions these reflexes may be exaggerated. From a clinical point of view it is important to know the level of the spinal cord at which each reflex is mediated. Some of the important stretch reflexes are described below. The spinal segments concerned are given in brackets.

(**1**) The **knee jerk** or **patellar tendon reflex** consists of extension of the leg by contraction of the quadriceps when the ligamentum patellae is tapped (L2, L3, L4).

(**2**) The **ankle jerk** or **Achilles tendon reflex** consists of plantar flexion of the foot on tapping the tendo calcaneus (L5, S1, S2).

(**3**) The **biceps tendon reflex** consists of flexion of the forearm on tapping the biceps tendon (C5, C6).

(**4**) The **triceps tendon reflex** consists of extension of the forearm on tapping the triceps tendon (C6, C7, C8).

(**5**) The **supinator jerk** (or **radial periosteal reflex**) consists of flexion of the forearm when the distal end of the radius is tapped (C7, C8). Note that the muscle responsible for this reflex is the brachioradialis, not the supinator. It is called the supinator jerk because the brachioradialis was at one time called the supinator longus. This is a periosteal reflex, not a tendon reflex. According to some authorities the spinal segments responsible for the reflex are C5, 6,7.

(**6**) The **wrist tendon reflex** consists of flexion of the fingers on percussion on wrist tendons (C8, T1).

(**7**) The **jaw** or **masseter reflex** is a myotatic reflex mediated through the trigeminal nerve (and not through the spinal cord). To elicit this reflex the patient is asked to open the mouth slightly. The examiner places his index finger over the middle of the patient's chin and taps it. This results in bilateral contraction of the masseter and temporalis muscles. Both afferent and efferent components of the reflex arc pass through the mandibular division of the trigeminal nerve, the nuclei concerned being located in the pons.

Superficial Reflexes

Stimulation of skin in certain regions of the body causes contraction of underlying muscles. This occurs reflexly, the reflex being mediated through the spinal cord. Some of these superficial reflexes are described below.

(**1**)The ***abdominal reflexes*** consist of contraction of underlying muscles on stroking the skin of the abdomen in its upper (T6,7), middle (T8,9) and lower (T10 to T12) parts.

(**2**)The ***cremasteric reflex*** consists of elevation of the scrotum on stroking the skin of the medial side of the thigh (T12 to L2).

(**3**)The ***gluteal reflex*** consists of contraction of the glutei on stroking the overlying skin (L4 to S1).

(**4**)The normal ***plantar reflex*** consists of plantar flexion of the toes on stroking the skin of the sole (L5 to S2). When there is an injury to the corticospinal system an abnormal response is obtained. There is extension (dorsiflexion) of the great toe and fanning out of other toes. This response is referred to as ***Babinski's sign.*** Such a response may also be seen in newborn infants, and sometimes in sleeping or intoxicated adults.

(**5**)The ***anal reflex*** consists of contraction of the external anal sphincter on stroking the perianal region (S4,5, coccygeal).

Other Important Spinal Levels

Movements of the head (through neck muscles) depend on segments C1 to C4; those of the diaphragm on segments C3 to C5; those of the upper extremity on segments C5 to T1; and those of the lower extremity on segments L1 to S2. Filling of the urinary bladder is mediated by segments T12 to L2, and evacuation by segments S3 to S5. Erection of the penis depends on segments S2 to S4, and ejaculation on segments L1 and L2 (smooth muscle), and also on S3 and S4 (striated muscle).

DEVELOPMENT OF THE SPINAL CORD

The spinal cord is developed from the caudal cylindrical part of the neural tube.

When this part of the neural tube is first formed, its cavity is in the form of a dorsoventral cleft. The lateral walls are thick, but the roof (dorsal), and the floor (ventral), are thin (Fig. 5.3A). The wall of the tube subdivides into the matrix cell or ependymal layer, the mantle layer and the marginal layer (Fig. 5.3B) as already described.

The mantle zone grows faster in the ventral part of the neural tube, and becomes thicker, than in the dorsal part. As a result, the ventral part of the lumen of the neural tube becomes compressed. The line separating the compressed ventral part, from the dorsal part, is called the ***sulcus limitans*** (Fig. 5.3C). With its formation, the lateral wall of the developing spinal cord can be divided into a dorsal part, called the dorsal or ***alar lamina***, and a ventral part, called the ventral or ***basal lamina***.

This division is of considerable functional importance. The basal lamina develops into structures that are motor in function, and the alar lamina into those that are sensory. The alar and basal laminae are also called the ***alar*** and ***basal plates*** respectively.

With continued growth in thickness of the mantle layer, the spinal cord gradually acquires its definitive form (Figs. 5.3D, E). With growth of the alar lamina, the dorsal part of the cavity within the cord becomes obliterated: the posterior median septum is formed in this situation. The ventral part of the cavity remains as the ***central canal.*** Further enlargement of the basal lamina causes it to project forwards on either side of the midline, leaving a furrow, the ***anterior median fissure***, between the projecting basal laminae of the two sides.

The nerve cells that develop in the mantle zone of the basal lamina become the ***neurons of the anterior grey column*** (Fig. 5.4). The axons of these cells grow out of the ventrolateral angle of the spinal cord to form the ***anterior nerve roots*** of the spinal nerves. The nerve cells that develop in the mantle layer of the alar lamina form the ***neurons of the posterior grey column***. These are sensory neurons of the second order. Their axons travel predominantly upwards in the marginal layer to form the ***ascending tracts*** of the spinal cord. Many of these cells form ***interneurons.***

The ***dorsal nerve roots*** are formed by the axons of cells that develop from the neural crest (Fig. 5.4). Groups of these cells collect on the dorsolateral aspect of the developing spinal cord to form the *dorsal nerve root ganglia* (or *spinal ganglia*). The axons of these cells divide into two. The central processes migrate towards the spinal cord, and establish contact with the dorsolateral aspect of the latter, thus forming the *dorsal nerve roots*. These axons finally synapse with neurons of the posterior grey column developing in the alar lamina. The peripheral processes of the cells of the dorsal nerve root ganglia grow outwards to form the sensory components of the spinal nerves.

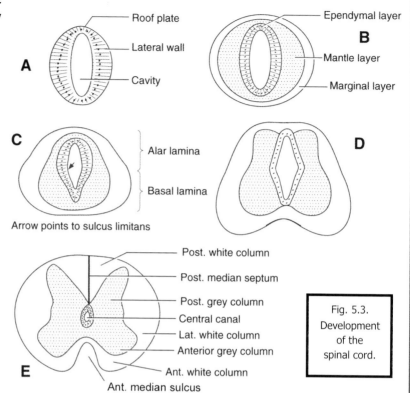

Arrow points to sulcus limitans

Fig. 5.3. Development of the spinal cord.

As stated above, the axons of neurons in the posterior grey column enter the marginal layer, to form the *ascending tracts* of the spinal cord. At the same time, axons of cells developing in various parts of the brain grow downwards to enter the marginal layer of the spinal cord and form its *descending tracts*. These ascending and descending tracts form the *white matter* of the spinal cord. As the mantle layer takes on the shape of the anterior and posterior *grey columns*, the white matter becomes subdivided into anterior, lateral and posterior *white columns*.

The phenomenon of *recession* of the spinal cord has already been discussed.

Related topics

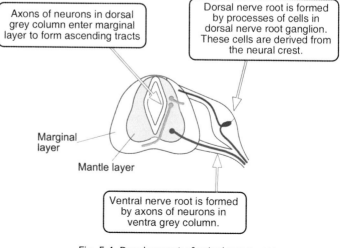

Fig. 5.4. Development of spinal nerve roots.

Gross Anatomy of the Brainstem

The brainstem consists (from above downwards) of the midbrain, the pons and the medulla (Figs 6.1, 6.2). The midbrain is continuous, above, with the cerebral hemispheres. The medulla is continuous, below, with the spinal cord. Posteriorly, the pons and medulla are separated from the cerebellum by the fourth ventricle (Fig. 6.3). The ventricle is continuous, below, with the central canal, which traverses the lower part of the medulla, and becomes continuous with the central canal of the spinal cord. Cranially, the fourth ventricle is continuous with the aqueduct, which passes through the midbrain. The midbrain, pons and medulla are connected to the cerebellum by the superior, middle and inferior cerebellar peduncles, respectively.

A number of cranial nerves are attached to the brainstem. The third and fourth nerves emerge from the surface of the midbrain; and the fifth from the pons. The sixth, seventh and eighth nerves emerge at the junction of the pons and medulla. The ninth, tenth, eleventh and twelfth cranial nerves emerge from the surface of the medulla.

The surface of the brainstem is intimately related to the meninges and to arteries and veins.

The Medulla: gross anatomy

The medulla is broad above, where it joins the pons; and narrows down below, where it becomes continuous with the spinal cord. Its length is about 3 cm and its width is about 2 cm at its upper end.

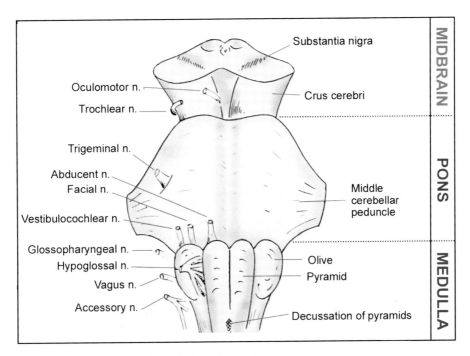

Fig. 6.1. Ventral aspect of the brainstem.

The junction of the medulla and cord is usually described as lying at the level of the upper border of the atlas vertebra. The transition is, in fact, not abrupt but occurs over a certain distance. The medulla is divided into a lower closed part, which surrounds the central canal; and an upper open part, which is related to the lower part of the fourth ventricle. The surface of the medulla is marked by a series of fissures or sulci that divide it into a number of regions. The ***anterior median fissure*** and the ***posterior median sulcus*** are upward continuations of the corresponding features seen on the spinal cord. On each side the ***anterolateral sulcus*** lies in line with the ventral roots of spinal nerves. The rootlets of the hypoglossal nerve emerge from this sulcus. The ***posterolateral sulcus*** lies in line with the dorsal nerve roots of spinal nerves, and gives attachment to rootlets of the glossopharyngeal, vagus and accessory nerves. The region between the anterior median sulcus and the anterolateral sulcus is occupied (on either side of the midline) by an elevation called the ***pyramid***. The elevation is caused by a large bundle of fibres that descend from the cerebral cortex to the spinal cord. Some of these fibres cross from one side to the other in the lower part of the medulla, obliterating the anterior median fissure. These crossing fibres constitute the ***decussation of the pyramids***.

Some other fibres emerge from the anterior median fissure, above the decussation, and wind laterally over the surface of the medulla. These are the ***anterior external arcuate fibres***. In the upper part of the medulla, the region between the anterolateral and posterolateral sulci shows a prominent, elongated, oval swelling named the ***olive***. This swelling is about half an inch long. It is produced by a large mass of grey matter called the ***inferior olivary nucleus***. The posterior part of the medulla, between the posterior median sulcus and the posterolateral sulcus, contains tracts that enter it from the posterior funiculus of the spinal cord. These are the ***fasciculus gracilis*** lying medially, next to the midline, and the ***fasciculus cuneatus*** lying laterally. These fasciculi end in rounded elevations called the ***gracile and cuneate tubercles***. These tubercles are produced by masses of grey matter called the ***nucleus gracilis*** and the ***nucleus cuneatus*** respectively. Just above these tubercles the

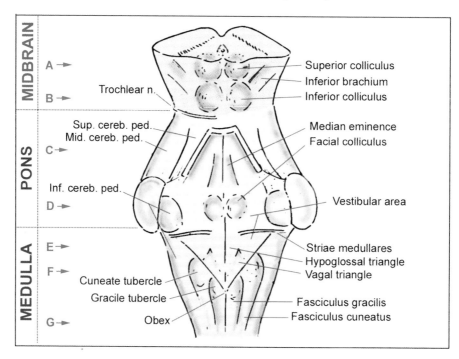

Fig. 6.2. Dorsal aspect of the brainstem. A transverse section showing the main features present at level A is shown in Fig. 6.10; at B in 6.9; at C in 6.7; at D in 6.8; at E in 6.6; at F in 6.5; and at G in 6.4.

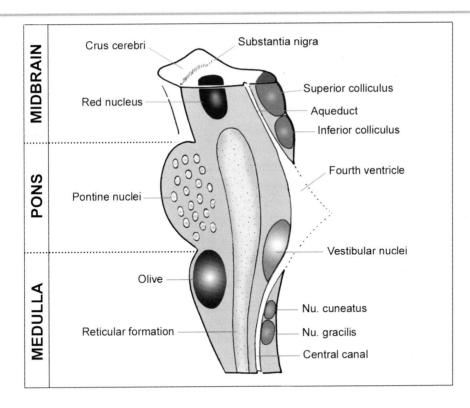

Fig. 6.3. Median section through the brainstem. Some important masses of grey matter are shown projected on to median plane.

posterior aspect of the medulla is occupied by a triangular fossa which forms the lower part of the floor of the fourth ventricle. This fossa is bounded on either side by the inferior cerebellar peduncle. The lower part of the medulla, immediately lateral to the fasciculus cuneatus, is marked by another longitudinal elevation called the ***tuberculum cinereum***. This elevation is produced by an underlying collection of grey matter called the ***spinal nucleus of the trigeminal nerve***. The grey matter of this nucleus is covered by a layer of nerve fibres that form the ***spinal tract of the trigeminal nerve***.

The Pons: gross anatomy

The pons shows a convex anterior surface, marked by prominent transversely running fibres. Laterally, these fibres collect to form a bundle, the middle cerebellar peduncle. The trigeminal nerve emerges from the anterior surface, and the point of its emergence is taken as a landmark to define the plane of junction between the pons and the middle cerebellar peduncle. The anterior surface of the pons is marked, in the midline, by a shallow groove, the ***sulcus basilaris***, which lodges the basilar artery. The line of junction between the pons and the medulla is marked by a groove through which a number of cranial nerves emerge. The abducent nerve emerges from just above the pyramid and runs upwards in close relation to the anterior surface of the pons. The facial and vestibulo-cochlear nerves emerge from the interval between the olive and the pons. The posterior aspect of the pons forms the upper part of the floor of the fourth ventricle.

On either side of the lower part of the pons there is a region called the ***cerebello-pontine angle***. This region lies near the lateral aperture of the fourth ventricle. The facial, vestibulo-cochlear and glossopharyngeal nerves, the nervus intermedius, and sometimes the labyrinthine arteries lie in this region.

The Midbrain: gross anatomy

When the midbrain is viewed from the anterior aspect, we see two large bundles of fibres, one on each side of the middle line. These are the ***crura*** of the midbrain. The crura are separated by a deep fissure. Near the pons the fissure is narrow, but broadens as the crura diverge to enter the corresponding cerebral hemispheres. The parts of the crura just below the cerebrum form the posterior boundary of a space called the ***interpeduncular fossa*** (Fig. 8.7). The oculomotor nerve emerges from the medial aspect of the crus (singular of crura) of the same side.

The posterior aspect of the midbrain is marked by four rounded swellings. These are the ***colliculi***, one superior and one inferior on each side. Each colliculus is related laterally to a ridge called the ***brachium***. The ***superior brachium*** (also called the superior quadrigeminal brachium, or brachium of superior colliculus) connects the superior colliculus to the lateral geniculate body. Similarly, the ***inferior brachium*** (also called the inferior quadrigeminal brachium or brachium of inferior colliculus) connects the inferior colliculus to the medial geniculate body. Just below the colliculi, there is the uppermost part of a membrane, the ***superior medullary velum***, which stretches between the two superior cerebellar peduncles, and helps to form the roof of the fourth ventricle. The trochlear nerve emerges from the velum, and then winds round the side of the midbrain to reach its ventral aspect.

In the description of the surface features of the brainstem, given above, reference has been made to the floor of the fourth ventricle. This is described in Chapter 20. It is important that this description be read at this stage, so as to obtain a complete idea of the posterior aspect of the pons and medulla.

Preliminary Review of the Internal Structure of the Brainstem

The following description is confined to those features of internal structure that can be seen with the naked eye. A detailed consideration of the internal structure of the brainstem will be taken up in Chapter 11.

The main features of the internal structure of the brainstem are most easily reviewed by examining transverse sections at various levels. These are illustrated in Figs. 6.4 to 6.8. The levels represented in these figures are indicated in Fig. 6.2.

The Medulla

A section at the level of the pyramidal decussation (Fig. 6.4) shows some similarity to sections through the spinal cord. The ***central canal*** is surrounded by ***central grey matter***. The ***ventral grey columns*** are present, but are separated from the central grey matter by ***decussating pyramidal fibres***. The region behind the central grey matter is occupied by the ***fasciculus gracilis***, medially; and by the ***fasciculus cuneatus*** laterally. Closely related to these fasciculi there are two tongue-shaped extensions of the central grey matter. The medial of these extensions is the ***nucleus gracilis***, and the lateral is the ***nucleus cuneatus***. More laterally, there is the ***spinal nucleus of the trigeminal nerve***. When traced inferiorly, this nucleus reaches the second cervical segment of the spinal cord, where it becomes continuous with the substantia gelatinosa. Above, the nucleus extends as far as the

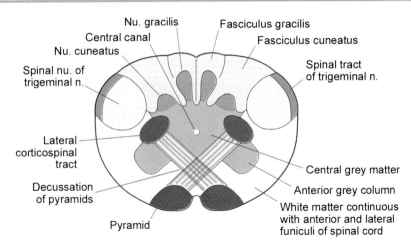

Fig. 6.4. Main features to be seen in a transverse section through the medulla at the level of the pyramidal decussation (Level G in Fig. 6.2).

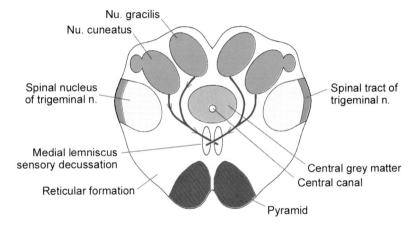

Fig. 6.5. Transverse section through the medulla to show the main features seen at the level of the sensory decussation (Level F in Fig. 6.2).

upper part of the pons. The spinal nucleus of the trigeminal nerve is related superficially to the **spinal tract** of the nerve. The ventral part of the medulla is occupied, on either side of the midline, by a prominent bundle of fibres: these fibres form the **pyramid**. The fibres of the pyramids are corticospinal fibres on their way from the cerebral cortex to the spinal cord. At this level in the medulla many of these fibres run backwards and medially to cross in the midline. These crossing fibres constitute the **decussation of the pyramids**. Having crossed the midline, the corticospinal fibres turn downwards to enter the lateral white column of the spinal cord. The anterolateral region of the medulla is continuous with the anterior and lateral funiculi of the spinal cord.

A section through the medulla at a somewhat higher level is shown in Fig. 6.5. The central canal surrounded by central grey matter, the nucleus gracilis, the nucleus cuneatus, the spinal nucleus of the trigeminal nerve, and the pyramids occupy the same positions as at lower levels. The nucleus gracilis and the nucleus cuneatus are, however, much larger and are no longer continuous with the central grey matter. The fasciculus gracilis and the fasciculus cuneatus are less prominent. The region just behind the pyramids is occupied by a prominent bundle of fibres, the **medial lemniscus**, on

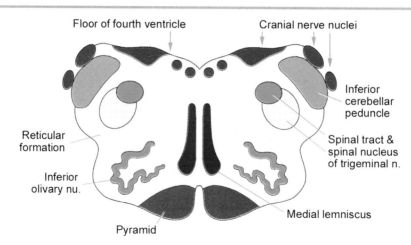

Fig. 6.6. Main features to be seen in a transverse section through the medulla at the level of the olive
(Level E in Fig. 6.2).

either side of the midline. The medial lemniscus is formed by fibres arising in the nucleus gracilis and the nucleus cuneatus. These fibres cross the midline and turn upwards in the lemniscus of the opposite side. The crossing fibres of the two sides constitute the **sensory decussation**. The region lateral to the medial lemniscus contains scattered neurons mixed with nerve fibres. This region is the **reticular formation**. More laterally there is a mass of white matter containing various tracts.

A section through the medulla at the level of the olive is shown in Fig. 6.6. The pyramids, the medial lemniscus, the spinal nucleus and tract of the trigeminal nerve, and the reticular formation are present in the same relative position as at lower levels. The medial lemniscus is, however, much more prominent and is somewhat expanded anteriorly. Lateral to the spinal nucleus (and tract) of the trigeminal nerve we see a large compact bundle of fibres. This is the **inferior cerebellar peduncle** which connects the medulla to the cerebellum. Posteriorly, the medulla forms the floor of the fourth ventricle. Here it is lined by a layer of grey matter in which are located several important cranial nerve nuclei (Chapter 10).

The **inferior olivary nucleus** forms a prominent feature in the anterolateral part of the medulla at this level. It is made up of a thin lamina of grey matter that is folded on itself like a crumpled purse. The nucleus has a hilum that is directed medially.

The Pons

The pons is divisible into a **ventral part** and a **dorsal part** (Fig. 6.7).

The ventral (or basilar) part contains numerous transverse and vertical fibres. Amongst the fibres are groups of cells that constitute the **pontine nuclei**. When traced laterally the transverse fibres form the **middle cerebellar peduncle**. The vertical fibres are of two types. Some of them descend from the cerebral cortex to end in the pontine nuclei. Others are corticospinal fibres that descend through the pons into the medulla where they form the pyramids.

The dorsal part (or tegmentum) of the pons may be regarded as an upward continuation of the part of the medulla behind the pyramids. Superiorly, it is continuous with the tegmentum of the midbrain. It is bounded posteriorly by the fourth ventricle. Laterally, it is related to the **superior cerebellar peduncles** in its upper part (Fig. 6.7); and to the inferior cerebellar peduncles in its lower part (Fig. 6.8). The spinal nucleus and tract of the trigeminal nerve lie just medial to these peduncles. The medial lemniscus forms a transversely elongated band of fibres just behind the ventral part of the pons.

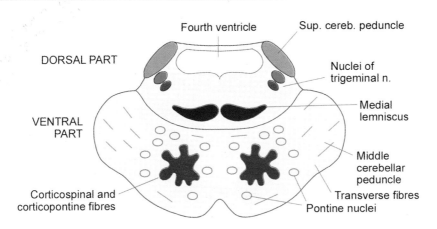

Fig. 6.7. Main features to be seen in a transverse section through the upper part of the pons (Level C in Fig. 6.2)

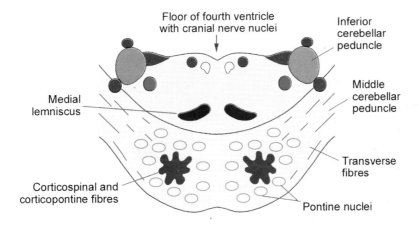

Fig. 6.8. Main features to be seen in a transverse section through the lower part of the pons. (Level D in Fig. 6.2).

The Midbrain

For convenience of description, the midbrain may be divided as follows (Fig. 6.9).

(i) The part lying behind a transverse line drawn through the cerebral aqueduct is called the *tectum*. It consists of the *superior and inferior colliculi* of the two sides.

(ii) The part lying in front of the transverse line is made up of right and left halves called the *cerebral peduncles*. Each peduncle consists of three parts. From anterior to posterior side these are the *crus cerebri* (or basis pedunculi), the *substantia nigra* and the *tegmentum*.

The crus cerebri consists of a large mass of vertically running fibres. These fibres descend from the cerebral cortex. Some of these pass through the midbrain to reach the pons, while others reach the spinal cord. The two crura are separated by a notch seen on the anterior aspect of the midbrain.

The substantia nigra is made up of pigmented grey matter and, therefore, appears dark in colour.

The tegmentum of the two sides is continuous across the midline. It contains important masses of grey matter as well as fibre bundles. The largest of the nuclei is the *red nucleus* (Fig. 6.10) present in the upper half of the midbrain. The tegmentum also contains the *reticular formation* which is

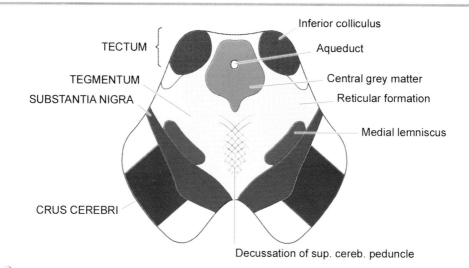

Fig. 6.9. Main features to be seen in a transverse section through the lower part of the midbrain. (Level B in Fig. 6.2)

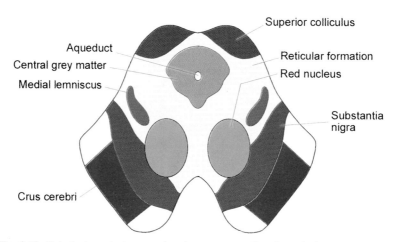

Fig. 6.10. Main features to be seen in a transverse section through the upper part of the midbrain. (Level A in Fig. 6.2)

continuous below with that of the pons and medulla. The fibre bundles of the tegmentum include the ***medial lemniscus*** which lies just behind the substantia nigra, lateral to the red nucleus. The lower part of the tegmentum is traversed by a large number of fibres that cross the midline from one side to the other. These are the fibres of the superior cerebellar peduncles that have their origin in the cerebellum and decussate before ending in the red nucleus (and in some other centres).

It may be noted that some authorities describe the corresponding half of the tectum as part of the cerebral peduncle.

SUBDIVISIONS OF NEURAL TUBE

DEVELOPMENT

We have seen earlier that even before the neural tube has completely closed, it is divisible into an enlarged cranial part and a caudal tubular part. The enlarged cranial part forms the brain. The caudal tubular part forms the spinal cord: it is at first short, but gradually gains in length as the embryo grows. The cavity of the developing brain soon shows three dilatations (Fig. 6.11B). Cranio-caudally, these are the ***prosencephalon, mesencephalon***, and ***rhombencephalon***. The prosencephalon becomes subdivided into the ***telencephalon*** and the ***diencephalon*** (Fig. 6.11C). The telencephalon consists of right and left ***telencephalic vesicles***. The rhombencephalon also becomes subdivided into a cranial part, the ***metencephalon***, and a caudal part, the ***myelencephalon***. The parts of the brain that are developed from each of these divisions of the neural tube are shown in Fig. 6.11.

Prosencephalon	Telencephalon	Cerebral cortex Corpus striatum	Cerebral hemisphere
	Diencephalon	Thalamus Hypothalamus Optic stalk Pars nervosa of hypophysis cerebri	
Mesencephalon		Midbrain	
Rhombencephalon	Metencephalon	Pons and cerebellum	
	Myelencephalon	Medulla oblongata	

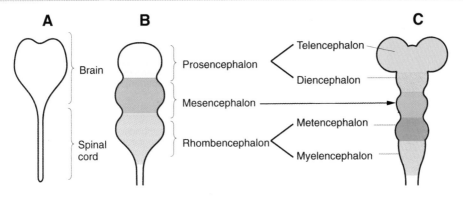

Fig. 6.11. Primary brain vesicles and their subdivisions.

The prosencephalon, mesencephalon and rhombencephalon are at first arranged cranio-caudally (Fig. 6.12A). Their relative position is greatly altered by the appearance of a number of flexures. These are:

(a)   the ***cervical flexure***, at the junction of the rhombencephalon and the spinal cord (Fig. 6.12B);
(b)   the ***mesencephalic flexure*** (or ***cephalic flexure***); in the region of the midbrain (Fig. 6.12C);
(c)   the ***pontine flexure***, at the middle of the rhombencephalon, dividing it into the metencephalon and myelencephalon (Fig. 6.12D); and
(d)   the ***telencephalic flexure***, that occurs much later, between the telencephalon and diencephalon.

These flexures lead to the orientation of the various parts of the brain as in the adult.

DEVELOPMENT

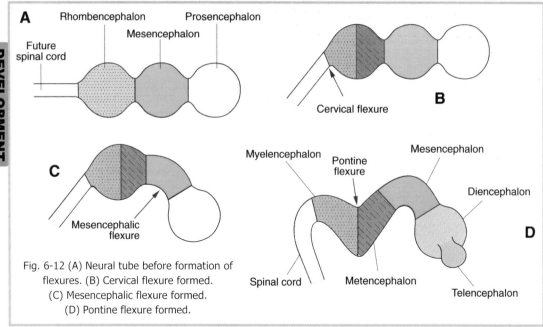

Fig. 6-12 (A) Neural tube before formation of
flexures. (B) Cervical flexure formed.
(C) Mesencephalic flexure formed.
(D) Pontine flexure formed.

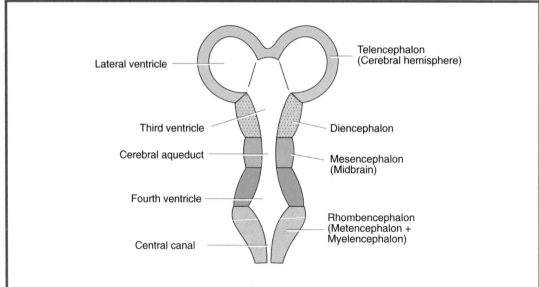

Fig. 6.13. Development of ventricles of the brain.

Each of the subdivisions of the developing brain encloses a part of the original cavity of the neural tube (Fig. 6.13). The cavity of each telencephalic vesicle becomes the *lateral ventricle*, and that of the diencephalon (along with the central part of the telencephalon), becomes the *third ventricle*. The cavity of the mesencephalon remains narrow, and forms the *aqueduct*, while the cavity of the rhombencephalon forms the *fourth ventricle*. Its continuation in the spinal cord is the *central canal*. For development of individual parts of the brainstem see Chapter 11.

THE BRAINSTEM IS DESCRIBED IN DETAIL IN CHAPTER 11. MANY RELEVANT TOPICS ARE GIVEN IN CHAPTERS 8, 9, 10, 12 AND 21

7 : Gross Anatomy of the Cerebellum

The cerebellum (or small brain) lies in the posterior cranial fossa. In the adult the weight of the cerebellum is about 150 g. This is about ten per cent of the weight of the cerebral hemispheres. Like the cerebrum, the cerebellum has a superficial layer of grey matter, the cerebellar cortex. Because of the presence of numerous fissures, the cerebellar cortex is much more extensive than the size of this part of the brain would suggest. It has been estimated that the surface area of the cerebellar cortex is about fifty per cent of the area of the cerebral cortex.

The cerebellum lies behind the pons and the medulla. It is separated from the cerebrum by a fold of dura mater called the **tentorium cerebelli.** Anteriorly, the fourth ventricle intervenes between the cerebellum (behind), and the pons and medulla (in front). Part of the cavity of the ventricle extends into the cerebellum as a transverse cleft. This cleft is bounded cranially by the superior (or anterior) medullary velum, a lamina of white matter (Fig. 20.13).

Subdivisions of the Cerebellum

The cerebellum consists of a part lying near the midline called the **vermis,** and of two lateral **hemispheres.** It has two surfaces, **superior** and **inferior.** On the superior aspect, there is no line of distinction between vermis and hemispheres. On the inferior aspect, the two hemispheres are separated by a deep depression called the **vallecula.** The vermis lies in the depth of this depression. On each side the vermis is separated from the corresponding cerebellar hemisphere by a **paramedian sulcus.** Anteriorly and posteriorly the hemispheres extend beyond the vermis and are separated by anterior and posterior **cerebellar notches.** (The falx cerebelli lies in the posterior notch).

The surface of the cerebellum is marked by a series of fissures that run more or less parallel to one another. The fissures subdivide the surface of the cerebellum into narrow leaf like bands or **folia.** The long axis of the majority of folia is more or less transverse. Sections of the cerebellum cut at right angles to this axis have a characteristic tree-like appearance to which the term **arbor-vitae** (tree of life) is applied.

Some of the fissures on the surface of the cerebellum are deeper than others. They divide the cerebellum into **lobes** within which smaller **lobules** may be recognised. To show the various subdivisions of the cerebellum in a single illustration it is usual to represent the organ as if it has been 'opened out' so that the superior and inferior aspects can both be seen. Such an illustration is shown in Fig. 7.1. This should be compared with Figs. 7.2 A and B which are more realistic drawings of the superior and inferior surfaces, and with Fig. 7.3 which is a midline section showing the subdivisions of the vermis.

The deepest fissures in the cerebellum are:

(i) the **primary fissure** (fissura prima) running transversely across the superior surface, and

(ii) the **posterolateral fissure** seen on the inferior aspect.

These fissures divide the cerebellum into three lobes. The part anterior to the primary fissure is the **anterior lobe.** The part between the two fissures is the **posterior lobe** (sometimes called the **middle lobe).** The remaining part is the **flocculonodular lobe.** The anterior and posterior lobes together form the **corpus cerebelli.**

The vermis is so called because it resembles a worm. Proceeding from above downwards in Fig. 7.1 it is seen to consist of the **lingula, central lobule** and **culmen** (in the anterior lobe); the **declive, folium (or folium vermis), tuber (or tuber vermis), pyramis (or pyramid)** and **uvula** (in the middle lobe); and the **nodule** (in the flocculonodular lobe).

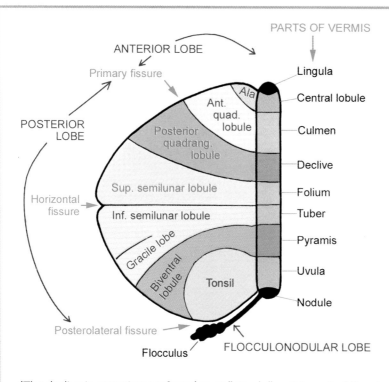

PARTS OF VERMIS

ANTERIOR LOBE

Primary fissure

ANTERIOR LOBE

POSTERIOR LOBE

Horizontal fissure

Posterolateral fissure

Ala

Ant. quad. lobule

Posterior quadrang. lobule

Sup. semilunar lobule

Inf. semilunar lobule

Gracile lobe

Biventral lobule

Tonsil

Flocculus

FLOCCULONODULAR LOBE

Lingula
Central lobule
Culmen
Declive
Folium
Tuber
Pyramis
Uvula
Nodule

Fig. 7.1. Scheme to show the subdivisions of the cerebellum. From Fig. 7.3 note that the vermis is curved on itself so that the lingula and nodule are in fact close to each other.

(The declive is sometimes referred to as "simple" as it is part of the simple lobule: see next para).

With the exception of the lingula each subdivision of the vermis is related laterally to a part of the hemisphere. In the anterior lobe, we have the ***ala*** lateral to the central lobule; and the ***anterior quadrangular lobule*** lateral to the culmen. (A very small part lateral to the lingula is called the wing of the lingula). In the middle lobe, we have the ***posterior quadrangular lobule*** lateral to the declive; the ***superior semilunar lobule*** lateral to the folium; the ***inferior semilunar lobule*** and the ***gracile (or paramedian) lobule*** lateral to the tuber; the ***biventral lobule*** lateral to the pyramid; and the ***tonsil*** (or tonsilla) lateral to the uvula. The nodule is continuous laterally with the flocculus through the inferior medullary velum.

Some other terms used are as follows. The biventral lobule is so called as it is partially divided into a ***lateral belly*** and a ***medial belly***. The posterior quadrangular lobule and the declive are collectively referred to as the ***simple lobule***. The tonsil and biventral lobule correspond to the ***paraflocculus*** of some other species.

The term ***accessory paraflocculus*** is applied to a small flower-like area between the tonsil and the flocculus.

The fissures separating the subdivisions of the cerebellum are shown in Fig. 7.1. We have seen that the ***primary fissure*** separates the anterior and posterior lobes. It, therefore intervenes between the anterior and posterior quadrangular lobules; and also separates the culmen and declive. The ***posterolateral fissure*** separates the posterior lobe from the flocculonodular lobe; and extends into the interval between the nodule and the uvula. The ***horizontal fissure*** (Figs. 7.1, 7.3) divides the cerebellum into upper and lower halves. The parts shown above this fissure in Fig. 7.1 are seen on the superior surface of the cerebellum (Fig. 7.2A), and those below it on the inferior surface (Fig. 7.2B). It intervenes between the superior and inferior semilunar lobules; and between the folium and the tuber.

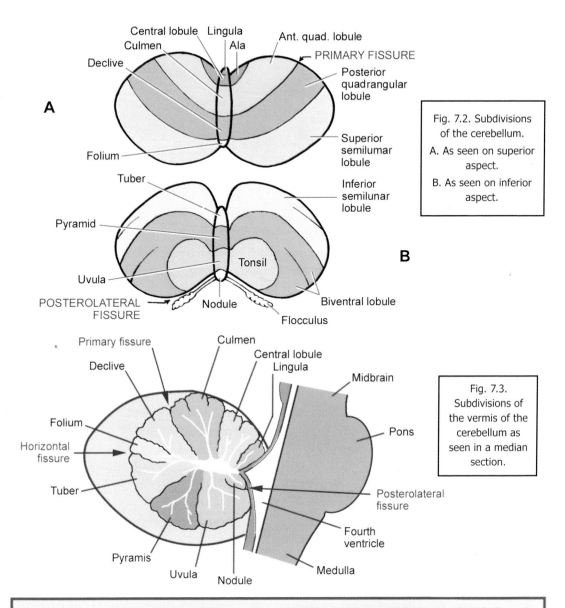

Fig. 7.2. Subdivisions of the cerebellum.

A. As seen on superior aspect.

B. As seen on inferior aspect.

Fig. 7.3. Subdivisions of the vermis of the cerebellum as seen in a median section.

Some other named fissures are as follows. The ***postlingual fissure*** separated the lingula from the central lobule. The ***postcentral fissure*** intervenes between the central lobule and culmen. The tuber is separated from the pyramis by the ***prepyramidal fissure,*** and the pyramis is separated from the uvula by the ***postpyramidal fissure***.

From developmental, phylogenetic and functional points of view the cerebellum is often divided into ***archicerebellum*** (oldest, black in Fig. 7.1); ***paleocerebellum*** (old, shaded in dots); and ***neocerebellum*** (new, unshaded). These correspond roughly (but not precisely) to the flocculonodular node, anterior and posterior lobes respectively. The connections of the archicerebellum are predominantly vestibular; and it is concerned with the maintenance of body equilibrium. The paleocerebellum is connected predominantly to the spinal cord. It is concerned mainly with maintenance of muscle tone and finer control of movements. The neocerebellum has extensive connections with the cerebral cortex (through pontine nuclei). It is usually regarded as being responsible for fine co-ordination of voluntary movements, but its precise role is not known.

From the point of view of its connections the cerebellar cortex may also be divided into a vermal part (vermis), paravermal (or paramedian) parts and lateral parts.

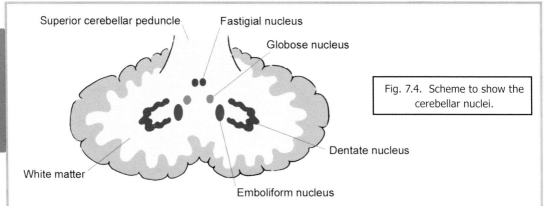

Fig. 7.4. Scheme to show the cerebellar nuclei.

Grey matter of the cerebellum

Most of the grey matter of the cerebellum is arranged as a thin layer covering the central core of white matter. This layer is the **cerebellar cortex**. The subdivisions of the cerebellar cortex correspond to the subdivisions of the cerebellum described above.

Embedded within the central core of white matter there are masses of grey matter which constitute the **cerebellar nuclei.** These are as follows (Fig. 7.4).

(1) The **dentate nucleus** lies in the centre of each cerebellar hemisphere. Cross sections through the nucleus have a striking resemblance to those through the inferior olivary nucleus. Like the latter it is made up of a thin lamina of grey matter that is folded upon itself so that it resembles a crumpled purse. Both the nuclei have a hilum directed medially.

(2) The **emboliform nucleus** lies on the medial side of the dentate nucleus.

(3) The **globose nucleus** lies medial to the emboliform nucleus.

(4) The **fastigial nucleus** lies close to the middle line in the anterior part of the superior vermis. For details of the connections of the cerebellar cortex and of cerebellar nuclei see Chapter 12.

White matter of the cerebellum

The central core of each cerebellar hemisphere is formed by white matter. The peduncles are continued into this white matter. The white matter of the two sides is connected by a thin lamina of fibres that are closely related to the fourth ventricle. The upper part of this lamina forms the superior medullary velum (see below), and its inferior part forms the inferior medullary velum. Both these take part in forming the roof of the fourth ventricle.

The white matter consists of:

(**a**)   Afferent fibres entering the cerebellum from outside.

(**b**)   Projection fibres from the cerebellar cortex to the cerebellar nuclei.

(**c**)   Association fibres interconnecting different parts of the cerebellar cortex.

(**d**)   Commissural fibres connecting the two cerebellar hemispheres.

(**e**)   Fibres from the cerebellar nuclei (and some from the cerebellar cortex) to centres outside the cerebellum.

Cerebellar Peduncles

The fibres entering or leaving the cerebellum pass through three thick bundles called the cerebellar peduncles: superior, middle and inferior.

Inferior cerebellar peduncle

This peduncle is also called the **restiform body**. This is a thick bundle of fibres that connects the posterolateral part of the medulla with the cerebellum. The peduncle passes upwards and laterally along the inferolateral margin of the rhomboid fossa (floor of fourth ventricle, Fig. 20.12). Near the upper end of the medulla the peduncle lies between the superior cerebellar peduncle (on its medial side) and the middle cerebellar peduncle (laterally). The inferior peduncle then turns sharply backwards to enter the while core of the cerebellum.

Over the medial part of the inferior cerebellar peduncle there are fibres that pass through the vestibular nuclei before entering the cerebellum. These fibres constitute the **juxtarestiform body**.

Middle cerebellar peduncle

The middle cerebellar peduncle begins as a lateral continuation of the ventral part of the pons. Its fibres, which arise in pontine nuclei, cross to the opposite side. The fibres of the peduncle form a thick bundle that passes laterally and backwards to enter the white core of the cerebellum through the horizontal fissure. On entering the cerebellum the fibres are placed lateral to those of the inferior peduncle (the superior peduncle being still more medial in position).

Superior cerebellar peduncle

The superior cerebellar peduncle consists mainly of fibres arising in cerebellar nuclei (mainly the dentate nucleus). The fibres pass forwards, upwards and medially, lying along the upper and lateral margin of the rhomboid fossa. The right and left peduncles are connected by a thin lamina of white matter, the **superior (or anterior) medullary velum**. Along with the velum the peduncles form the upper part of the roof of the fourth ventricle (Fig. 20.13). The fibres of the peduncle enter the midbrain and cross to the opposite side before ending (mainly) in the red nucleus. Many of the fibres ascend to the thalamus.

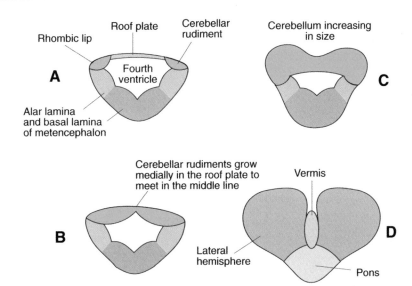

Fig. 7.5. Some stages in the development of the cerebellum. (A) Cerebellar rudiments appear from alar lamina of metencephalon. (B) They grow into the roof plate of the metencephalon to meet in the midline. (C) Cerebellum enlarges and bulges out of the fourth ventricle. (D) Lateral hemispheres and vermis can be distinguished.

DEVELOPMENT OF THE CEREBELLUM

The cerebellum develops from the dorsolateral part of the alar lamina of the metencephalon (Fig. 7.5A). Obviously, there are at first two primordia of the cerebellum, right and left. These extend medially in the roof plate of the metencephalon to eventually fuse across the midline (Figs. 7.5B, C). As the cerebellum increases in size, fissures appear on its surface. The lateral lobes and vermis can soon be distinguished, as a result of differential growth.

The developing cerebellum can be divided into: (a) an ***intraventricular part*** that bulges into the cavity of the developing fourth ventricle, and (b) an ***extraventricular part*** that is seen as a bulging on the surface (Fig. 7.5C). At first the intraventricular part is the larger of the two, but at a later stage, the extraventricular part becomes much larger than the intraventricular part and constitutes almost the whole of the organ (Fig. 7.5D).

The cerebellum, at first, consists of the usual matrix cell, mantle and marginal layers. Some cells of the mantle layer migrate into the marginal layer to form the cerebellar cortex. The cells of the mantle layer that do not migrate into the cortex, develop into the ***dentate, emboliform, globose*** and ***fastigal nuclei***.

The ***superior cerebellar peduncle*** is formed chiefly by the axons growing out of the dentate nucleus. The ***middle cerebellar peduncle*** is formed by axons growing into the cerebellum from the cells of the pontine nuclei, while the ***inferior cerebellar peduncle*** is formed by fibres that grow into the cerebellum from the spinal cord and medulla.

DEVELOPMENT

FOR FURTHER DETAILS ABOUT THE CEREBELLUM
SEE CHAPTER 12.

8 : Gross Anatomy of The Cerebral Hemispheres

Exterior of the Cerebral Hemispheres

Poles, Surfaces, and Borders

The cerebrum consists of two cerebral hemispheres that are partially connected with each other. When viewed from the lateral aspect each cerebral hemisphere has the appearance shown in Fig. 8.1. Three somewhat pointed ends or *poles* can be recognised. These are the *frontal pole* anteriorly, the *occipital pole* posteriorly, and the *temporal pole* that lies between the frontal and occipital poles, and points forwards and somewhat downwards.

A coronal section through the cerebral hemispheres (Fig. 8.2) shows that each hemisphere has three borders: *superomedial, inferolateral* and *inferomedial.* These borders divide the surface of the hemisphere into three large surfaces: *superolateral, medial* and *inferior.* The inferior surface is further subdivided into an anterior *orbital* part and a posterior *tentorial* part. (Fig. 8.3).

Corresponding to these subdivisions, the inferomedial border is divided into an anterior part called the *medial orbital border* and a posterior part called the *medial occipital border.* The orbital part of the inferolateral border is called the *superciliary border* (as it lies just above the level of the eyebrows).

The surfaces of the cerebral hemisphere are not smooth. They show a series of grooves or *sulci* which are separated by intervening areas that are called *gyri.*

Lobes

For convenience of description each cerebral hemisphere is divided into four major subdivisions or *lobes.* To consider the boundaries of these lobes reference has to be made to some sulci and other features to be seen on each hemisphere (Fig. 8.1).

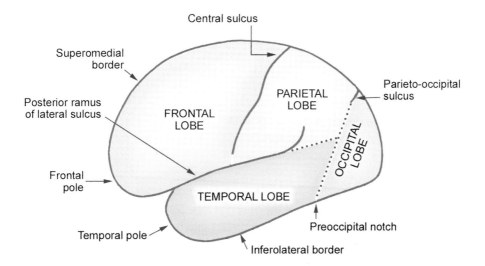

Fig. 8.1. Lateral aspect of cerebral hemisphere to show borders, poles and lobes.

BASIC

(a) On the superolateral surface of the hemisphere there are two prominent sulci. One of these is the **posterior ramus of the lateral sulcus** which begins near the temporal pole and runs backwards and slightly upwards. Its posteriormost part curves sharply upwards. The second sulcus that is used to delimit the lobes is the **central sulcus.** It begins on the superomedial margin a little behind the midpoint between the frontal and occipital poles, and runs downwards and forwards to end a little above the posterior ramus of the lateral sulcus.

(b) On the medial surface of the hemisphere, near the occipital pole, there is a sulcus called the **parietooccipital sulcus** (Fig. 8.5). The upper end of this sulcus reaches the superomedial border and a small part of it can be seen on the superolateral surface (Fig. 8.1).

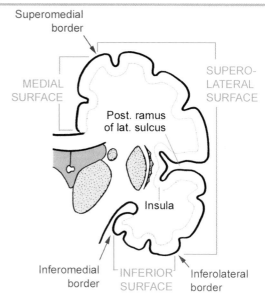

Fig. 8.2. Coronal section through a cerebral hemisphere to show its borders and surfaces.

(c) A little anterior to the occipital pole the inferolateral border shows a slight indentation called the **preoccipital notch (or preoccipital incisure).**

To complete the subdivision of the hemisphere into lobes we now have to draw two imaginary lines. The first imaginary line connects the upper end of the parieto-occipital sulcus to the preoccipital notch. The second imaginary line is a backward continuation of the posterior ramus of the lateral sulcus (excluding the posterior upturned part) to meet the first line. We are now in a position to define the limits of the various lobes as follows.

(**1**) The **frontal lobe** lies anterior to the central sulcus, and above the posterior ramus of the lateral sulcus.

(**2**) The **parietal lobe** lies behind the central sulcus. It is bounded below by the posterior ramus of the lateral sulcus and by the second imaginary line; and behind by the upper part of the first imaginary line.

(**3**) The **occipital lobe** is the area lying behind the first imaginary line.

(**4**) The **temporal lobe** lies below the posterior ramus of the lateral sulcus and the second imaginary line. It is separated from the occipital lobe by the lower part of the first imaginary line.

Before going on to consider further subdivisions of each of the lobes named above, attention has to be directed to details of some structures already mentioned.

(**a**) The upper end of the central sulcus winds round the superomedial border to reach the medial surface. Here its end is surrounded by a gyrus called the **paracentral lobule** (Fig. 8.5). The lower end of the central sulcus is always separated by a small interval from the posterior ramus of the lateral sulcus (Fig. 8.1).

(**b**) The lateral sulcus begins on the inferior aspect of the cerebral hemisphere where it lies between the orbital surface and the anterior part of the temporal lobe (Fig. 8.7). It runs laterally to reach the superolateral surface. On reaching this surface it divides into three rami (branches). These rami are **anterior (or anterior horizontal), ascending (or anterior ascending)** and **posterior** (Fig. 8.4). The anterior and ascending rami are short and run into the frontal lobe in the directions indicated by their names. The posterior ramus has already been considered. Unlike most other sulci, the lateral sulcus is very deep. Its walls cover a fairly large area of the surface of the hemisphere called the *insula* (Fig. 8.2).

Further Subdivisions of the Superolateral Surface

The subdivisions of the superolateral surface are described below and are shown in Fig. 8.4.

Frontal lobe

The frontal lobe is further subdivided as follows. The *precentral sulcus* runs downwards and forwards parallel to and a little anterior to the central sulcus. The area between it and the central sulcus is the *precentral gyrus.* In the region anterior to the precentral gyrus there are two sulci that run in an anteroposterior direction. These are the *superior* and *inferior frontal sulci.* They divide this region into *superior, middle* and *inferior*

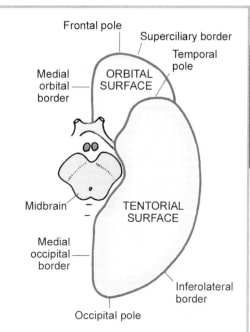

Fig. 8.3. Inferior aspect of a cerebral hemisphere to show its borders, poles and surfaces.

frontal gyri. The anterior and ascending rami of the lateral sulcus extend into the inferior frontal gyrus dividing it into three parts. The part below the anterior ramus is the *pars orbitalis*; that between the anterior and ascending rami is the *pars triangularis*; and the part posterior to the ascending ramus is the *pars opercularis.*

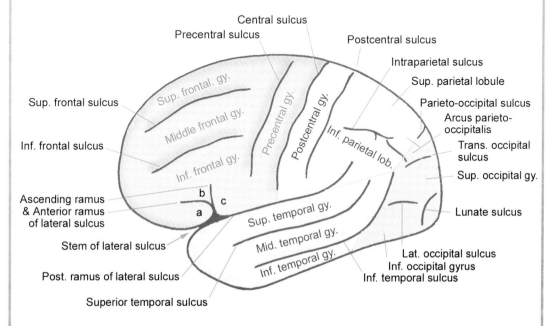

Fig. 8.4. Simplified presentation of sulci and gyri on the superolateral surface of the cerebral hemisphere. (a = pars orbitalis; b = pars triangularis; c = pars opercularis).

Temporal lobe

The temporal lobe has two sulci that run parallel to the posterior ramus of the lateral sulcus. They are termed the ***superior and inferior temporal sulci.*** They divide the superolateral surface of this lobe into ***superior, middle and inferior temporal gyri.***

Parietal lobe

The parietal lobe shows the following subdivisions. The ***postcentral sulcus*** runs downwards and forwards parallel to and a little behind the central sulcus. The area between these two sulci is the ***postcentral gyrus.*** The rest of the parietal lobe is divided into a ***superior parietal lobule*** and an ***inferior parietal lobule*** by the ***intraparietal sulcus.*** The upturned posterior end of the posterior ramus of the lateral sulcus extends into the inferior parietal lobule. The posterior ends of the superior and inferior temporal sulci also turn upwards to enter this lobule. The upturned ends of these three sulci divide the inferior parietal lobule into three parts. The part that arches over the upturned posterior end of the posterior ramus of the lateral sulcus is called the ***supramarginal gyrus.*** The part that arches over the superior temporal sulcus is called the ***angular gyrus.*** The part that arches over the posterior end of the inferior temporal sulcus is called the ***arcus temporooccipitalis.***

Occipital lobe

The occipital lobe shows three rather short sulci. One of these, the ***lateral occipital sulcus*** lies horizontally and divides the lobe into ***superior and inferior occipital gyri.*** The ***lunate sulcus*** runs downwards and slightly forwards just in front of the occipital pole. The vertical strip just in front of it is the ***gyrus descendens.*** The ***transverse occipital sulcus*** is located in the uppermost part of the occipital lobe. The upper end of the parieto-occipital sulcus (which just reaches the superolateral surface from the medial surface) is surrounded by the ***arcus parieto-occipitalis.*** As its name suggests, it belongs partly to the parietal lobe and partly to the occipital lobe.

Insula

In the depth of the stem and posterior ramus of the lateral sulcus there is a part of the cerebral hemisphere called the insula (insula = hidden). It is surrounded by a ***circular sulcus.*** During development of the cerebral hemisphere this area grows less than surrounding areas which, therefore, come to overlap it and occlude it from surface view. These surrounding areas are called ***opercula*** (= lids). The ***frontal operculum*** lies between the anterior and ascending rami of the lateral sulcus. The ***frontoparietal operculum*** lies above the posterior ramus of the lateral sulcus. The ***temporal operculum*** lies below this sulcus. The temporal operculum has a superior surface hidden in the depth of the lateral sulcus (Figs. 8.2, 8.15B). On this surface are located two gyri called the ***anterior and posterior transverse temporal gyri.*** The surface of the insula itself is divided into a number of gyri.

Medial Surface of Cerebral Hemisphere

When the two cerebral hemispheres are separated from each other by a cut in the midline the appearances seen are shown in Figs. 8.5 and 8.6.

The structures seen are as follows.

The ***corpus callosum*** is a prominent arched structure consisting of commissural fibres passing from one hemisphere to the other (Fig. 8.6). It consists of a central part called the ***trunk,*** a posterior end or ***splenium,*** and an anterior end or ***genu.*** A little below the corpus callosum we see the third

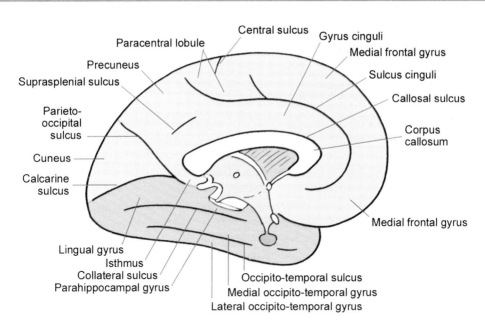

Fig. 8.5. Simplified presentation of sulci and gyri on the medial aspect of the cerebral hemisphere. The medial surface (pink) and the tentorial surface (green) are seen. The corpus callosum and some other structures connecting the two hemispheres have been cut across.

ventricle of the brain. A number of structures can be identified in relation to this ventricle. The *interventricular foramen* through which the third ventricle communicates with the lateral ventricle can be seen in the upper and anterior part. Posteroinferiorly, the ventricle is continuous with the *cerebral aqueduct.* The lateral wall of the ventricle is formed in greater part by a large mass of grey matter called the *thalamus.* The right and left thalami are usually interconnected (across the midline) by a strip of grey matter called the *interthalamic connexus.* The anteroinferior part of the lateral wall of the third ventricle is formed by a collection of grey matter that constitutes the *hypothalamus.*

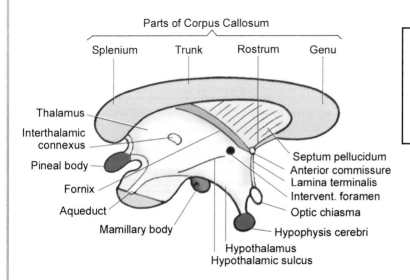

Fig. 8.6. Enlarged view of part of Fig. 8.5 to show some structures to be seen on the medial aspect of the cerebral hemisphere.

Above the thalamus there is a bundle of fibres called the ***fornix.*** Posteriorly, the fornix is attached to the under surface of the corpus callosum, but anteriorly it disappears from view just in front of the interventricular foramen. Extending between the fornix and the corpus callosum there is a thin lamina called the ***septum pellucidum (or septum lucidum)***, which separates the right and left lateral ventricles from each other. Removal of the septum pellucidum brings the interior of the lateral ventricle into view.

In the anterior wall of the third ventricle there are the ***anterior commissure*** and the ***lamina terminalis.*** The anterior commissure is attached to the genu of the corpus callosum through a thin lamina of fibres that constitutes the ***rostrum*** of the corpus callosum. Below, the anterior commissure is continuous with the ***lamina terminalis*** which is a thin lamina of nervous tissue. The lower end of the lamina terminalis is attached to the optic chiasma. Just in front of the lamina terminalis there are the ***paraterminal gyrus*** and the ***parolfactory gyrus*** (Fig. 16.10). Posteriorly, the third ventricle is related to the ***pineal body (or pineal gland)*** and inferiorly to the ***hypophysis cerebri.***

Above the corpus callosum (and also in front of and behind it) we see the sulci and gyri of the medial surface of the hemisphere (Fig. 8.5). The most prominent of the sulci is the ***cingulate sulcus*** which follows a curved course parallel to the upper convex margin of the corpus callosum. Anteriorly, it ends below the rostrum of the corpus callosum. Posteriorly, it turns upwards to reach the superomedial border a little behind the upper end of the central sulcus. The area between the cingulate sulcus and the corpus callosum is called the ***gyrus cinguli.*** It is separated from the corpus callosum by the ***callosal sulcus.***

The part of the medial surface of the hemisphere between the cingulate sulcus and the superomedial border consists of two parts. The smaller posterior part which is wound around the end of the central sulcus is called the ***paracentral lobule***. The large anterior part is called the ***medial frontal gyrus.*** These two parts are separated by a short sulcus continuous with the cingulate sulcus.

The part of the medial surface behind the paracentral lobule and the gyrus cinguli shows two major sulci that cut off a triangular area called the ***cuneus.*** The triangle is bounded anteriorly and above by the ***parieto-occipital sulcus;*** inferiorly by the ***calcarine sulcus;*** and posteriorly by the superomedial border of the hemisphere. The calcarine sulcus extends forwards beyond its junction with the parieto-occipital sulcus and ends a little below the splenium of the corpus callosum. The small area separating the splenium from the calcarine sulcus is called the ***isthmus.*** Between the parieto-occipital sulcus and the paracentral lobule there is a quadrilateral area called the ***precuneus.*** Anteroinferiorly the precuneus is separated from the posterior part of the gyrus cinguli by the ***suprasplenial (or subparietal) sulcus.***

The precuneus and the posterior part of the paracentral lobule form the medial surface of the parietal lobe.

Although the parieto-occipital and calcarine sulci appear to be continuous with each other on surface view, they are separated by the ***cuneate gyrus*** (or ***cuneolingual gyrus***) which lies in the depth of the area where the two sulci meet. The parts of the calcarine sulcus anterior and posterior to the junction with the parieto-occipital sulcus are separated by a deeply situated ***anterior cuneolingual gyrus.***

Inferior Surface of Cerebrum

When the cerebrum is separated from the hindbrain by cutting across the midbrain, and is viewed from below, the appearances seen are shown in Fig. 8.7. Posterior to the midbrain we see the under surface of the splenium of the corpus callosum. Anterior to the midbrain there is a depressed area

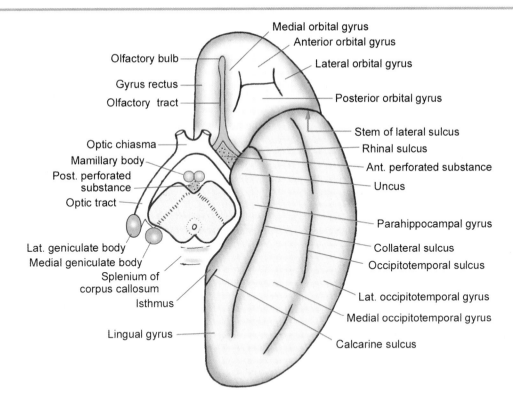

Fig. 8.7. Structures to be seen on the inferior aspect of the cerebrum.
The midbrain has been cut across.

called the ***interpeduncular fossa***. The fossa is bounded in front by the ***optic chiasma*** and on the sides by the right and left ***optic tracts***. The optic tracts wind round the sides of the midbrain to terminate on its posterolateral aspect. In this region two swellings, the ***medial and lateral geniculate bodies***, can be seen. Certain structures are seen within the interpeduncular fossa. These are closely related to the floor of the third ventricle (see also Fig. 8.6). Anterior and medial to the crura of the midbrain there are two rounded swellings called the ***mamillary bodies.*** Anterior to these bodies there is a median elevation called the ***tuber cinereum,*** to which the infundibulum of the hypophysis cerebri is attached. The triangular interval between the mamillary bodies and the midbrain is pierced by numerous small blood vessels and is called the ***posterior perforated substance.*** A similar area lying on each side of the optic chiasma is called the ***anterior perforated substance***. The anterior perforated substance is bounded anterolaterally by the lateral olfactory stria and posterolaterally by the uncus. The anterior perforated substance is connected to the insula by a band of grey matter called the ***limen insulae*** which lies in the depth of the stem of the lateral sulcus.

In addition to these structures we see the sulci and gyri on the orbital and tentorial parts of the inferior surface of the each cerebral hemisphere. These parts are separated from each other by the stem of the lateral sulcus.

Sulci and gyri on orbital surface

Close to the medial border of the orbital surface there is an anteroposterior sulcus: it is called the ***olfactory sulcus*** because the olfactory bulb and tract lie superficial to it. The area medial to this sulcus is called the *gyrus rectus*. The rest of the orbital surface is divided by an H-shaped *orbital sulcus* into *anterior*, *posterior*, *medial* and *lateral orbital gyri.*

Sulci and gyri on tentorial surface

The tentorial surface is marked by two major sulci that run in an anteroposterior direction. These are the *collateral sulcus* medially, and the *occipito-temporal sulcus* laterally. The posterior part of the collateral sulcus runs parallel to the calcarine sulcus: the area between them is the *lingual gyrus.* Anteriorly, the lingual gyrus becomes continuous with the *parahippocampal gyrus* which is related medially to the midbrain and to the interpeduncular fossa. The anterior end of the parahippocampal gyrus is cut off from the curved temporal pole of the hemisphere by a curved *rhinal sulcus.* This part of the parahippocampal gyrus forms a hook-like structure called the *uncus,* details of which are considered later. Posteriorly, the parahippocampal gyrus becomes continuous with the gyrus cinguli through the isthmus (Fig. 8.5). The area between the collateral sulcus and the rhinal sulcus medially, and the occipitotemporal sulcus laterally, is the *medial occipitotemporal gyrus.* The area lateral to the occipitotemporal sulcus is called the *lateral occipitotemporal gyrus.* This gyrus is continuous (around the inferolateral margin of the cerebral hemisphere) with the inferior temporal gyrus.

AN INTRODUCTION TO SOME STRUCTURES WITHIN THE CEREBRAL HEMISPHERES

The surface of the cerebral hemisphere is covered by a thin layer of grey matter called the *cerebral cortex*. The cortex follows the irregular contour of the sulci and gyri of the hemisphere and extends into the depths of the sulci. As a result of this folding of the cerebral surface, the cerebral cortex acquires a much larger surface area than the size of the hemispheres would otherwise allow.

The greater part of the cerebral hemisphere deep to the cortex is occupied by white matter within which are embedded certain important masses of grey matter. Immediately lateral to the third ventricle

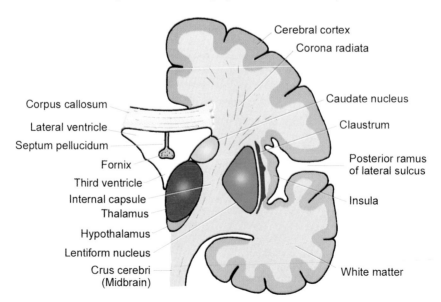

Fig. 8.8. Coronal section through a cerebral hemisphere to show important masses of grey matter and some other structures within the hemisphere.

there are the ***thalamus*** and ***hypothalamus*** (and certain smaller masses) derived from the diencephalon. More laterally there is the ***corpus striatum*** which is derived from the telecephalon. It consists of two masses of grey matter, the ***caudate nucleus*** and the ***lentiform nucleus***. A little lateral to the lentiform nucleus we see the cerebral cortex in the region of the insula. Between the lentiform nucleus and the insula there is a thin layer of grey matter called the ***claustrum.*** The caudate nucleus, the lentiform nucleus, the claustrum and some other masses of grey matter (all of telencephalic origin) are referred to as ***basal nuclei*** or as ***basal ganglia.***

The white matter that occupies the interval between the thalamus and caudate nucleus medially, and the lentiform nucleus laterally, is called the ***internal capsule.*** It is a region of considerable importance as major ascending and descending tracts pass through it. The white matter that radiates from the upper end of the internal capsule to the cortex is called the ***corona radiata.***

The two cerebral hemispheres are interconnected by fibres passing from one to the other. These fibres constitute the ***commissures*** of the cerebrum. The largest of these is the ***corpus callosum*** which is seen just above the lateral ventricles in Fig. 8.8.

DEVELOPMENT OF THE CEREBRAL HEMISPHERE

The layout of structures in the cerebral hemisphere is better understood by a knowledge of its development (Fig. 8.9).

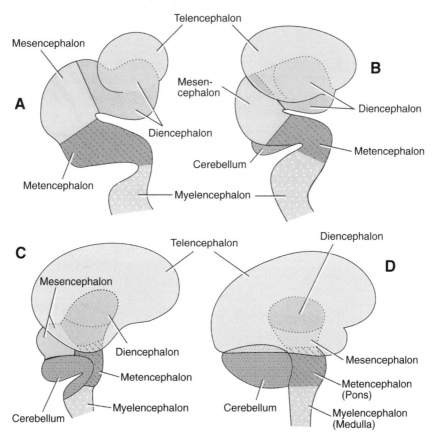

Fig. 8.9. Development of external form of the human brain. Note progressive overlapping of diencephalon and mesencephalon by the expanding telencephalon.

The cerebrum is a derivative of the prosencephalon. We have seen that the prosencephalon is divisible into a median *diencephalon* and two lateral *telencephalic vesicles* (Fig. 6.11C). The telencephalic vesicles give origin, on either side, to the *cerebral cortex* and the *corpus striatum*. The diencephalon gives rise to the *thalamus*, *hypothalamus* and related structures. The telencephalic vesicles are at first small, but rapidly increase in size extending upwards, forwards and backwards. As a result of this enlargement, the telencephalon comes to completely cover the lateral surface of the diencephalon and eventually fuses with it. Thus, the cerebral cortex and corpus striatum come to lie lateral to the thalamus and hypothalamus.

With further upward, forward and backward extension of the telencephalic vesicles, the vesicles of the two sides come into apposition with each other above, in front of, and behind the diencephalon.

The cavity of the diencephalon forms the *third ventricle*, while the cavities of the two telencephalic vesicles form the *lateral ventricles* (Fig. 6.13).

Each lateral ventricle is at first a spherical space within the telencephalic vesicle. With the forward and backward growth of the vesicle, the ventricle becomes elongated anteroposteriorly. The posterior end of the telencephalic vesicle now grows downwards and forwards, to form the temporal lobe, and the cavity within it becomes the *inferior horn*. The ventricle thus becomes C-shaped. Finally, as a result of backward growth, the occipital pole of the hemisphere becomes established, the part of the ventricle within it becoming the *posterior horn*.

Important Functional Areas of the Cerebral Cortex

Some areas of the cerebral cortex can be assigned specific functions. These areas can be defined in terms of sulci and gyri described in preceding pages. However, some areas are commonly referred to by numbers and it is necessary to know what these numbers mean. Various workers who have studied the microscopic structure of the cerebral cortex have found that there is considerable variation from region to region. They have also found that these variations do not necessarily follow the boundaries of sulci and gyri, but often cut across them. Various authors have worked out 'maps' of the cerebral cortex indicating areas of differing structure. The best known scheme is that of Brodmann who represented different areas by numbers. Although the functional significance of the areas is open to question, areas of the cortex are very frequently referred to by Brodmann's numbers. It is, therefore, necessary to be familiar with them. The numbers most commonly referred to are indicated in Fig. 8.10 A, B.

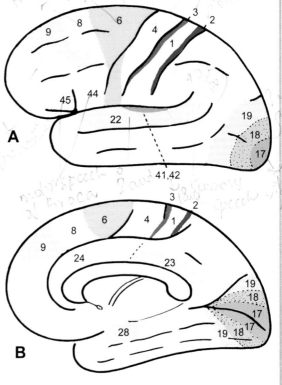

Fig. 8.10. Location of some of the areas of Brodmann on the superolateral aspect (A), and on the medial aspect of the cerebral hemisphere (B).

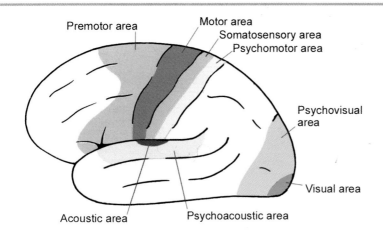

Premotor area | Motor area | Somatosensory area | Psychomotor area | Psychovisual area | Visual area | Psychoacoustic area | Acoustic area

Fig. 8.11. Traditional concept of functional areas on the superolateral aspect of the cerebral hemisphere.

The concepts regarding the different functional areas of the cerebral cortex have undergone considerable modification in recent years, but in clinical work reference continues to be made to classical subdivisions which are as follows.

Motor area

The motor area of classical description is located in the precentral gyrus on the superolateral surface of the hemisphere (Fig. 8.11), and in the anterior part of the paracentral lobule on the medial surface. It corresponds to area 4 of Brodmann (and possibly to the part of area 6 which lies in the precentral gyrus, Fig. 8.10). Specific regions within the area are responsible for movements in specific parts of the body.

Stimulation of the paracentral lobule produces movement in the lower limbs. The trunk and upper limb are represented in the upper part of the precentral gyrus, while the face and head are represented in the lower part of the gyrus.

Another feature of interest is that the area of cortex representing a part of the body is not proportional to the size of the part, but rather to intricacy of movements in the region. Thus relatively large areas of cortex are responsible for movements in the hands or in the lips.

Premotor area

The premotor area is located just anterior to the motor area. It occupies the posterior parts of the superior, middle and inferior frontal gyri (Fig. 8.11). The part of the premotor area located in the superior and middle frontal gyri corresponds to areas 6 and 8 of Brodmann (Fig. 8.10). The part in the inferior frontal gyrus corresponds to areas 44 and 45 and constitutes the ***motor speech area (of Broca).*** Stimulation of the premotor area results in movements, but these are somewhat more intricate than those produced by stimulation of the motor area.

Closely related to the premotor area there are two specific areas of importance. One is the motor speech area of Broca, mentioned above; and the other is the frontal eye field.

Motor Speech Area

The motor speech area of Broca lies in the inferior frontal gyrus (areas 44 & 45, Figs. 8.10A, 15.4). Injury to this region results in inability to speak (***aphasia***) even though the muscles concerned are not paralysed. These effects occur only if damage occurs in the left hemisphere in right handed persons; and in the right hemisphere in left handed persons. In other words motor control of speech is confined to one hemisphere: that which controls the dominant upper limb.

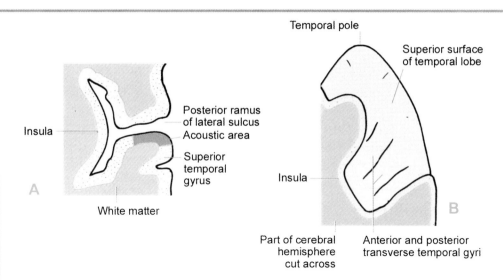

Fig. 8.12. A. Location of the acoustic area in relation to the superior temporal gyrus.
B. Upper surface of the superior temporal gyrus to show transverse temporal gyri.

Frontal Eye Field

The frontal eye field lies in the middle frontal gyrus just anterior to the precentral gyrus (Fig. 15.4). It includes parts of areas 6, 8, and 9. Stimulation of this area causes both eyes to move to the opposite side. These are called **conjugate movements.** Movements of the head and dilatation of the pupil may also occur. This area is connected to the cortex of the occipital lobe that is concerned with vision. It is also connected to the thalamus (medial dorsal nucleus).

Sensory Area

The sensory area of classical description is located in the postcentral gyrus (Fig. 8.11). It corresponds to areas 1, 2, and 3 of Brodmann. It also extends onto the medial surface of the hemisphere where it lies in the posterior part of the paracentral lobule. Responses can be recorded from the sensory area when individual parts of the body are stimulated.

A definite representation of various parts of the body can be mapped out in the sensory area. It corresponds to that in the motor area in that the body is represented upside down. The area of cortex that receives sensations from a particular part of the body is not proportional to the size of that part, but rather to the complexity of sensations received from it. Thus the digits, the lips and the tongue have a disproportionately large representation.

Visual Areas

The areas concerned with vision are located in the occipital lobe, mainly on the medial surface, both above and below the calcarine sulcus (area 17). Area 17 extends into the cuneus, and into the lingual gyrus (Fig. 8.10). Posteriorly, it may extend onto the superolateral surface where it is limited (anteriorly) by the lunate sulcus. Area 17 is continuous, both above and below, with area 18 and beyond this with area 19. Areas 18 and 19 are responsible mainly for interpretation of visual impulses reaching area 17: they are often described as **psychovisual areas**.

Acoustic (auditory) Area

The acoustic area, or the area for hearing, is situated in the temporal lobe. It lies in that part of the superior temporal gyrus which forms the inferior wall of the posterior ramus of the lateral sulcus

(Fig. 8.12A). In this situation there are two short oblique gyri called the anterior and posterior *transverse temporal gyri* (areas 41, 42 and 52: Figs. 8. 12B). The acoustic area lies in the anterior transverse temporal gyrus (area 41) and extends to a small extent onto the surface of the hemisphere in the superior temporal gyrus (See areas 41, 42 in Fig. 8.10).

WHITE MATTER OF CEREBRAL HEMISPHERES

Deep to the cerebral cortex the greater part of each cerebral hemisphere is occupied by nerve fibres that constitute the white matter. These fibres may be:

(**a**) *Association fibres* that interconnect different regions of the cerebral cortex.

(**b**) *Projection fibres* that connect the cerebral cortex with other masses of grey matter; and *vice versa.*

(**c**) *Commissural fibres* that interconnect identical areas in the two hemispheres.

Association Fibres

These may be short and may connect adjoining gyri. Alternatively, they may be long and may connect distant parts of the cerebral cortex. Many of the association fibres form bundles that can be seen by gross dissection. Some of these are shown in Fig. 8.13. Some association fibres pass through commissures to connect *dissimilar* areas in the two cerebral hemispheres.

Projection Fibres

These fibres connect the cerebral cortex to centres in the brainstem and spinal cord, in both directions. Fibres to the cortex are often referred to as *corticopetal fibres*, while those going away from the cortex are referred to as *corticofugal fibres.* Fibres connecting the cortex with the thalamus, the hypothalamus and the basal ganglia, are also projection fibres. Many of the major projection fibres pass through the internal capsule, which is considered below.

The Internal Capsule

We have seen that a large number of nerve fibres interconnect the cerebral cortex with centres in the brainstem and spinal cord, and with the thalamus. Most of these fibres pass through the interval between the thalamus and caudate nucleus medially, and the lentiform nucleus laterally. This region

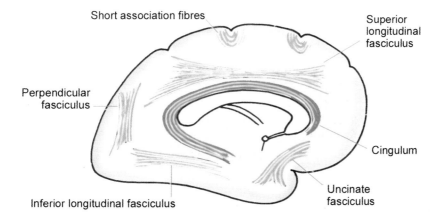

Fig. 8.13. Some large bundles of fibres present within the cerebral hemisphere.

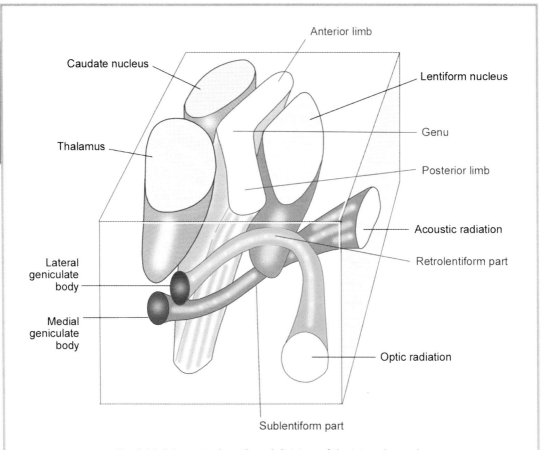

Fig. 8.14. Scheme to show the subdivisions of the internal capsule.

is called the ***internal capsule.*** Above, the internal capsule is continuous with the corona radiata; and, below, with the crus cerebri (of the midbrain).

The internal capsule may be divided into the following parts (Fig. 8.14).

(**a**) The ***anterior limb*** lies between the caudate nucleus medially, and the anterior part of the lentiform nucleus laterally.

(**b**) The ***posterior limb*** lies between the thalamus medially, and the posterior part of the lentiform nucleus on the lateral side.

(**c**) In transverse sections through the cerebral hemisphere the anterior and posterior limbs of the internal capsule are seen to meet at an angle open outwards. This angle is called the ***genu*** (genu = bend).

(**d**)   Some fibres of the internal capsule lie behind the posterior end of the lentiform nucleus. They constitute its ***retrolentiform part.***

(**e**)   Some other fibres pass below the lentiform nucleus (and not medial to it). These fibres constitute the ***sublentiform part*** of the internal capsule.

Details of the fibres passing through the internal capsule are considered in Chapter 17.

Corpus Callosum

The corpus callosum is made up of a large mass of nerve fibres that connects the two cerebral hemispheres (Fig. 8.6). It is subdivided into a central part or ***trunk,*** an anterior end that is bent on itself to form the ***genu***, and an enlarged posterior end called the ***splenium.*** A thin lamina of nerve

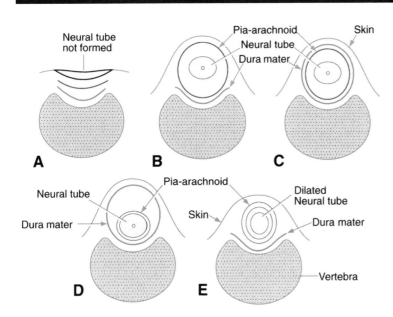

Fig. 8.15. Anomalies of the
neural tube.
(A) Posterior rachischisis.
(B), (C) and (E) Varieties of
meningo-myelocoele.
(D) Meningocoele.

BASIC

fibres connects the genu to the upper end of the lamina terminalis. These fibres form the ***rostrum*** of the corpus callosum. The corpus callosum is intimately related to the lateral ventricles. Its under surface gives attachment to the septum pellucidum (Figs. 8.6, 13.1).

The fibres of the corpus callosum interconnect the corresponding regions of almost all parts of the cerebral cortex of the two hemispheres. The fibres of the genu run forwards into the frontal lobes, the fibres of the two sides forming a fork-like structure called the ***forceps minor***. Many fibres of the splenium run backwards into the occipital lobe to form a similar structure called the ***forceps major***. (Each half of the forceps major bulges into the posterior horn of the corresponding lateral ventricle, forming the bulb of the posterior horn).

The fibres of the trunk of the corpus callosum (and some from the splenium) run laterally and as they do so they intersect the fibres of the corona radiata. As they pass laterally, some fibres of the trunk and of the splenium of the corpus callosum, form a flattened band called the ***tapetum***. The tapetum is closely related to the posterior and inferior horns of the lateral ventricle.

As mentioned above all fibres passing through the corpus callosum are not strictly commissural. Some fibres that interconnect dissimilar areas in the two hemispheres are really association fibres.

Blood Supply of the Brain

A consolidated account of the blood supply of all parts of the brain is given in Chapter 21.

ANOMALIES OF THE BRAIN AND THE SPINAL CORD

Non-closure of Neural Tube

1. ***Posterior rachischisis:*** The whole length of the neural tube remains unclosed (Figs. 8.15A).

2. ***Anencephaly:*** The neural tube remains open in the region of the brain. The exposed brain tissue degenerates.

3. Non fusion of the neural tube is of necessity associated with non-closure of the cranium (***cranium bifidum***) or of the vertebral canal (***spina bifida***, Fig. 8.15A.).

Note the following facts about anencephaly.

CLINICAL

(a) It is a serious defect incompatiable with life.
(b) It can be diagnosed before birth by ultrasonography.
(c) The level of alpha-fetoprotein in amniotic fluid is raised.
(d) An anencephalic fetus cannot swallow amniotic fluid. This can lead to excessive amount of amniotic fluid (hydramnios).

Outward Bulging of Neural Tube and Covering Membranes

As a result of non-fusion of the neural tube, or of overlying bones (e.g. spina bifida), neural tissue may lie outside the cranial cavity or vertebral canal. When this happens in the region of the brain the condition is called *encephalocoele*, and when it occurs in the spinal region it is called *myelocoele* (Figs. 8.15B, C).

1. When the condition is due to non-closure of the neural tube, nervous tissue is exposed on the surface, as in anencephaly, and in rachischisis (Fig. 8.15A).

2. When the neural tube has closed, and the outward bulging is a result of a defect in the overlying bones, the neural tissue is covered by bulging skin and membranes (*meningo-mylocoele*) (Figs. 8.15B, C, E). The corresponding condition in the region of the skull is *meningo-encephalocoele*

3. Occasionally the bulging is caused by the membranes alone (*meningocoele*), the neural tissue being normally located (Fig. 8.15D). Some varieties of these conditions are illustrated in Figs. 8.15B to E.

When a meningoencephalocoele is present, the medulla oblongata, and the tonsils of the cerebellum, are displaced caudally into the foramen magnum causing obstruction to the flow of cerebrospinal fluid. This leads to hydrocephalus. These conditions together constitute the *Arnold Chiari deformity*.

Congenital Hydrocephalus

An abnormal quantity of cerebrospinal fluid may accumulate in the ventricular system of the brain (*hydrocephalus*). This may be due to a blockage to its flow or to excessive production. The ventricles become very large and the infant is born with a large head. The pressure of the fluid causes degeneration of nervous tissue. Similar enlargement of the spinal cord is called *hydromyelia*; the enlargement of the central canal being called *syringocoele*. This condition may be associated with the formation of abnormal cavities near the central canal (*syringomyelia*). Destruction of nervous tissue at this site results in a characteristic syndrome.

In one form of hydrocephalus resulting from blockage of the median and lateral apertures of the fourth ventricle, the enlargement is predominantly in the posterior cranial fossa, and the cerebellum is abnormal (*Dandy Walker syndrome*). Obstruction to flow of cerebrospinal fluid may also be caused by stenosis or malformation of the cerebral aqueduct.

Faulty Development

The brain may be too small (*microcephaly*) or too large (*macrocephaly*). Gyri may be absent or may be poorly formed. Faulty development of the cerebral cortex may lead to impaired intelligence or in congenital paralysis.

Absence of Parts of the Nervous System

Parts of the nervous system may be absent. Absence of the corpus callosum, spinal cord or cerebellum is documented.

FURTHER DETAILS ABOUT VARIOUS PARTS OF THE CEREBRAL HEMISPHERES ARE GIVEN IN CHAPTERS 13 TO 17. FOR BLOOD SUPPLY SEE CHAPTER 21.

9 : Tracts of Spinal Cord and Brainstem

We have seen that a collection of nerve fibres within the central nervous system, that connects two masses of grey matter, is called a tract. A tract may be defined as a collection of nerve fibres having the same origin, course, and termination. Tracts may be ascending or descending. They are usually named after the masses of grey matter connected by them. Thus, a tract beginning in the cerebral cortex and descending to the spinal cord is called the corticospinal tract, while a tract ascending from the spinal cord to the thalamus is called the spinothalamic tract. We have noted that tracts are sometimes referred to as fasciculi (= bundles) or lemnisci (=ribbons). The major tracts passing through the spinal cord and brainstem are shown schematically in Fig. 9.1. The position of the tracts in a transverse section of the spinal cord is shown in Fig. 9.2, and at ascending levels of the brainstem in Figs. 11.1 to 11.3, 11.5, and 11.7 to 11.9. It will be a useful exercise for the student to follow the course of each tract described below by noting its position in each of these figures proceeding from Figs. 11.1 to 11.9 in the case of ascending tracts, and in the reverse order for descending tracts. In studying these figures it must be remembered that in actual fact the boundaries of areas occupied by the fibres of each tract are not clear cut. There is considerable overlap of the territories of various tracts. The lines of demarcation shown in the diagrams are, therefore, approximate and artificial. It may also be remembered that the position of a particular tract varies at different levels of the spinal cord; and that some of the tracts shown in Fig. 9.2 are present only in the upper part of the cord.

Descending Tracts ending in the Spinal Cord

CORTICOSPINAL TRACTS

The corticospinal tracts are made up, predominantly, of axons of neurons lying in the motor area of the cerebral cortex (area 4). Some fibres also arise from the premotor area (area 6) and some from the somatosensory area (areas 3, 2, 1) (Figs. 9.3, 8.10 and 15.4). A few fibres arise in the parietal cortex (area 5). From this origin fibres pass through the corona radiata to enter the internal capsule where they lie in the posterior limb (Figs. 9.3 and 17.2A). After passing through the internal capsule the fibres enter the crus cerebri (of the midbrain): they occupy the middle two-thirds of the crus. The fibres then descend through the ventral part of the pons to enter the pyramids in the upper part of the medulla.

Near the lower end of the medulla about 80 percent of the fibres cross to the opposite side. (The crossing fibres of the two sides constitute the decussation of the pyramids.)

The fibres that have crossed in the medulla enter the lateral funiculus of the spinal cord and descend as the ***lateral corticospinal tract*** (Fig. 9.2). The fibres of this tract terminate in grey matter at various levels of the spinal cord. Most of them end by synapsing with internuncial neurons in the bases of the dorsal and ventral grey columns (laminae IV to VII). The internuncial neurons carry the impulses brought by fibres of the tract to ventral horn cells. Some fibres of the tract terminate directly on ventral horn cells (lamina IX, dorsolateral, central and ventrolateral groups).

The corticospinal fibres that do not cross in the pyramidal decussation enter the anterior funiculus of the spinal cord to form the ***anterior corticospinal tract.*** On reaching the appropriate level of the

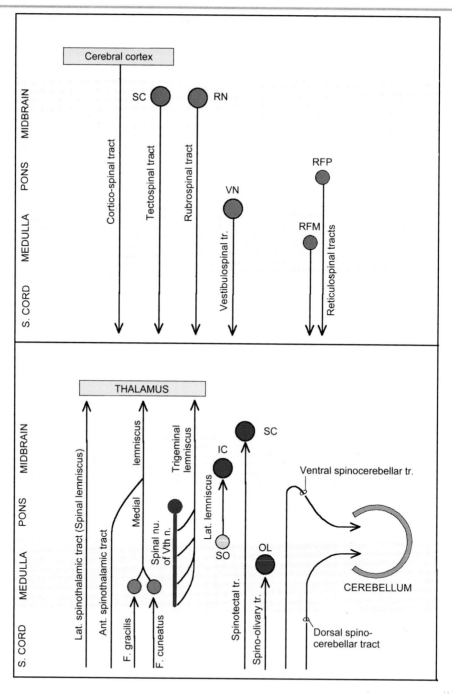

Fig. 9.1. Scheme to show the major tracts passing through the brainstem. SC = superior colliculus. RN = red nucleus. VN = vestibular nuclei. RFP = reticular formation of pons. RFM = reticular formation of medulla. IC = inferior colliculus. SO = superior olivary nucleus

spinal cord the fibres of this tract cross the midline (through the anterior white commissure) to reach grey matter on the opposite side of the cord. Their manner of termination is similar to that of fibres of the lateral corticospinal tract. In this way the corticospinal fibres of both the lateral and anterior tracts

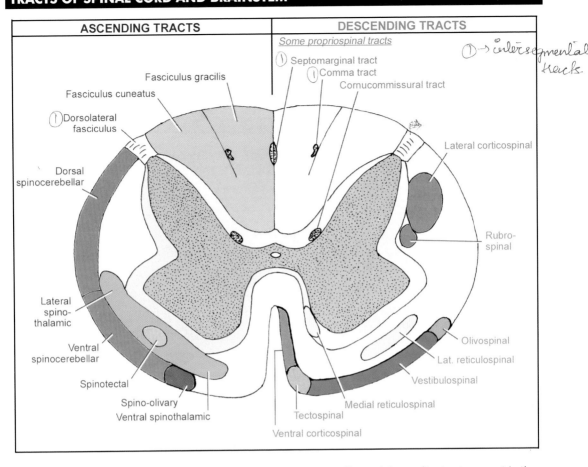

Fig. 9.2. Simplified scheme to show the positions of the main ascending and descending tracts present in the spinal cord. Note that the positions of the tracts vary at different levels of the cord; and that the areas occupied by the fibres of different tracts overlap considerably.

ultimately connect the cerebral cortex of one side with ventral horn cells in the opposite half of the spinal cord.

The cerebral cortex controls voluntary movement through the corticospinal tract. Interruption of the tract anywhere in its course leads to paralysis of the muscles concerned. As the fibres are closely packed in their course through the internal capsule and brainstem small lesions here can cause widespread paralysis.

The neurons that give origin to the fibres of the corticospinal tracts are often referred to as **upper motor neurons** in distinction to the ventral horn cells and their processes which constitute the **lower motor neurons**. Interruption of either of these neurons leads to paralysis, but the nature of the paralysis is distinctive in each case.

Having considered the basic facts about the corticospinal tracts we may now consider some additional features of interest.

(**1**) The majority of fibres constituting the corticospinal tracts (70%) are myelinated. Most of the fibres are of small diameter (1 to 4 μm) while about 20% of fibres are of large diameter (11 to 22 μm). The latter arise from the giant pyramidal neurons (cells of Betz) lying in the motor area of the cerebral cortex.

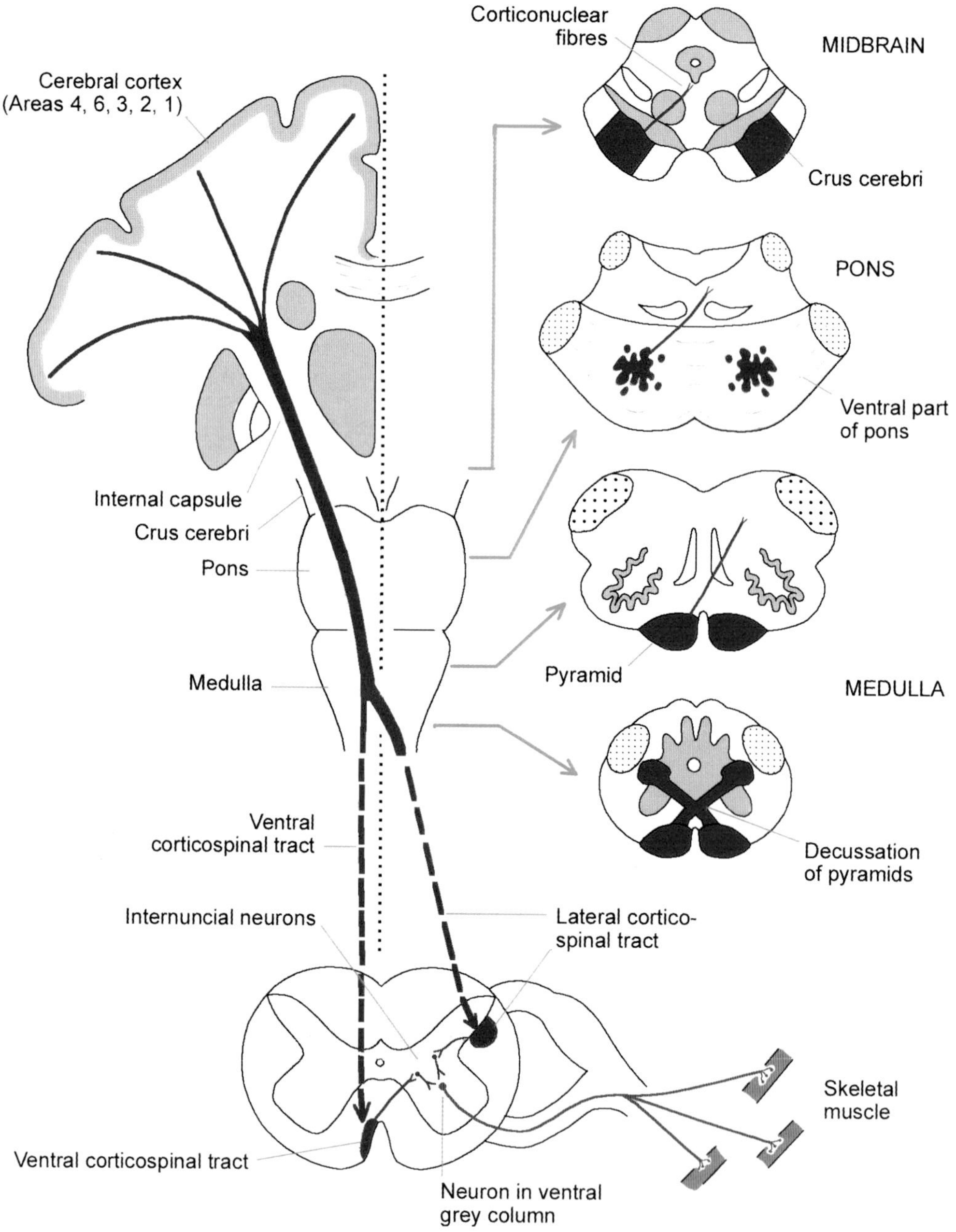

Fig. 9.3. Scheme to show the course of the corticospinal tracts. Note the position of the tracts at various levels of the brainstem.

Fibres of the corticospinal tract are unmyelinated at birth. Myelination begins in the second postnatal week and gradually extends down the axons. It is completed in the second year. The infant acquires proper motor control only after myelination of the corticospinal tracts is completed.

(2) The proportion of fibres crossing in the decussation of the pyramids is variable (75 to 90%). Very rarely all corticospinal fibres may descend in the anterior corticospinal tract. Conversely, this tract may be absent. Some fibres may descend in the lateral funiculus of the same side. According to some authorities such fibres form a separate *anterolateral corticospinal tract.* These fibres terminate on the same side of the spinal cord.

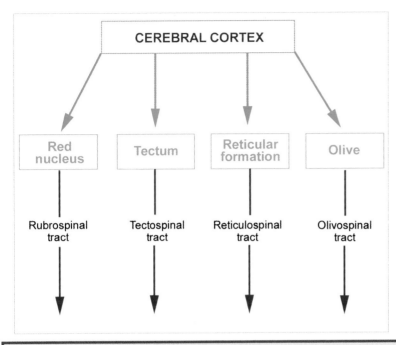

Fig. 9.4. Indirect pathways through which the cerebral cortex may influence the spinal cord. These are often described as extrapyramidal tracts. The presence of olivospinal fibres is doubtful.

(3) The lateral corticospinal tract extends to the lowest segments of the spinal cord, but the anterior tract extends only to the midthoracic level.

(4) The longest fibres of the tract (for lowest segments of the spinal cord) lie most superficially within the tract; while the shortest fibres lie most medially. Fibres of the corticospinal tracts are arranged somatotropically (This term means that within the tract the fibres meant for control of muscles in different parts of the body are arranged in a definite sequence).

(5) Corticospinal fibres are usually described as ending (directly, or through internuncial neurons) in relation to alpha neurons, in contrast to some other descending tracts which are said to end in relation to gamma neurons. However, recent work shows that corticospinal fibres end in relation to both alpha and gamma neurons.

(6) The influence of this tract is said to be facilitatory for flexors and inhibitory for extensors.

(7) Apart from their motor functions, corticospinal fibres influence conduction in ascending tracts. This influence is mediated through axons of cells lying in the parietal lobe, which end predominately in laminae IV to VI.

(8) For effects of damage to corticospinal tracts see page 103.

Rubrospinal tract

This tract is made up of axons of neurons lying in the red nucleus (which lies in the upper part of the midbrain). The fibres of the tract cross to the opposite side in the lower part of the tegmentum of the midbrain. The crossing fibres constitute the ***ventral tegmental decussation*** (Fig. 11.9). The tract descends through the pons and medulla to enter the lateral funiculus of the spinal cord (Fig. 9.2). Here the tract lies just in front of the lateral corticospinal tract. The fibres of the rubrospinal tract end by synapsing with ventral horn cells through internuncial neurons located in laminae V to VII of the spinal grey matter.

The tract is believed to be facilitatory to flexors and inhibitory to extensors. The rubrospinal tract is much better developed in some other species than in man. In man, the tract reaches only the upper three cervical segments of the spinal cord.

BASIC

Tectospinal tract

The fibres of this tract arise from neurons in the superior colliculus (midbrain). The fibres cross to the opposite side in the upper part of the tegmentum of the midbrain. The crossing fibres form ***the dorsal tegmental decussation*** (Fig. 11.9). The tract descends through the pons and medulla into the anterior funiculus of the spinal cord. The fibres terminate by synapsing with ventral horn cells in cervical segments of the cord, through internuncial neurons located in laminae VI to VIII of the spinal grey matter.

Vestibulospinal tracts

There are two vestibulospinal tracts, lateral and medial.

Lateral vestibulospinal tract

The neurons of origin of the lateral vestibulospinal tract lie in the lateral vestibular nucleus. This tract is uncrossed and lies in the anterior funiculus of the spinal cord (Fig. 9.2) (shifting medially as it descends). Its fibres end in relation to neurons in the ventral grey column (laminae VII and VIII). This tract is an important efferent path for equilibrium.

The fibres of the lateral vestibulospinal tract are somatotropically arranged. Fibres to cervical segments arise from the cranio-ventral part of the lateral vestibular nucleus, and those to the thoracic segments from the central part, and those to the lumbosacral segments from the dorsocaudal parts of the nucleus.

Medial vestibulospinal tract

The medial vestibulospinal tract arises mainly from the medial vestibular nucleus (with some fibres from the inferior and lateral nuclei). The tract descends through the anterior funiculus (within the sulcomarginal fasciculus). The fibres are partly crossed and partly uncrossed. They end in cervical segments of the cord in laminae VII and VIII.

ADVANCED

The lateral vestibulospinal tract is facilitatory to motor neurons supplying extensor muscles (of the neck, back and limbs); and is inhibitory to flexor muscles. The medial tract is inhibitory to muscles of the neck and back.

Olivospinal tract

This tract is generally described as arising from the inferior olivary nucleus (medulla) and terminating in relation to ventral horn cells of the spinal cord. However, recent research suggests that fibres do not descend from the inferior olive to the spinal cord.

Reticulospinal tracts

The reticular formation is connected to spinal grey matter through the medial and lateral reticulospinal tracts.

Medial reticulospinal tract

Fibres arise from the medial part of the reticular formation of both the pons and the medulla (mainly from the nucleus gigantocellularis reticularis of the medulla, and the oral and caudal reticular nuclei of the pons). The fibres which are crossed and uncrossed descend in the anterior funiculus (near the anterior median fissure). The fibres reach all levels of the spinal cord. They end directly, or through interneurons, on alpha and gamma motor neurons. The tract is facilitatory to muscles of the trunk and

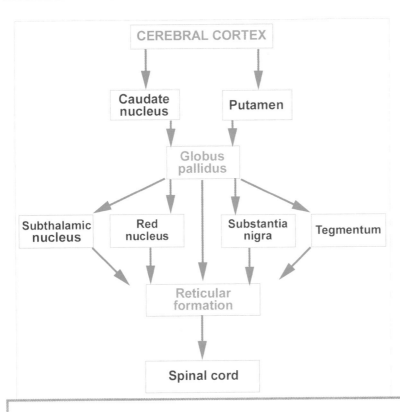

CEREBRAL CORTEX

Caudate nucleus

Putamen

Globus pallidus

Subthalamic nucleus

Red nucleus

Substantia nigra

Tegmentum

Reticular formation

Spinal cord

Fig. 9.5.
Indirect pathways through which the corpus striatum may influence the spinal cord.

BASIC

limbs, but some fibres are inhibitory to neck muscles. The tract is concerned with postural adjustments of the head, trunk and limbs.

Lateral reticulospinal tract

This tract is constituted by fibres arising in the ventrolateral part of the reticular formation of the pons (caudal and oral pontine reticular nuclei). The fibres cross to the opposite side in the medulla and run down in the lateral funiculus.

ADVANCED

Reticulospinal fibres terminate widely in spinal grey matter, but the exact laminae in which they end are controversial. They possibly terminate in all laminae other than II and III, with the majority ending in laminae VI to VIII. Some fibres reach the lateral cervical nucleus. Apart from control of motor function, the reticulospinal tracts may influence transmission of pain through ascending tracts.

Descending Autonomic Fibres

Hypothalamospinal fibres begin (mainly) in the paraventricular nucleus of the hypothalamus, and descend uncrossed in the dorsolateral funiculus. The axons end in relation to sympathetic and parasympathetic preganglionic neurons located in the intermediolateral grey column (and other regions) of spinal grey matter. The neuromediators demonstrated in these fibres include dopamine, oxytocin and vasopressin.

Some fibres (noradrenergic) descend into the cord from the locus coeruleus. These fibres are widely distributed in spinal grey matter, but the greatest number end in relation to preganglionic parasympathetic neurons in sacral segments of the spinal cord. Some adrenergic fibres also descend from the medulla to the intermediolateral grey column.

Some groups of neurons located in the brainstem give off serotoninergic fibres that descend into the spinal cord as two bundles, lateral and ventral. The lateral fibres end in laminae I, II and V and

ADVANCED

probably influence pain perception. The ventral fibres reach laminae VIII and IX. They are facilitatory to motor neurons.

Other descending tracts

In addition to the better known descending tracts described above, fibres may also descend to the spinal cord from the interstitial nucleus (located near the third ventricle), the tegmentum of the midbrain, and from the nucleus of the solitary tract.

BASIC

Significance of Descending tracts

The various descending tracts described above, that end in relation to ventral horn cells, influence their activity, and thereby have an effect on contraction and tone of skeletal muscle. Although a small number of the fibres of these tracts may synapse directly with ventral horn cells, most of them influence these cells through intervening internuncial neurons. This influence is exerted both on alpha neurons and gamma neurons. We have already seen that gamma neurons indirectly influence the activity of alpha neurons via muscle spindles. Hence, all these influences ultimately reach the alpha neurons. Such influences may be either facilitatory or inhibitory. The corticospinal and rubrospinal tracts are described as being facilitatory to flexors and inhibitory to extensors, while the vestibulospinal tract is said to have the opposite effect. The medial reticulospinal tract is generally regarded as facilitatory and the lateral tract as inhibitory. However, motor control is far more complex than such simple statements may suggest.

The corticospinal tracts are often referred to as *pyramidal tracts.* Traditionally all other descending tracts projecting on motor neurons have been collectively referred to as *extrapyramidal tracts.* It has often been presumed that the pyramidal and extrapyramidal tracts act in opposition to each other. It has also been said that the pyramidal fibres end in relation to alpha neurons, and extrapyramidal fibres in relation to gamma neurons. However, it is now recognised that such a distinction is artificial and of little significance either physiological or clinical.

We have seen that autonomic nerve fibres arise from neurons located in the general visceral efferent nuclei of the brainstem, and from the intermediolateral region of the spinal grey matter. These regions are under control from higher centres through descending autonomic pathways described above.

In addition to their influence on motor activity, it has been relatively recently recognised that descending tracts may influence the transmission of afferent impulses through ascending tracts.

Descending Tracts
ending in the Brainstem

Corticonuclear tracts

The nuclei of cranial nerves that supply skeletal muscle (i.e., somatic efferent and special visceral efferent nuclei) are functionally equivalent to ventral horn cells of the spinal cord. They are under cortical control through fibres that are closely related in their origin and course to corticospinal fibres. At various levels of the brainstem these fibres cross to the opposite side to end by synapsing with cells in cranial nerve nuclei, either directly or through interneurons.

Cortico-ponto-cerebellar pathway

Fibres arising in the cerebral cortex of the frontal, temporal, parietal and occipital lobes descend through the corona radiata and internal capsule to reach the crus cerebri. The frontopontine fibres occupy the medial one sixth of the crus; and the temporopontine fibres (along with occipitopontine and parietopontine fibres) occupy the lateral one sixth of the crus (Fig. 11.8). These fibres enter the ventral part of the pons to end in pontine nuclei of the same side.

Axons of neurons in the pontine nuclei form the transverse fibres of the pons. These fibres cross the middle line and pass into the middle cerebellar peduncle of the opposite side. The fibres of this peduncle reach the cerebellar cortex.

The cortico-ponto-cerebellar pathway forms the anatomical basis for control of cerebellar activity by the cerebral cortex.

Other fibres ending in the Brainstem

The cerebral cortex also exercises control on various masses of grey matter (other than cranial nerve nuclei and pontine nuclei) of the brainstem. Fibres from the cortex end in the red nucleus, the tectum, the substantia nigra, the inferior olivary nucleus (?), the interstitial nucleus and the reticular formation. These centres can also be influenced by the cortex indirectly through the striatum (caudate nucleus and putamen of lentiform nucleus) and the globus pallidus (Figs 9.4, 9.5). In turn these centres influence the spinal cord directly through tracts descending from them (rubrospinal, tectospinal, olivospinal, reticulospinal); and indirectly through the reticular formation and the reticulospinal tracts. These connections are often described as part of the extrapyramidal pathways referred to above.

Disorders of Motor Function

Inability to move a part of the body is referred to as *paralysis.* This can be produced by interruption of motor pathways anywhere between the motor area of the cerebral cortex and the muscles themselves. We have seen that the pathway from cortex to muscle involves at least two neurons. The first of these is located in the cerebral cortex. Its axon terminates in the spinal cord or in motor cranial nerve nuclei in the brainstem. From a physiological and clinical point of view this neuron is referred to as the *upper motor neuron*. The second neuron is located in the anterior grey column of the spinal cord (or in motor nuclei of the brainstem) and sends out an axon that travels through a peripheral nerve to innervate muscle. This neuron is referred to as the *lower motor neuron.* (For the present purpose we may ignore interneurons present in the pathway). When lower motor neurons are destroyed, or their continuity interrupted, the muscles supplied by them lose their tone (i.e., they become flaccid); and in course of time the muscles undergo atrophy. Changes in electrical responses of the muscles also take place. These alterations constitute the *reaction of degeneration.* In addition, because of interruption of the efferent part of reflex pathways tendon reflexes are abolished.

Destruction or interruption of the upper motor neuron is not followed by any of these changes. On the other hand it is usually accompanied by an increase in muscle tone, and exaggeration of tendon reflexes. It is, therefore, possible to distinguish between an upper motor neuron paralysis (often called *spastic paralysis*) and a lower motor neuron (or *flaccid*) paralysis. Paralysis may be confined to one limb (*monoplegia*) or to both limbs on one side of the body (*hemiplegia*). Paralysis of both lower limbs is called *paraplegia,* and that of all four limbs is called *quadriplegia.* Paralysis of muscles supplied by one or more cranial nerves may occur in isolation, or in combination with hemiplegia. Destruction of a particular region often destroys lower motor neurons situated at that level resulting in a localised flaccid paralysis of muscles supplied from that level. This lesion may at the same time interrupt descending tracts (representing upper motor neurons), resulting in a spastic paralysis below the level of the lesion. *The presence of a localised flaccid paralysis can thus serve as a pointer to the level of lesion.*

It is also important to remember that the fibres of upper motor neurons meant for the limbs cross the midline in the lower part of the medulla (in the decussation of the pyramids); and those for the cranial nerves cross just above the level of their termination. A lesion above the level of crossing produces a paralysis in the opposite half of the body, and a lesion below this level produces paralysis on the same side.

Keeping the considerations discussed above in mind we may now consider the effects of lesions of the motor pathways at various levels.

(**1**) Because of the large extent of the ***motor areas of the cerebral cortex*** lesions here produce a relatively localised paralysis e.g., a monoplegia.

(**2**) A lesion in the ***internal capsule*** is capable of producing widespread paralysis on the opposite half of the body (hemiplegia) which may also involve the lower part of the face and the tongue. (The cranial nerves having a bilateral corticonuclear supply are spared). A lesion in the internal capsule is most likely to result from thrombosis or rupture of one of the arteries supplying the capsule. The artery most often involved is Charcot's artery of cerebral haemorrhage (Chapter 21).

(**3**) Lesions of corticospinal fibres at various levels in the ***brainstem***, above the level of the pyramidal decussation, can produce contralateral hemiplegia. If the lesion crosses the midline symptoms can be bilateral. Involvement of motor cranial nerve nuclei (or of fibres arising from them) may result in various combinations. For example, a lesion in the upper part of the midbrain can produce a paralysis of muscles supplied by the oculomotor nerve on the side of lesion, along with a hemiplegia on the opposite side (***Weber's syndrome***). A similar lesion in the pons, results in a paralysis of the lateral rectus muscle (abducent nerve) on the side of lesion with hemiplegia on the opposite side (***Raymond's syndrome***). Alternatively, facial paralysis of one side can be combined with contralateral hemiplegia (***Millard Gubler syndrome***). Various such combinations may result depending on the level of lesion.

(**4**) Lesions affecting the lateral corticospinal tract in the spinal cord produce an upper motor neuron paralysis of muscles on the same side of the body. Lesions above the fifth cervical segment result in paralysis of both upper and lower extremities; while lesions below the first thoracic segment affect only the lower limbs. As in the brainstem, lesions in the spinal cord may be bilateral. Involvement of lower motor neurons at the level of lesion produces a flaccid paralysis of muscles supplied from that level, along with spastic paralysis below the level of injury. A knowledge of muscles supplied by individual spinal segments can thus help in locating the level of a lesion in the spinal cord.

In some diseases (e.g., ***poliomyelitis***) damage may be confined to lower motor neurons, and the resulting paralysis may be purely flaccid. Such lesions are accompanied by muscular wasting , muscle twitchings (fasciculation) and contracture of opposing muscles.

Lesions of extrapyramidal tracts are marked by great rgidity (of the clasp knife type). The rigidity leads to greatly reduced mobility. Tendon reflexes are exaggerated.

In the above description we have (for sake of simplicity) considered involvement of motor neurons in isolation. However, disease at any level can involve other structures resulting in sensory and other disturbances.

Rigidity

Muscle tone has been described on page 55. When tone is excessive the body becomes rigid. Distinctive types of rigidity are recognised. (a) If we try to flex a rigid limb, and there is sudden loss of resistance, the rigidity is described as clasp knife rigidity. (b) When the resistance is uniform over the range of movement the condition is called lead pipe rigidity. When resistance is intermittent the rigidity is said to be of the cog wheel type.

Ascending Tracts

Introductory Remarks

The ascending tracts of the spinal cord and brainstem represent one stage of multineuron pathways by which afferent impulses arising in various parts of the body are conveyed to different parts of the brain. The ***first order neurons*** of these pathways are usually located in spinal (dorsal nerve root) ganglia (Fig. 3.3). We have seen that the neurons in these ganglia are unipolar (pseudounipolar). Each neuron gives off a peripheral process and a central process. The peripheral processes of the neurons form the afferent fibres of peripheral nerves. They end in relation to sensory end organs (receptors) situated in various tissues. The central processes of these neurons enter the spinal cord through the dorsal nerve roots. Having entered the cord the central processes, as a rule, terminate by synapsing with cells in spinal grey matter. Some of them may run upwards in the white matter of the cord to form ascending tracts (Fig. 9.6). The majority of ascending tracts are, however, formed by axons of cells in spinal grey matter. These are ***second order*** sensory neurons (Fig. 9.8). In the case of pathways that convey sensory information to the cerebral cortex the second order neurons end by synapsing with neurons in the thalamus. ***Third order*** sensory neurons located in the thalamus carry the sensations to the cerebral cortex. The following additional points may now be noted.

(**1**) Having entered the spinal cord, the central processes of the first order neurons may ascend or descend to end in higher or lower segments of the cord. Alternatively, they may divide into ascending and descending branches.

(**2**) The axons of the second order neurons may enter white matter on the same side, forming an uncrossed tract; or on the opposite side, forming a crossed tract.

(**3**) Internuncial neurons may be interposed between the main neurons of the pathway.

(**4**) The fibres of the tract may give collaterals to various masses of grey matter.

(**5**) In the case of the head (and other parts supplied by cranial nerves) the first order neurons are located in sensory ganglia situated on the cranial nerves. (In some of these ganglia *viz.,* cochlear and vestibular, the neurons are bipolar, not unipolar as in most ganglia). The central processes of these neurons end in relation to afferent nuclei of cranial nerves. The neurons in these nuclei constitute second order neurons.

(**6**) The neurons of the mesencephalic nucleus of the trigeminal nerve are believed to be first order sensory neurons.

They are exceptional in being the only such neurons that lie within the brain.

(**7**) Only those afferent impulses which reach the cerebral cortex are consciously perceived. One exception to this may be perception of some degree of pain in the thalamus. Afferent impulses ending in the cerebellum or in the brainstem influence the activities of these centres.

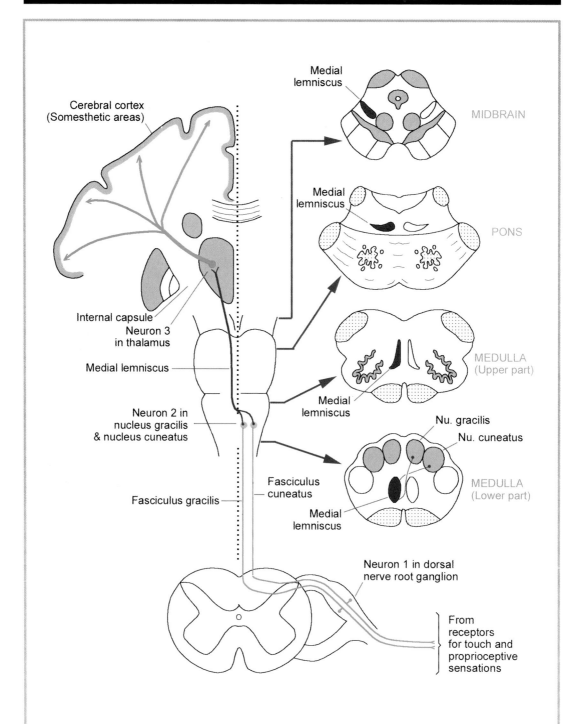

Fig. 9.6. Scheme to show the main features of the posterior column medial lemniscus pathway. Note the position of the medial lemniscus at various levels of the brainstem.

PATHWAYS CONNECTING THE SPINAL CORD TO THE CEREBRAL CORTEX

The Posterior Column – Medial Lemniscus Pathway

(a) Fasciculus gracilis and fasciculus cuneatus:

These tracts occupy the posterior funiculus of the spinal cord and are, therefore, often referred to as the **posterior column tracts** (Fig. 9.2). They are unique in that they are formed predominantly by central processes of neurons located in dorsal nerve root ganglia i.e., by first order sensory neurons (Fig. 9.6). The fibres derived from the lowest ganglia are situated most medially; while those from the highest ganglia are most lateral. The fasciculus gracilis, which lies medially is, therefore, composed of fibres from the coccygeal, sacral, lumbar and lower thoracic ganglia; while the fasciculus cuneatus which lies laterally consists of fibres from upper thoracic and cervical ganglia. The fibres of these fasciculi extend upwards as far as the lower part of the medulla. Here the fibres of the gracile and cuneate fasciculi terminate by synapsing with neurons in the nucleus gracilis and nucleus cuneatus respectively.

It has recently been shown that the fasciculus gracilis and the fasciculus cuneatus also contain some fibres that originate in the dorsal grey column (laminae III, IV) i.e., second order sensory neurons.

Some afferents from spinal ganglia pass through the dorsal funiculus to reach the dorsal nucleus and other areas of spinal grey matter.

(b) Medial Lemniscus

The neurons of the gracile and cuneate nuclei are second order sensory neurons. Their axons run forwards and medially (as **internal arcuate fibres**) to cross the middle line. The crossing fibres of the two sides constitute the **sensory decussation (or lemniscal decussation).** Having crossed the middle line, the fibres turn upwards to form a prominent bundle called the **medial lemniscus** (Fig. 9.6). The medial lemniscus runs upwards through the medulla, pons and midbrain to end in the thalamus (ventral posterolateral nucleus).

(c) Third order sensory neurons located in the thalamus give off axons that pass through the internal capsule and the corona radiata to reach the somatosensory areas of the cerebral cortex.

The pathway described above carries:

(**i**) Some components of the sense of touch. These include deep touch and pressure, the ability to localise exactly the part touched (tactile localisation), the ability to recognise as separate two points on the skin that are touched simultaneously (tactile discrimination), and the ability to recognise the shape of an object held in the hand (stereognosis).

(**ii**) Proprioceptive impulses that convey the sense of position and of movement of different parts of the body.

(**iii**) The sense of vibration.

Some further facts of interest about the fasciculus gracilus and fasciculus cuneatus are as follows.

1. Nerve fibres carrying proprioceptive impulses through the fasciculus gracilis predominantly end in the dorsal nuclei (in the posterior grey column of thoracic segments of the spinal cord) and, therefore, do not reach cervical levels. Hence, most of the fibres passing through the fasciculus in upper cervical segments are from cutaneous receptors.

BASIC

ADVANCED

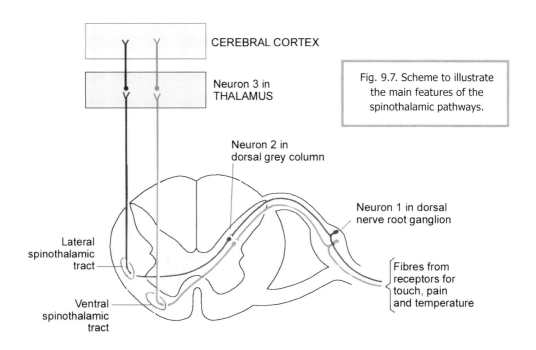

CEREBRAL CORTEX

Neuron 3 in
THALAMUS

Fig. 9.7. Scheme to illustrate
the main features of the
spinothalamic pathways.

Neuron 2 in
dorsal grey column

Neuron 1 in dorsal
nerve root ganglion

Lateral
spinothalamic
tract

Fibres from
receptors for
touch, pain
and temperature

Ventral
spinothalamic
tract

2. In contrast to the fasciculus gracilis, the fasciculus cuneatus carries numerous proprioceptive fibres (as well as those for cutaneous sensations) throughout its extent.

3. Both the fasciculi are made up predominantly of myelinated fibres.

4. In experimental animals it has been shown that the fibres of these fasciculi are grouped in terms of the dermatomes they carry impulses from. At higher levels the fibres change position and come to be arranged somatotropically (i.e., in accordance with parts of the body). This somatotropic organisation is maintained in the gracile and cuneate nuclei. The fibres from the lower limb are most medial (in nucleus gracilis) followed by those from the trunk and upper limbs (in nucleus cuneatus).

5. The nucleus gracilis and cuneatus receive descending fibres from the cerebral cortex, the cerebellum, and from the reticular formation. These afferents may facilitate or inhibit transmission through these nuclei.

Spinothalamic Pathways

Anterior and Lateral spinothalamic tracts

(**a**) The first order neurons of this pathway are located in spinal ganglia. The central processes of these neurons enter the spinal cord and terminate in relation to spinal grey matter. They may ascend in the dorsolateral tract (situated near the tip of the dorsal grey column, Fig. 9.2) for one or more segments before ending in grey matter.

(**b**) The second order neurons of this pathway, are located mainly in laminae IV, V, VI and VII. The axons of these neurons constitute the anterior and lateral spinothalamic tracts. They cross to the opposite side of the spinal cord in the white commissure (but some fibres may remain on the same side). The crossing of the fibres is oblique. The fibres for the lateral spinothalamic tract cross within the same segment of the cord, while those of the anterior spinothalamic tract may ascend for one or more segments before they cross to the opposite side. The tracts also carry some uncrossed fibres (about 10 per cent).

The fibres for the anterior spinothalamic tract enter the anterior funiculus (Figs. 9.2, 9.7) where they lie medial to emerging fibres of ventral nerve roots. The fibres for the lateral spinothalamic tract enter the lateral funiculus. The two tracts form one continuous band that runs up the spinal cord. On reaching the medulla the two tracts separate. The anterior spinothalamic tract joins the medial lemniscus and travels through it to the thalamus. The lateral spinothalamic tract runs through the brainstem as a separate bundle called the ***spinal lemniscus*** which (like the anterior tract) ends in the thalamus. All spinothalamic fibres end in the ventral posterolateral nucleus.

Traditionally it has been said that the anterior spinothalamic tract carries sensations of crude touch and pressure, while the lateral tract has been said to carry sensations of pain and temperature. It is now realised that although different fibres within the spinothalamic tracts carry different types of sensations, the anterior and lateral spinothalamic tracts constitute a single functional unit.

According to some authorities the anterior spinothalamic tract does not join the medial lemniscus, but travels along with the lateral spinothalamic tract in the spinal lemniscus.

Studies in experimental animals (monkeys) have brought out some interesting facts regarding the location of neurons giving rise to the spinothalamic tracts.

1. The neurons are not uniformly distributed through the length of the cord. As many as 30% of all neurons are present in the first three cervical segments; and another 20% in the lower cervical segments. Lumbar segments account for another 20%, the remaining 30% being from thoracic and sacrococcygeal segments.

2. About ten per cent of neurons are ipsilateral, and of these 50% are in the upper three cervical segments.

3. The neurons are widely distributed in spinal grey matter, but the laminae involved vary at different levels of the spinal cord. In the upper three cervical segments most neurons lie in laminae VI and VII. Some neurons lie in laminae I, IV, and V. Ipsilateral neurons lie mainly in lamina VIII.

In the lower cervical segments, and also in the lumbar region, the neurons lie in laminae 1, V, VII and VIII. In thoracic segments they are confined to laminae V and VII.

Dorsolateral spinothalamic tract

In addition to the anterior and lateral spinothalamic tracts a separate dorsolateral spinothalamic tract has been described. The fibres of this tract arise from neurons in lamina I, cross to the opposite side, and ascend in the dorsolateral fasciculus to reach the ventral posterolateral nucleus of the thalamus. The tract carries impulses arising in skin (mainly pain and temperature). Relief of pain observed after dorsolateral cordotomy may be a result of the cutting of these fibres.

Spino-cervico-thalamic pathway

This is yet another pathway through which cutaneous sensations (touch, pressure, pain and temperature) reach the thalamus. Axons arising from neurons located in laminae III to V of spinal grey matter collect to form a ***spinocervical tract*** that ascends through the dorsolateral fasciculus. They end in the ***lateral cervical nucleus*** (which is a small collection of neurons lying amongst the fibres of the lateral funiculus in spinal segments C1 and C2). New fibres arising here project to the ventral posterolateral nucleus of the thalamus.

ASCENDING PATHWAYS ENDING IN THE BRAINSTEM

A number of tracts arising in spinal grey matter, and ending in masses of grey matter in the brainstem, are described. Some of them are as follows.

Spinoreticular Tracts

Spinoreticular fibres begin from spinal neurons mainly in lamina VII (also V and VIII). The fibres are partly crossed and partly uncrossed. The fibres ascend in the ventrolateral part of the spinal cord, intermingling with spinothalamic tracts. They end in the reticular formation of the medulla and pons. The tract probably carries pain.

Spino-olivary tract

The **spino-olivary tract** is also a crossed tract. It lies at the junction of the anterior and lateral funiculi of the spinal cord. The fibres of the tract end in accessory olivary nuclei.

Spinomesencephalic tracts

A number of tracts travel from spinal cord to different areas in the midbrain. They are collectively referred to as spinomesencephalic tracts.

The **spinotectal tract** connects the spinal grey matter to the superior colliculus. It is a crossed tract. It carries impulses that regulate reflex movements of the head and eyes in response to stimulation of some parts of the body. According to some authorities the tract may carry sensations of pain and temperature. Other spinal fibres reach the pretectal nuclei, and some nuclei in the reticular formation of the midbrain. Spinal cells projecting to the midbrain are located mainly in lamina I. They also lie in laminae IV to VII. Most of the fibres cross the midline and ascend in the anterior part of the spinal cord. Painful stimuli may pass through these fibres.

Sensory Disorders

Interruption of ascending pathways carrying various sensations results in loss of sensory perception (**anaesthesia**) over parts of the body concerned. In case of peripheral nerves the area of anaesthesia following injury is often much less than the area of distribution of the nerve. This is so because of considerable overlap in the areas supplied by different nerves. The area of skin supplied from one spinal segment is called a **dermatome.** Dermatomes for adjoining segments overlap, a given area of skin being innervated by two or more segments.

In the case of spinal cord lesions, the level of disease can be inferred from the level of sensory loss. In this connection it must be remembered that the finer modalities of touch are carried by the posterior column tracts which are uncrossed. Crude touch, pain and temperature are carried by the spinothalamic tracts which are crossed. Thus, a unilateral lesion in the spinal cord can result in loss of the power of tactile localisation, tactile discrimination and of stereognosis on the side of lesion; with loss of crude touch, pain and temperature on the opposite side. Because of a double pathway for touch, loss of sensations of pain and temperature is often more obvious than interference with touch. We have seen that, while crossing the midline, fibres of the spinothalamic tracts do not run horizontally. They ascend as they cross so that their path is oblique. The degree of obliquity is greater in the case of fibres carrying touch as compared to those carrying pain and temperature. Because of this there can be a difference of a few segments in the level at which (or below which) these sensations are lost when the crossing fibres are interrupted by a lesion. In a disease called **syringomyelia**, the region of the spinal cord near the central canal undergoes degeneration with formation of cavities. Fibres of spinothalamic tracts crossing in this region are interrupted. Sensations of pain and temperature are lost over the part of the skin from which fibres are interrupted, but touch is retained as there is an additional pathway for it through the posterior column tracts. This phenomenon is called **dissociated anaesthesia.**

Sensory disturbances can also result from lesions in the brainstem because of damage to the medial lemniscus or to the spinal and trigeminal lemnisci. Lesions of the thalamus can produce bizarre sensory disturbances. Lesions in the internal capsule can cause sensory loss in the entire opposite half of the body as thalamocortical fibres pass through this region. Pressure on sensory areas of the cerebral cortex can result in various abnormal sensations, or in anaesthesia over certain regions. Damage to pathways carrying special sensations of smell, vision and hearing can result in various defects.

Some other terms are used to describe sensory disturbances. Reduced perception for touch is *hypoaesthesia*, for pain it is *hypoalgesia*. Increased perception for touch is *hyperaesthesia*. Abnormal sensations are referred to as *paraesthesias*.

Referred Pain

It sometimes happens that when one of the viscera is diseased pain is not felt in the region of the organ itself, but is felt in some part of the skin and body wall. This phenomenon is called *referred pain.* This pain is usually (but not always) referred to areas of skin supplied by the same spinal segments which innervate the viscus. Some classical examples of referred pain are as follows.

(**1**) Pain arising in the diaphragm, or diaphragmatic pleura, is referred to the shoulder (C4).

(**2**) Pain arising in the heart is referred to the lower cervical and upper thoracic segments. It is felt in the chest wall and along the medial side of the left arm. It may also be referred to the neck or jaw.

(**3**) Referred pain from the stomach is felt in the epigastrium (T6 to T9); and that from the intestines is felt in the epigastrium and around the umbilicus (T7 to T10). Pain from the ileocaecal region is felt in the right iliac region. Pain from the appendix is felt in the umbilical region.

(**4**) Pain from the gall bladder is referred to the epigastrium. It may also be referred to the back just below the inferior angle of the right scapula.

(**5**) Pain arising in the area of distribution of one division of the trigeminal nerve may be referred along other branches of the same division, or even along branches of other divisions.

Thalamic syndrome

1. Threshold for appreciation of touch pain or temperature is lowered.
2. Sensation that are normal may appear to be exaggerated or unpleasant.
3. There may be spontaneous pain.
4. Emotions may be abnormal.

Cordotomy

Sometimes a patient may be in severe pain that cannot be controlled by drugs. As an extreme measure pain may be relieved by cutting the spinothalamic tracts. The operation is called cordotomy.

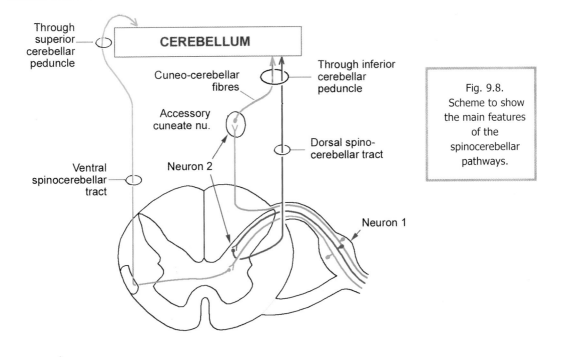

Fig. 9.8. Scheme to show the main features of the spinocerebellar pathways.

The ligamentum denticulatum serves as a guide to the surgeon. For relief of pain the incision is placed anterior to this ligament (**anterolateral cordotomy**).

Pain can also be relieved by cutting the posterior nerve roots in the region. This operation is called **posterior rhizotomy**.

Spinocerebellar Pathways

These pathways carry proprioceptive impulses arising in muscle spindles, Golgi tendon organs, and other receptors to the cerebellum. They constitute the afferent component of reflex arcs involving the cerebellum, for control of posture. Recent investigations have shown that some exteroceptive sensations (e.g., touch) may reach the cerebellum through these pathways.

(**a**) The first order neurons of these pathways are located in dorsal nerve root ganglia. Their peripheral processes end in relation to muscle spindles, Golgi tendon organs and other proprioceptive receptors. Some fibres are related to end organs concerned with exteroceptive sensations (touch, pressure). The central processes of the neurons concerned ascend in the posterior funiculi for varying distances before ending in spinal grey matter. Some of them ascend all the way to the medulla and end in the accessory cuneate nucleus.

(**b**) The second order neurons of the pathway are arranged in a number of groups.

(**i**) Neurons located in the dorsal nucleus (situated on the medial side of the base of the dorsal grey column in segments C8 to L3 of the spinal cord: Fig. 5.2) give origin to fibres of the **dorsal (posterior) spinocerebellar tract.** This is an uncrossed tract lying in the lateral funiculus (Fig. 9.2). It begins in the lumbar segments of the spinal cord and ascends to the medulla where its fibres become incorporated in the inferior cerebellar peduncle and pass through it to reach the vermis of the cerebellum (Fig. 9.8).

(**ii**) The neurons giving origin to the **ventral (anterior) spinocerebellar tract** are probably located in the junctional area between the ventral and dorsal grey columns (laminae V, VI, VII) in the lumbar and sacral segments of the cord. Some of the neurons concerned may lie in the ventral grey column (spinal border cells). The fibres of this tract are predominantly crossed. They ascend in the lateral funiculus, anterior to the fibres of the dorsal spinocerebellar tract (Fig. 9.2), and pass through the medulla and pons. At the upper end of the pons the fibres turn downwards to enter the superior cerebellar peduncle through which they reach the vermis of the cerebellum (Fig. 9.8).

From a functional point of view both the ventral and dorsal spinocerebellar tracts are concerned mainly with the lower limbs and trunk. The dorsal tract is believed to carry impulses concerned with fine co-ordination of muscles controlling posture, and with movements of individual muscles. On the other hand the ventral tract is concerned with movements of the limb as a whole.

(**iii**) We have seen that the central processes of some first order neurons (related to cervical segments) reach the accessory cuneate nucleus (also called the lateral or external cuneate nucleus) in the medulla. Second order neurons lying in this nucleus give origin to **posterior external arcuate fibres** which enter the inferior cerebellar peduncle (of the same side) to reach the cerebellum. This **cuneocerebellar tract** carries impulses from the upper limb. It may be regarded as the forelimb equivalent of the dorsal spinocerebellar tract.

(iv) *Rostral spinocerebellar pathway:* This tract is believed to arise from spinal grey matter in cervical regions of the spinal cord. The neurons of origin lie in the lower four cervical segments (lamina VII). These neurons constitute the *nucleus centrobasalis*.

Most fibres of the pathway are uncrossed. They reach the cerebellum through the inferior and superior cerebellar peduncles. This pathway is regarded, functionally, as the forelimb equivalent of the ventral spinocerebellar tract.

From the above account of spinocerebellar pathways it will be seen that these are two neuron pathways in contrast to three neuron pathways to the cerebral cortex.

(v) Impulses from the spinal cord may reach the cerebellum indirectly by traveling through the spino-olivary tract, and through olivocerebellar fibres. Similarly, impulses may reach the cerebellum after traveling through spinoreticular and reticulocerebellar fibres.

(vi) A *cervicocerebellar pathway* carrying proprioceptive impulses from neck muscles has been described in some animals. The neurons of origin lie in the same region as those of the rostral cerebellar pathway, but in the upper four cervical segments. The fibres pass through the superior cerebellar peduncle to reach the cerebellum.

Spinocerebellar fibres reaching the cerebellum end as mossy fibres. Representation in the cerebellar cortex is somatotropic (i.e., fibres carrying sensations from different parts of the body end in definite areas of cortex). Conduction in the spinocerebellar tracts can be inhibited or facilitated under the influence of descending tracts (corticospinal, reticulospinal, rubrospinal).

Disorders of Equilibrium

We have seen that the maintenance of equilibrium, and of correct posture, is dependent on reflex arcs involving various centres including the spinal cord, the cerebellum, and the vestibular nuclei. Afferent impulses for these reflexes are carried by the posterior column tracts (fasciculus gracilis and fasciculus cuneatus), the spinocerebellar tracts, and others. Efferents reach neurons of the ventral grey column (anterior horn cells) through rubrospinal, vestibulospinal, and other 'extrapyramidal' tracts. Interruption of any of these pathways; or lesions in the cerebellum, the vestibular nuclei and other centres concerned; can result in various abnormalities involving maintenance of posture and coordination of movements.

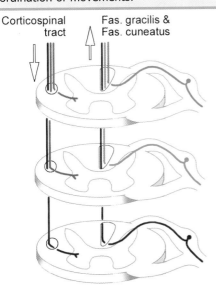

Fig. 9.9. Scheme to show the pattern of lamination of the corticospinal and posterior column tracts.

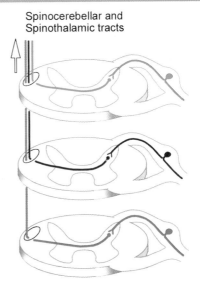

Fig. 9.10. Scheme to show the pattern of lamination of the spinocerebellar and spinothalamic tracts.

Inability to maintain the equilibrium of the body, while standing, or while walking, is referred to as *ataxia.* This may occur as a result of the interruption of afferent proprioceptive pathways (*sensory ataxia*). Disease of the cerebellum itself, or of efferent pathways, results in more severe disability. Lack of proprioceptive information can be compensated to a considerable extent by information received through the eyes. The defects are, therefore, much more pronounced with the eyes closed (*Romberg's sign*). (See Chapter 12).

Propriospinal tracts

In addition to the various ascending and descending tracts described in preceding sections, the white matter of the spinal cord contains numerous fibres that interconnect neurons in different segments of the cord. These fibres, that are both ascending and descending, constitute the propriospinal or intersegmental tracts. These tracts are present in the anterior, lateral and posterior funiculi and occupy areas adjacent to spinal grey matter. In addition to intersegmental fibres this region is also believed to contain some reticulospinal and descending autonomic fibres.

Nerve fibres in propriospinal tracts are classified as long, intermediate or short. Neurons from which they arise lie in laminae V to VIII. They are interneurons, but can carry impulses arising in one segment to distant regions. Some propriospinal tracts that have been given special names are as follows.

1. The *dorsolateral fasciculus* (*or tract of Lissauer*) contains many propriospinal fibres. It also contains ascending and descending branches of axons entering the spinal cord through dorsal nerve roots. Many fibres are axons of cells in the substantia gelatinosa.

2. Several relatively discrete bundles of fibres have been described in the dorsal funiculi. These are the *comma tract* (also called the *semilunar tract* or *interfascicular fasciculus*); the *septomarginal tract* and the *cornu commissural tract* (Fig. 9.2).

Lamination of fibres in tracts

An interesting aspect of the larger tracts of the spinal cord is that the fibres entering or leaving the tracts at various levels of the cord appear to be arranged in layers. This is spoken of as *lamination.* Lamination in individual tracts is easily remembered once the reason for it is understood. From Fig. 9.9 (left half) it will be clear that in the case of any descending tract located lateral to the grey matter in which the fibres of the tract terminate, the fibres for the lowest segments of the cord must be placed most laterally if intercrossing of fibres is to be avoided. This explains the arrangement seen in the lateral corticospinal tract. In the case of an ascending tract the arrangement of fibres depends on whether the incoming fibres approach the tract from the medial or lateral side. In the case of the posterior column tracts the fibres (derived from the dorsal nerve roots) enter from the lateral side. Hence as shown in Fig. 9.9 (right half) the lowest fibres are situated most medially. On the contrary in the case of spinothalamic and spinocerebellar tracts, the fibres arise in the spinal grey matter and enter the tracts from the medial side. Hence, as shown in Fig. 9.10 the lowest fibres are most lateral.

Control of conduction through ascending tracts

There are observations to show that conduction through ascending tracts can be controlled (inhibited or facilitated) under the influence of axons descending from higher centres to the neurons which give origin to the tracts.

Stimulation of certain regions in the brainstem reticular formation inhibits transmission of pain through spinothalamic tracts. The centres of the reticular formation concerned are said to constitute and *endogenous analgesic system*.

Transmission of painful impulses can also be inhibited by stimulation of areas of cerebral hemisphere involved in transmission or perception of the same (i.e., thalamus, parts of cerebral cortex). Conversely, stimulation of some other areas can increase transmission of painful stimuli.

Corticospinal fibres also inhibit neurons giving rise to spinocerebellar tracts. On the other hand vestibulospinal and rubrospinal fibres stimulate the neurons.

Control of conduction of different impulses is believed to be produced mainly by presynaptic inhibition in spinal grey matter. A gate mechanism that determines whether noxious stimuli should be allowed to pass has been postulated and it has been suggested that the substantia gelatinosa may play an important role in this regard. Although the existence of some kind of gate mechanism is accepted, its exact nature, and the role of the substantia gelatinosa are not established.

Involvement of Spinal Cord in Disease

CLINICAL

Trauma

1. The spinal cord can be injured by fractures of the spine. These are most common in the thoracic region. Complete damage at this level leads to paraplegia. Sensations are also lost below the level of lesion.

2. Brown Sequard syndrome. This is produced by a lesion cutting through one half (right or left) of the spinal cord. The effects are as follows.

Effects on the side of lesion

(a) Cutting of pyramidal tracts produces spastic paralysis below the level of lesion.

(b) Cutting of posterior column tracts (fasciculus gracilis and cuneatus) causes loss of propioceptive sensations and of fine touch.

Effects on side opposite to that of lesion

Cutting of spinothalamic tracts causes loss of pain and temperature sensation. Touch is spared as the pathways for it are bilateral.

Tumours

A tumour in the vertebral canal can press upon the spinal cord at any level. The effects will depend upon the tracts and nerve roots pressed upon.

Prolapsed intervertebral disc

The spinal cord may be pressed upon by a central prolapse of the nucleus pulposus of an intervertebral disc (Note that a lateral prolapse causes pressure on nerve roots).

Tabes Dorsalis

In this condition, caused by syphilis, the posterior column tracts are affected. There is numbness, paraesthesias and severe pains in some parts of the body, while there is hypersensitivity in others. Maintenence of posture is affected. Romberg's sign is positive.

Arterial thrombosis

Thrombosis in the anterior spinal artery, or in one of the arteries supplying the medulla can interrupt tracts with serious consequences. See anterior spinal artery syndrome, and medial and lateral medullary syndromes in Chapter 21.

10 : Cranial Nerve Nuclei

The seven functional components to which the fibres of a cranial nerve may belong are as follows. **(1)** Somatic efferent. **(2)** General visceral efferent. **(3)** Special visceral efferent. **(4)** General somatic afferent. **(5)** Special somatic afferent. **(6)** General visceral afferent. **(7)** Special visceral afferent.

Each functional component has its own nuclei of origin (in the case of efferent fibres) or of termination (in the case of afferent fibres). In the embryo the nuclei related to the various components are arranged in vertical rows (or columns) in a definite sequence in the grey matter related to the floor of the fourth ventricle (Fig. 10.1). The sequence is easily remembered if the following facts are kept in mind.

(**a**) Each half of the floor of the ventricle is divided into a medial part and a lateral part by the ***sulcus limitans. Efferent nuclei*** lie in the medial part (called the ***basal lamina***) and ***afferent nuclei*** in the lateral part (called the ***alar lamina***).

(**b**) In each part (medial or lateral) ***visceral nuclei*** lie nearer the sulcus limitans than ***somatic nuclei.***

(**c**) Within each category (e.g., visceral efferents, somatic afferents etc.) the ***general nucleus*** lies nearer the sulcus limitans than the ***special nucleus.***

Thus in proceeding laterally from the midline the sequence of nuclear columns is as follows.

1. Somatic efferent (SE). This column is not subdivided into general and special parts.
2. Special visceral (or branchial) efferent (SVE).   **3.**   General visceral efferent (GVE).
4. General visceral afferent (GVA).   **5**. Special visceral afferent (SVA).
6. General somatic afferent (GSA). **7**. Special somatic afferent (SSA).

As development proceeds parts of these columns disappear so that each of them no longer extends the whole length of the brainstem, but is represented by one or more discrete nuclei. These nuclei are shown schematically in the lower half of Fig. 10.1. Some nuclei retain their original positions in relation to the floor of the fourth ventricle, but some others migrate deeper into the brainstem. The position of the nuclei relative to the posterior surface of the brainstem is illustrated in Fig. 10.2. The positions of the nuclei as seen in transverse sections of the brainstem are shown in Fig. 10.3.

In the description that follows the nuclei of the third to twelfth cranial nerves are considered as they are located in the brainstem. The third and fourth nerves belong to the midbrain; the fifth, sixth, seventh (and part of eighth) to the pons; and the remaining to the medulla.

Somatic Efferent Nuclei

The somatic efferent column consists of the following nuclei that supply striated (skeletal) muscle of somatic origin.

1. The ***oculomotor nucleus*** is situated in the upper part of the midbrain at the level of the superior colliculus (Figs. 10.1, 10.2 and 10.3F). The nuclei of the two sides form a single complex that lies in the central grey matter, ventral to the aqueduct.

2. The ***trochlear nucleus*** is situated in the lower part of the midbrain at the level of the inferior colliculus (Figs. 10.1, 10.2 and 10.3E). The nucleus lies ventral to the aqueduct in the central grey matter.

3. The ***abducent nucleus*** is situated in the lower part of the pons. It lies in the grey matter lining the floor of the fourth ventricle near the midline (Figs. 10.1, 10.2 and 10.3C)

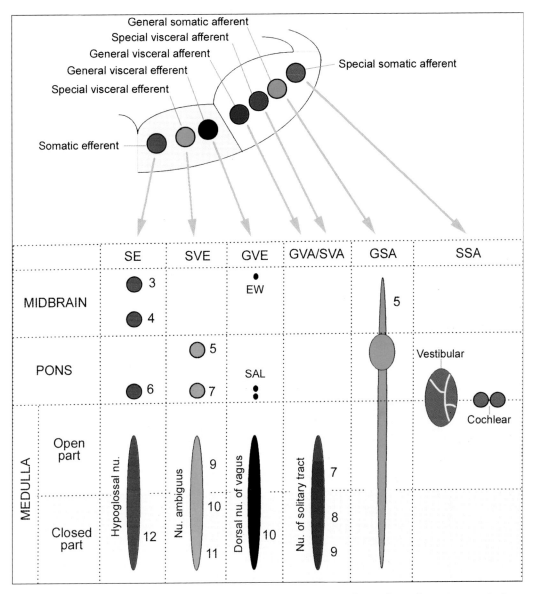

Fig. 10.1. Functional classification of cranial nerve nuclei. The upper figure shows the arrangement of nuclear columns in the brainstem of the embryo. The lower figure shows the nuclei derived from each column. Numbers indicate the cranial nerves connected to the nuclei.

4. The ***hypoglossal nucleus*** lies in the medulla. It is an elongated column extending into both the open and closed parts of the medulla. Its upper part lies deep to the hypoglossal triangle in the floor of the fourth ventricle. When traced downwards it lies next to the midline in the central grey matter ventral to the central canal (Figs. 10.1, 10.2 and 10.3 A,B).

Special Visceral Efferent Nuclei

These nuclei are also called branchial efferent or branchiomotor nuclei. They supply striated (skeletal) muscle derived from branchial arches.

BASIC

1. The *motor nucleus of the trigeminal nerve* lies in the upper part of the pons, in its dorsal part (Figs. 10.1, 10.2, and 10.3D). It is situated in the lateral part of the reticular formation, medial to the main sensory nucleus of the trigeminal nerve (see below).

2. The *nucleus of the facial nerve* lies in the lower part of the pons and occupies a position similar to that of the motor nucleus of the trigeminal nerve. The spinal nucleus and tract of the trigeminal nerve lie lateral to it. (Figs. 10.1, 10.2 and 10.3C).

3. The *nucleus ambiguus* lies in the

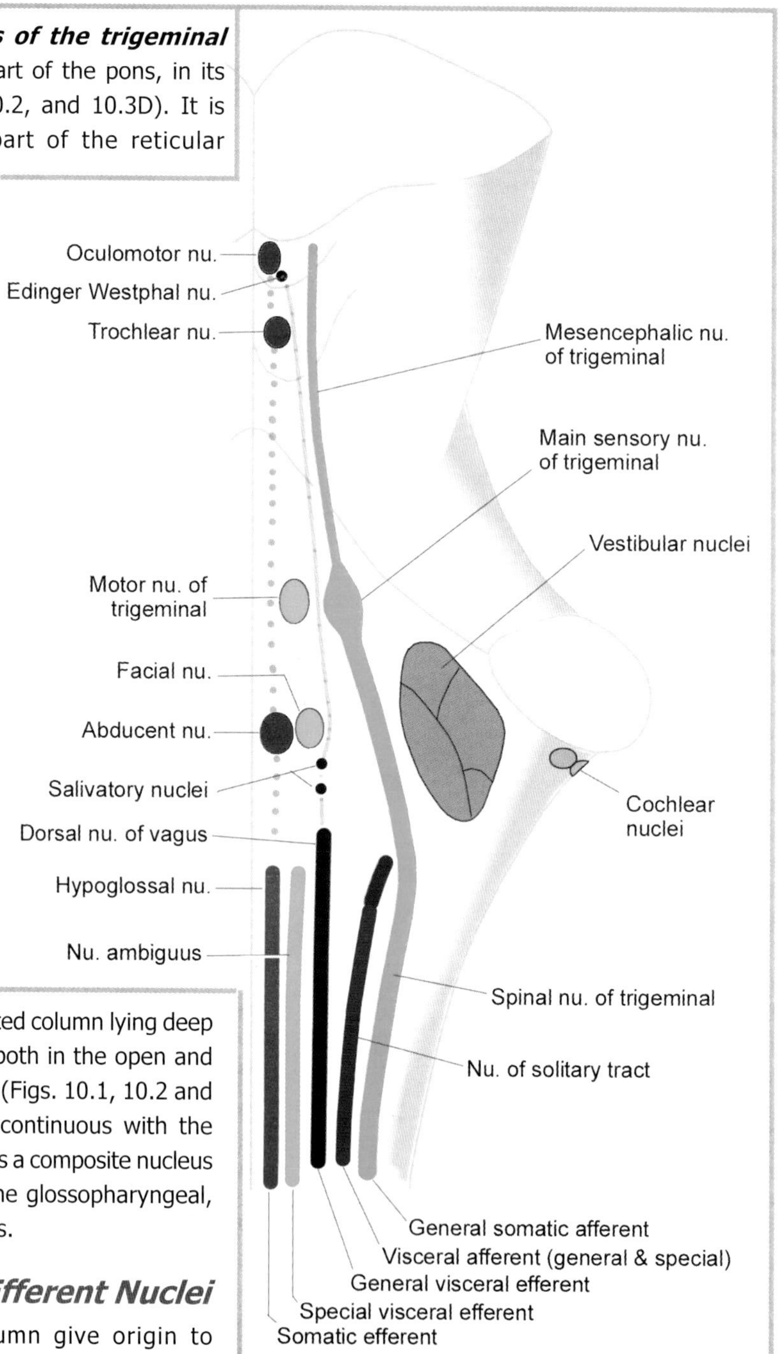

Fig. 10.2. Cranial nerve nuclei as projected onto the dorsal aspect of the brainstem.

Oculomotor nu.
Edinger Westphal nu.
Trochlear nu.
Mesencephalic nu. of trigeminal
Main sensory nu. of trigeminal
Vestibular nuclei
Motor nu. of trigeminal
Facial nu.
Abducent nu.
Cochlear nuclei
Salivatory nuclei
Dorsal nu. of vagus
Hypoglossal nu.
Nu. ambiguus
Spinal nu. of trigeminal
Nu. of solitary tract
General somatic afferent
Visceral afferent (general & special)
General visceral efferent
Special visceral efferent
Somatic efferent

medulla. It forms an elongated column lying deep in the reticular formation, both in the open and closed parts of the medulla (Figs. 10.1, 10.2 and 10.3A, B). Inferiorly, it is continuous with the spinal accessory nucleus. It is a composite nucleus and contributes fibres to the glossopharyngeal, vagus and accessory nerves.

General Visceral Efferent Nuclei

The nuclei of this column give origin to preganglionic fibres that constitute the cranial parasympathetic outflow. These fibres end in peripheral ganglia. Postganglionic fibres arising in these ganglia supply smooth muscle or glands. The nuclei are as follows.

1. The *Edinger-Westphal nucleus* (or *accessory oculomotor nucleus*) lies in the midbrain (Figs. 10.1, 10.2 and 10.3F). It is closely related to the oculomotor complex. Fibres arising in this nucleus pass through the oculomotor nerve. They relay in the ciliary ganglion to supply the sphincter pupillae and the ciliaris muscle.

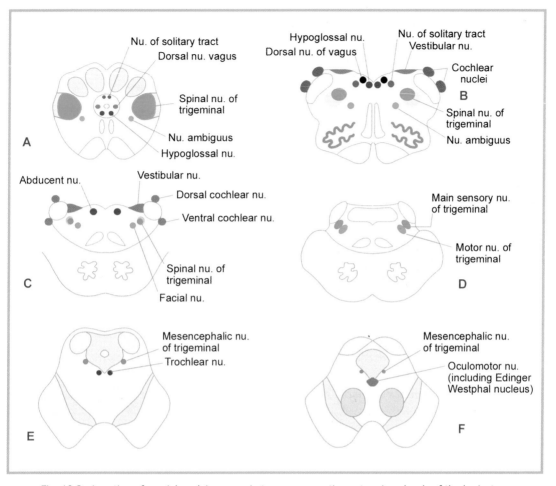

Fig. 10.3. Location of cranial nuclei as seen in transverse sections at various levels of the brainstem.

2. The *salivary* (or *salivatory*) *nuclei* (superior and inferior) lie in the dorsal part of the pons, just above its junction with the medulla (Figs. 10.1, 10.2). They are located just above the upper end of the dorsal nucleus of the vagus nerve (see below). The superior nucleus sends fibres into the facial nerve. These relay in the submandibular ganglion to supply the submandibular and sublingual salivary glands. The inferior nucleus sends fibres into the glossopharyngeal nerve. These fibres relay in the otic ganglion to supply the parotid gland. (The parotid gland may also receive some fibres from the superior salivatory nucleus, through the submandibular ganglion).

Other neurons probably located near the salivary nuclei send out fibres that supply the lacrimal gland, after relaying in the pterygopalatine ganglion. These fibres travel through the facial nerve.

3. The *dorsal (motor) nucleus of the vagus* (or *dorsal vagal nucleus*) lies in the medulla. It is a long nucleus lying vertically. Its upper end lies deep to the vagal triangle in the floor of the fourth ventricle. When traced downwards it extends into the closed part of the medulla where it lies in the lateral part of the central grey matter (Figs. 10.1, 10.2 and 10.3 A,B). Fibres arising in this nucleus supply the heart, lungs, bronchi, oesophagus, stomach, small intestine and large intestine up to the right two-thirds of the transverse colon. They end in ganglia (or nerve plexuses) closely related to these organs. Postganglionic fibres arise in these ganglia, and run a short course to supply smooth muscle and glands in these organs.

BASIC

Subdivisions of the nucleus (supplying different regions) have been described.

Some general visceral efferent fibres arise from the ***retrofacial nucleus*** which is a small collection of neurons located near the upper end of the nucleus ambiguus.

General and Special Visceral Afferent Nuclei

Both these columns are represented by the ***nucleus of the solitary tract***, present in the medulla (Figs. 10.1, 10.2). Like other cranial nerve nuclei of the medulla, the cells of this nucleus form an elongated column lying deep in the reticular formation. Its upper part lies ventrolateral to the dorsal nucleus of the vagus (Fig. 10.3B). When traced downwards it extends into the closed part of the medulla: here it lies dorsomedial to the vagal nucleus (Fig. 10.3A). The lower ends of the nuclei of the two sides fuse to form the ***commissural nucleus*** of the vagus. The nucleus solitarius receives fibres carrying general visceral sensations through the vagus and glossopharyngeal nerves. Through these afferents, and through connections with the reticular formation, the nucleus plays an important role in reflex control of respiratory and cardiovascular functions.

Fibres of taste (SVA) carried by the facial, glossopharyngeal and vagus nerves end in the upper part of the nucleus of the solitary tract which is sometimes called the ***gustatory nucleus.***

According to some authorities some general visceral afferent fibres end in the dorsal vagal nucleus.

General Somatic Afferent Nuclei

The general somatic afferent column is represented by the sensory nuclei of the trigeminal nerve. These are as follows.

1. The ***main*** (or ***superior***) ***sensory nucleus*** lies in the upper part of the pons, in the lateral part of the reticular formation. It lies lateral to the motor nucleus of the trigeminal (Figs 10.1, 10.2 and 10.3D). It is mainly concerned in mediation of proprioceptive impulses, touch and pressure (from the region to which the trigeminal nerve is distributed).

2. The ***spinal nucleus*** extends from the main nucleus down into the medulla (Figs 10.1, 10.2 and 10.3 A,B,C) and into the upper two segments of the spinal cord. Its lower end is continuous with the substantia gelatinosa of the cord. In addition to fibres of the trigeminal nerve, the nucleus also receives general somatic sensations carried by the facial, glossopharyngeal and vagus nerves.

The spinal nucleus is concerned mainly with the mediation of pain and thermal sensibility. Different parts of the nucleus correspond to different areas innervated. The spinal nucleus is divisible (cranio-caudally) into three sub-nuclei, ***oralis, interpolaris, and caudalis***.

3. The ***mesencephalic nucleus*** of the trigeminal nerve extends cranially from the upper end of the main sensory nucleus into the midbrain. Here it lies in the central grey matter lateral to the aqueduct (Fig. 10.3 E,F). Functionally, this nucleus appears to be similar to sensory ganglia of cranial nerves, and to the spinal ganglia, rather than to afferent nuclei. The neurons in it are unipolar. The peripheral processes of these neurons are believed to carry proprioceptive impulses from muscles of mastication, and possibly also from muscles of the eyeballs, face tongue and teeth. The central processes of the neurons in the nucleus probably end in the main sensory nucleus of the trigeminal nerve.

The mesencephalic nucleus is the centre for the jaw jerk.

Special Somatic Afferent Nuclei

These are the ***cochlear*** and ***vestibular nuclei***.

The cochlear nuclei are two in number, dorsal and ventral. They are placed dorsal and ventral, respectively, to the inferior cerebellar peduncle (Fig. 10.3 B,C) at the level of the junction of the pons and medulla. The two nuclei are continuous, being separated only by a layer of nerve fibres. Their connections are shown in Fig. 10.7.

The vestibular nuclei lie in the grey matter underlying the lateral part of the floor of the fourth ventricle (Fig.10.3 B,C). They lie partly in the medulla and partly in the pons. Four distinct nuclei are recognized: these are medial, lateral, inferior, and superior. The lateral nucleus is also called *Dieter's nucleus*. The connections of the vestibular nuclei are shown in Fig.10.8.

Other Connections of Cranial Nerve Nuclei

1. The somatic efferent and special visceral efferent nuclei of cranial nerves supply striated (skeletal) muscle. Their connections are, therefore, similar to those of ventral horn cells of the spinal cord (Fig. 10.4).

(a) These nuclei are under cortical control through corticonuclear fibres. Cortical control of the hypoglossal nucleus is contralateral (i.e., from the opposite cerebral hemisphere). Corticonuclear fibres to the part of the facial nucleus innervating the lower part of the face is contralateral; but fibres for the rest of the nucleus are bilateral. The trochear nucleus receives ipsilateral fibres (i.e., from the same side). All other nuclei are influenced by both cerebral hemispheres, but the fibres to the abducent nerve are predominantly crossed. Corticonuclear fibres probably terminate by synapsing with interneurons

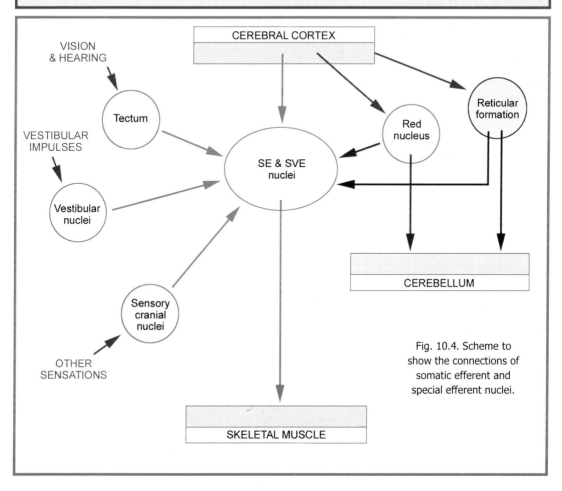

Fig. 10.4. Scheme to show the connections of somatic efferent and special efferent nuclei.

present in, or near, the nuclei. Some corticonuclear fibres follow an aberrant path in the brainstem and travel through the medial lemniscus.

(**b**) The nuclei are also influenced by other centres, namely the tectum, the red nucleus, and the reticular formation. The cerebellum, the diencephalon and the corpus striatum can influence the nuclei through these centres.

(**c**) The motor nuclei also receive afferents from sensory nuclei of the brainstem including the nucleus solitarius and the spinal nucleus of the trigeminal nerve. The motor nucleus of the trigeminal nerve receives some fibres from the mesencephalic nucleus. These fibres form part of the pathway for the jaw jerk.

(**d**) Motor nuclei may be connected to each other. The nuclei of the third, fourth and sixth cranial nerves are connected to each other, and to some other nuclei, through the medial longitudinal bundle. Fibres from the oculomotor, trochlear and abducent nuclei represent the final output of an elaborate system that controls eye movements.

2. The general visceral efferent nuclei innervate smooth muscle and glands. Their central connections are less well known.

(**a**) They receive afferents from sensory cranial nerve nuclei; in particular from the nucleus of the solitary tract.

(**b**) Visceral sensations may also reach these nuclei through collaterals from ascending tracts. The exact pathways are not known.

(**c**) The nuclei are connected with the reticular formation. Higher control is probably exercised by the hypothalamus. The cerebral cortex (specially the limbic lobe) and the thalamus may influence the nuclei through the hypothalamus.

3. The nucleus of the solitary tract (GVA, SVA) receives afferents from the viscera supplied by nerves connected to it. The nucleus also receives fibres from the cerebral cortex and from the cerebellum. These afferents may modify the transmission of sensory impulses.

Fibres arising in this nucleus carry visceral impulses to the hypothalamus and the thalamus through the ***solitario-hypothalamic*** and ***solitario-thalamic*** tracts respectively. The nucleus of the solitary tract also sends fibres to the reticular formation, the general visceral efferent nuclei and to the spinal cord.

4. The main afferents of the nuclei of the general somatic afferent column (made up of the main and spinal nuclei of the trigeminal nerve) are central processes of neurons in the trigeminal ganglion. After entering the pons, many of these processes

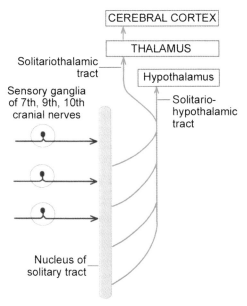

Fig. 10.5. Connections of the nucleus of the solitary tract.

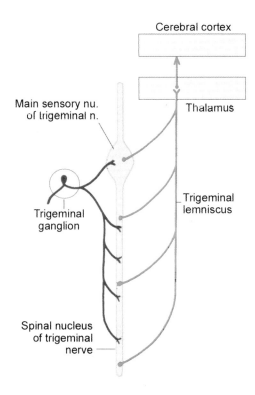

Fig. 10.6. Connections of the sensory nuclei of the trigeminal nerve.

divide into ascending and descending branches; while others ascend or descend. The ascending fibres end in the main sensory nucleus. Those that descend form a large bundle of fibres that constitutes the *spinal tract of the trigeminal nerve* (Fig. 10.6). The tract is closely related to the dorsolateral aspect of the spinal nucleus of the trigeminal nerve. The tract descends from the pons into the medulla, and then into the upper part of the spinal cord. (Apart from trigeminal fibres the tract also carries general somatic afferent fibres from the facial, glossopharyngeal and vagus nerves).

The fibres ending in the main sensory nucleus are concerned, predominantly, with touch; and those ending in the spinal nucleus are concerned, predominantly, with sensations of pain and temperature. However, the functional distinction between the two nuclei is by no means clear cut. These nuclei also receive descending fibres from the cerebral cortex: these fibres may influence the conduction of sensory impulses.

The lowest part of the spinal nucleus of the trigeminal nerve (nucleus caudalis) is of particular importance in pain reception. It receives nerve fibres from the nucleus raphe magnus that modulate pain transmission. (These nerve fibres contain enkephalin, noradrenaline and serotonin).

The neurons in the main sensory and spinal nuclei of the trigeminal nerve are second order neurons. Their axons are comparable to the fibres of the spinothalamic tracts. The axons cross to the opposite side and form a bundle called the *trigeminal lemniscus* (Fig. 10.6). This lemniscus ascends to the thalamus (ventral posteromedial nucleus). Some fibres in the lemniscus may be uncrossed. Third order neurons located in the thalamus carry the sensations to the sensory areas of the cerebral cortex. In the pons and midbrain the trigeminal lemniscus lies immediately lateral to the medial lemniscus (Figs. 11.5, 11.7 to 11.9). Its fibres are closely related to those of the spinal lemniscus (lateral spinothalamic tract).

A separate bundle of more dorsally situated trigeminothalamic fibres is also described.

In addition to the efferents to the thalamus, the trigeminal nuclei probably send fibres to other cranial nerve nuclei, reticular formation, cerebellum, and hypothalamus.

5. The special somatic afferent nuclei (cochlear and vestibular) have important connections (Figs. 10.7, 10.8). The cochlear nuclei form part of the pathway for hearing which is described below. The vestibular nuclei have numerous connections which are also considered below.

Pathway of Hearing & Connections of Cochlear Nuclei

The cochlear nuclei are cell stations in the pathway of hearing. The first neurons of this pathway are located in the spiral ganglion, present in intimate relationship to the cochlea. These neurons are bipolar. Their peripheral processes reach the hair cells in the spiral organ of Corti (which is the end organ for hearing). The central processes of the neurons form the cochlear nerve, and terminate in the dorsal and ventral cochlear nuclei. The neurons in these nuclei are, therefore, second order neurons. Their axons pass medially in the dorsal part of the pons. Most of them cross to the opposite side, but some remain uncrossed.

The crossing fibres of the two sides form a conspicuous mass of fibres called the *trapezoid body.* Some crossing fibres run separately in the dorsal part of the pons and do not form part of the trapezoid body. (These fibres constitute the so called *intermediate acoustic striae* and *dorsal acoustic striae*).

The large majority of fibres from the cochlear nuclei terminate in the superior olivary complex (made up of a number of nuclei). Third order neurons arising in this complex form an important ascending bundle called the *lateral lemniscus.* Some cochlear fibres that do not relay in the superior olivary nucleus join the lemniscus after relaying in scattered groups of cells lying within the trapezoid body:

BASIC

these cells constitute the ***trapezoid nucleus (nucleus of the trapezoid body).*** Still other cochlear fibres relay in cells that lie within the lemniscus itself: these neurons form the ***nucleus of the lateral lemniscus.*** The fibres of the lateral lemniscus ascend to the midbrain and terminate in the inferior colliculus. Fibres arising in the colliculus enter the inferior brachium to reach the medial geniculate body. Some fibres in the lemniscus reach this body without relay in the inferior colliculus. Fibres arising in the medial geniculate body form the ***acoustic radiation*** which ends in the acoustic area of the cerebral cortex. It may be stressed that each lateral lemniscus carries impulses arising in both the right and left cochleae.

ADVANCED

Some further facts about the auditory pathway are as follows.

(**a**) The spiral ganglion contains two types of cells, type I and type II. Type I cells form about 95% of the population. They innervate inner hair cells. The outer hair cells are innervated by type II cells.

(**b**) The cochlear nuclei contain many types of neurons. The number of neurons in these nuclei greatly exceeds that of cochlear nerve fibres (which are about 25,000). This is explained by the fact that one nerve fibre may synapse with several neurons; and by the view that many neurons of the nuclei are interneurons. This may also be correlated with the observation that the number of fibres in the lateral lemniscus is much greater than that in the cochlear nerve.

Neurons receiving fibres from different parts of the spiral organ are arranged in a definite sequence (in the ventral nucleus).

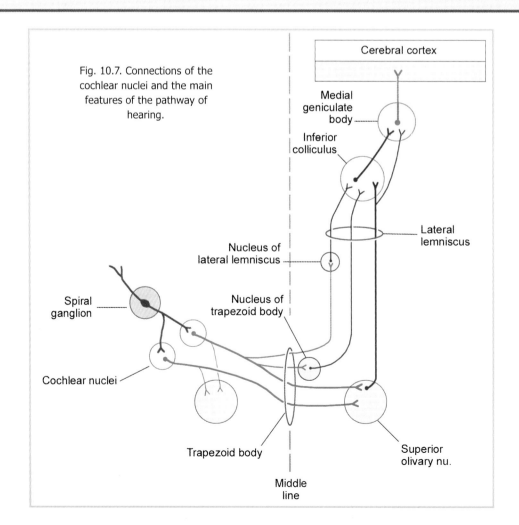

Fig. 10.7. Connections of the cochlear nuclei and the main features of the pathway of hearing.

Cerebral cortex

Medial geniculate body

Inferior colliculus

Lateral lemniscus

Nucleus of lateral lemniscus

Spiral ganglion

Nucleus of trapezoid body

Cochlear nuclei

Trapezoid body

Superior olivary nu.

Middle line

(**c**) The cochlear nerves may also carry efferent fibres. These fibres take origin in the pons in the vicinity of the superior olivary complex and travel to the spiral ganglion where they end in relation to both type I and type II cells. Such fibres could have an inhibitory or excitatory influence on transmission of auditory impulses.

(**d**) Fibres arising in the dorsal cochlear nucleus pass mainly through the dorsal and intermediate acoustic striae. They project directly to the inferior colliculus of the opposite side. Fibres from the ventral cochlear nucleus pass through the trapezoid body to reach the superior olivary complex.

(**e**) The superior olivary complex is made up of several nuclei. The main nuclei are the lateral superior olivary nucleus and the medial (or accessory) superior olivary nucleus. A retro-olivary group of nuclei is also described. The medial nucleus receives fibres from both cochleae and may play a role in localising the direction of sound (by calculating the time difference in arrival of inputs from the right and left cochleae). The retro-olivary group is believed to be the source of efferent fibres to the spiral ganglion. This group receives descending fibres from the inferior colliculus.

(**f**) Some fibres beginning in the trapezoid nuclei may reach some cranial nerve nuclei through the medial longitudinal fasciculus (see below); and may be involved in reflex control of the stapedius, the tensor tympani, and the muscles that move the eyeballs.

(**g**) Some fibres from the nucleus of the lateral lemniscus reach the superior colliculus. They help to coordinate visual and auditory stimuli.

Connections of Vestibular Nuclei

The vestibular nuclei receive the following afferents (Fig. 10.8).

(**1**) The main afferents are central processes of bipolar neurons of the vestibular ganglion. These fibres constitute the vestibular part of the vestibulo-cochlear nerve. They convey impulses from end organs in the semicircular ducts, the utricle and the saccule: these are necessary for maintenance of equilibrium.

After entering the medulla the fibres of the vestibular nerve divide into ascending and descending branches. The descending branches end in the medial, lateral and inferior vestibular nuclei. The ascending branches reach the superior vestibular nucleus.

(**2**) The vestibular nuclei also receive fibres from some parts of the cerebellum.

The efferents from the vestibular nuclei are as follows.

(**a**) Vestibulo-cerebellar fibres pass through the inferior cerebellar peduncle. The vestibulocerebellar fibres form a separate bundle, the ***juxtarestiform body***, within the peduncle. Some fibres of the vestibular nerves by-pass the vestibular nuclei and go straight to the cerebellum.

(**b**) Fibres arising in the vestibular nuclei establish connections with cranial nerve nuclei responsible for movements of the eyes (third, fourth, sixth) and of the neck (eleventh). These fibres form the ***medial longitudinal fasciculus (or bundle).*** (See below).

(**c**) Fibres from the lateral vestibular nucleus descend to the spinal cord as the vestibulospinal tract. Fibres from the medial (and other) nuclei descend to the spinal cord through the medial longitudinal fasciculus. These fibres are sometimes named the ***medial vestibulospinal tract.*** Some fibres reach the pontine reticular formation.

(**d**) Some fibres from the vestibular nuclei enter the lateral lemniscus.

(**e**) Some vestibular impulses reach the thalamus (ventro-posterior nucleus) and are relayed to the cerebral cortex. A vestibular centre is present in the parietal lobe just behind the postcentral gyrus.

Medial Longitudinal Fasciculus

The medial longitudinal fasciculus consists of fibres that lie near the midline of the brainstem. Above, it reaches up to the level of the third ventricle. (The ascending fibres end in the interstitial nucleus of Cajal, the nucleus of the posterior commissure, and the nucleus of Darkschewitsch).

Below, the medial longitudinal bundle becomes continuous with the anterior intersegmental tract of the spinal cord (Fig. 9.2). The fasciculus is closely related to the nuclei of the third, fourth, sixth and twelfth cranial nerves (all of the somatic efferent column and lying next to the midline). It is also related to the fibres of the seventh nerve (as they wind round the abducent nucleus), and to some fibres arising from the cochlear nuclei. In the spinal cord it establishes connections with ventral horn cells that innervate the muscles of the neck (Figs. 11.1 to 11.3, and 11.7 to 11.9).

The fibres that constitute the fasciculus are as follows.

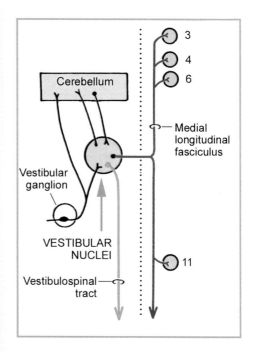

Fig. 10.8. Connections of the vestibular nuclei.

(**a**) Fibres arising in the vestibular nuclei of the same side as well as those of the opposite side. These fibres ascend or descend in the fasciculus to reach nuclei supplying the muscles of the eyeball and neck. These connections ensure harmonious movements of the eyes and head in response to vestibular stimulation.

(**b**) Some fibres of the fasciculus are connected to some nuclei of the auditory pathway. These are the nucleus of the trapezoid body and the nucleus of the lateral lemniscus. Some fibres arising in the dorsal cochlear nucleus are closely related to the fasciculus. Through these connections movements of the head and of the eyes can take place in response to auditory stimuli.

(**c**) The medial longitudinal fasciculus affords a pathway for fibres interconnecting the nuclei related to it. Connections between the facial and hypoglossal nuclei may facilitate simultaneous movements of the lips and tongue as in speech.

(**d**) Fibres from the medial (and other) vestibular nuclei descend in the fasciculus to the spinal cord. These fibres form the ***medial vestibulospinal tract.***

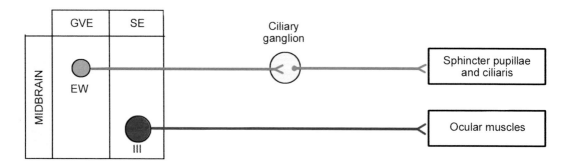

Fig. 10.9. Scheme to show the functional components of the oculomotor nerve.

BASIC

Functional Components of Individual Cranial Nerves

Having considered the cranial nerve nuclei and their connections it is now possible to work out the functional components of each cranial nerve.

I. Olfactory nerve

This is the nerve of smell. As the olfactory mucosa is derived from ectoderm (of the nasal placodes) this nerve is classified as **special somatic afferent** (along with vision and hearing). However, in view of the close relationship between the sensations of smell and taste, some authorities classify this nerve as special visceral afferent.

II. Optic nerve

This is the nerve of vision. Its fibres are regarded as **special somatic afferent**. From the point of view of its structure and development this nerve is to be regarded as a tract of the brain rather than as a peripheral nerve.

III. Oculomotor nerve

This nerve has the following components (Fig. 10.9).

(a) **Somatic efferent** fibres arising in the oculomotor nucleus supply all extrinsic muscles of the eyeball except the lateral rectus and the superior oblique.

(b) **General visceral efferent** fibres (preganglionic) arise in the Edinger-Westphal nucleus and terminate in the ciliary ganglion. Postganglionic fibres arising in this ganglion supply the sphincter pupillae and the ciliaris muscle.

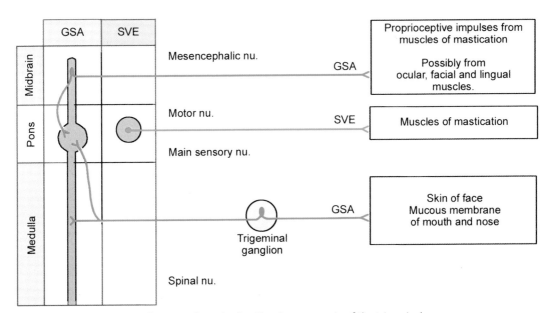

Fig. 10.10. Scheme to show the functional components of the trigeminal nerve

IV. Trochlear nerve

This nerve is made up of ***somatic efferent*** fibres arising in the trochlear nucleus and supplying the superior oblique muscle of the eyeball.

V. Trigeminal nerve

This nerve contains the following components (Fig. 10.10).

(a) ***Special visceral efferent*** fibres arise from the motor nucleus of the nerve and supply the muscles of mastication.

(**b**) ***General somatic afferent*** fibres of the nerve are peripheral processes of unipolar neurons in the trigeminal ganglion. They carry exteroceptive sensations from the skin of the face, and the mucous membrane of the mouth and nose. The central processes of the neurons in the ganglion constitute the sensory root of the nerve. They terminate in the main sensory nucleus and in the spinal nucleus of the nerve.

Another group of general somatic afferent neurons carry proprioceptive impulses from the muscles of mastication (and possibly from ocular, facial and lingual muscles). These fibres are believed to be peripheral processes of unipolar neurons located in the mesencephalic nucleus of this nerve.

VI. Abducent nerve

This nerve consists of ***somatic efferent*** fibres that arise from the abducent nucleus and supply the lateral rectus muscle of the eyeball.

VII. Facial nerve

The components of this nerve are as follows (Fig. 10.11).

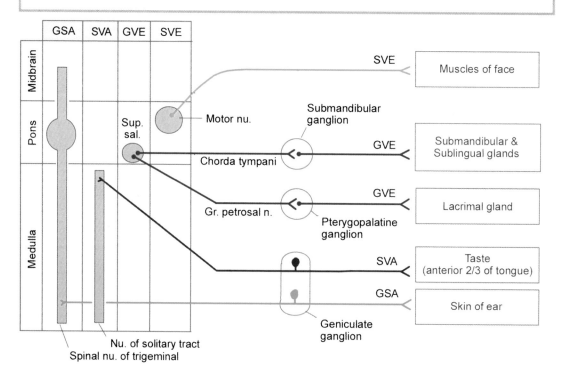

Fig. 10.11. Scheme to show the functional components of the facial nerve

(a) *Special visceral efferent* fibres begin from the motor nucleus and supply the various muscles to which the nerve is distributed.

(b) *General visceral efferent* fibres (preganglionic) arise in the superior salivary nucleus. They relay in the submandibular ganglion from which postganglionic fibres arise to supply the submandibular and sublingual salivary glands.

The facial nerve also carries general visceral efferent fibres for the lacrimal gland. The preganglionic neurons concerned are said to be located near the salivary nuclei. Their axons terminate in the pterygopalatine ganglion, from which postganglionic fibres arise to supply the gland.

(c) *Special visceral afferent* fibres are peripheral processes of cells in the geniculate ganglion of the nerve. They supply taste buds in the anterior two-thirds of the tongue (and some in the soft palate). The central processes of the ganglion cells carry these sensations to the upper part of the nucleus of the solitary tract.

(d) *General somatic afferent* fibres are also peripheral processes of some cells of the geniculate ganglion. They innervate a part of the skin of the external ear. The central processes of these cells end in the spinal nucleus of the trigeminal nerve.

VIII. Vestibulocochlear nerve.

Both the cochlear and vestibular divisions of this nerve are made up of *special somatic afferent* fibres. The fibres of the cochlear nerve are central processes of bipolar cells in the spiral ganglion. The peripheral processes of these neurons supply the organ of Corti. The fibres of the vestibular nerve are central processes of bipolar neurons in the vestibular ganglion. The peripheral processes of these neurons innervate the semicircular ducts, the utricle and the saccule of the internal ear.

In the past this nerve has also been called the auditory or stato-acoustic nerve.

IX. Glossopharyngeal nerve

The components of this nerve are as follows.

(a) *Special visceral efferent* fibres arise in the nucleus ambiguus and supply the stylopharyngeus muscle.

(b) *General visceral efferent* fibres (preganglionic) begin from the inferior salivary nucleus and travel to the otic ganglion. Postganglionic fibres arising in the ganglion supply the parotid gland.

(c) *General visceral afferent* fibres are peripheral processes of neurons in the inferior ganglion of the nerve. They carry general sensations (touch, pain, temperature) from the pharynx and the posterior part of the tongue to the ganglion. They also carry inputs from the carotid sinus and carotid body. Central processes of the neurons carry these sensations to the nucleus of the solitary tract. Some fibres from the carotid sinus and body reach the paramedian reticular formation of the medulla.

(d) *Special visceral afferent* fibres are also peripheral processes of neurons in the inferior ganglion. They carry sensations of taste from the posterior one-third of the tongue to the ganglion. The central processes carry these sensations to the nucleus of the solitary tract.

X. Vagus nerve

The components of this nerve are as follows (Fig. 10.12).

(a) *Special visceral efferent* fibres are processes of neurons in the nucleus ambiguus and supply the muscles of the pharynx and larynx.

(b) *General visceral efferent* fibres arise in the dorsal (motor) nucleus of the vagus. These are preganglionic parasympathetic fibres. They are distributed to thoracic and abdominal viscera. The postganglionic neurons concerned are situated in ganglia close to or within the walls of the viscera supplied.

(**c**) *General visceral afferent* fibres are peripheral processes of neurons located in the inferior ganglion of the nerve. They bring sensations from the pharynx, larynx, trachea, and oesophagus; and from abdominal and thoracic viscera. These are conveyed by central processes of the ganglion cells to the nucleus of the solitary tract. According to some authorities some of these fibres terminate in the dorsal nucleus of the vagus.

(**d**) *Special visceral afferent* fibres are also peripheral processes of neurons in the inferior ganglion. They carry sensations of taste from the posteriormost part of the tongue and from the epiglottis. The central processes of the neurons concerned terminate in the upper part of the nucleus of the solitary tract.

(**e**) *General somatic afferent* fibres are peripheral processes of neurons in the superior ganglion and are distributed to the skin of the external ear. The central processes of the ganglion cells terminate in relation to the spinal nucleus of the trigeminal nerve.

XI. Accessory nerve

This nerve consists, predominantly, of *special visceral efferent* fibres which arise from:

(**a**) the nucleus ambiguus to supply striated muscle of the pharynx, the soft palate, and the larynx (along with the vagus); and

(**b**) the lateral part of the anterior grey column of the upper five or six cervical segments of the spinal cord, to supply the trapezius and sternocleidomastoid muscles.

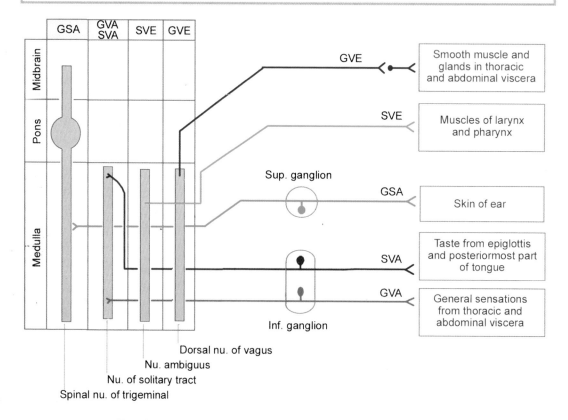

Fig. 10.12. Scheme to show the functional components of the vagus nerve.

XII. Hypoglossal nerve

This nerve is made up of the following components.

(a) *Somatic efferent* fibres are processes of neurons in the hypoglossal nucleus. They supply the muscles of the tongue.

(b) *General somatic afferent* fibres carry proprioceptive impulses from muscles of the tongue. The location of the cells of origin of these fibres is uncertain. In the embryo a small ganglion is present in relation to the nerve, but cannot be identified in the adult. Some unipolar cells can, however, be identified on the roots of the hypoglossal nerve.

Groups of neurons innervating individual muscles of the tongue can be recognised in the hypoglossal nucleus.

The functional components of cranial nerves enumerated above are those on which there is wide agreement. The presence of some additional components is described by some workers. The oculomotor, trochlear and abducent nerves may carry proprioceptive impulses (GSA) from ocular muscles; and the facial nerve from the muscles of the face, but as stated above most authorities believe that these impulses are carried by the trigeminal nerve. Some workers describe a GVE component in the accessory nerve (for supply of thoracic and abdominal viscera) and a GSA component (for skin of the ear, and for proprioceptive impulses from the stylopharyngeus) in the glossopharyngeal nerve.

Damage to Cranial Nerves and Testing

For detailed description of cranial nerves see the author's TEXTBOOK OF ANATOMY. Here we will consider how these nerves are tested during clinical examination, and some important features arising from damage to these nerves.

Olfactory nerve

The olfactory nerve is tested by asking the patient to recognize various odours. The right and left nerves can be tested separately by closing one nostril and putting the substance near the open nostril.

Optic nerve and visual pathway

Testing the optic nerve:

To test the optic nerve first ask the patient if his vision is normal. Acuity (sharpness) of vision can be tested by making the patient read letters of various sizes printed on a chart from a fixed distance. It must of course be remembered that loss of acuity of vision can be caused by errors of refraction, or by the presence of opacities in the cornea or the lens (cataract).

As part of a normal clinical examination the field of vision can be tested as follows. Ask the patient to sit opposite you (about half a meter away) and look straight forwards at you. As one eye to be tested at a time ask the patient to place a hand on one eye so that he can see only with the other eye. Stretch out one of your arms laterally so that your hand is about equal distance from your face and that of the patient. In this position you will probably not be able to see your hand. However, you may notice it if you move a finger. Keep moving your index finger and gradually bring the hand towards yourself until you can just see the movements of the finger. This gives you an idea of the extent of your own visual field in that direction. By asking the patient to tell you as soon as he can see the moving finger (making sure that he does not turn his head) you can get an idea of the patients field of vision in the direction of your hand. By repeating the test placing your hand in different directions a good idea of the field of vision of the patient can be obtained. If an abnormality is suspected detailed testing can be done using a procedure called perimetry.

If there is any doubt about the integrity of optic nerve the retina is examined using an ophthalmoscope. With this instrument we can see the interior of the eye through the pupil of the eye. The optic disc and blood vessels radiating from it can be seen.

Effects of injury to visual pathway

Injuries to different parts of the visual pathway can produce various kinds of defects. Loss of vision in one half (right or left) of the visual field is called hemianopia. If the same half of the visual field is lost in both eyes the defect is said to be homonymous and if different halves are lost the defect is said to be heteronymous. Note that the hemianopia is named in relation to the visual field and not to the retina.

Injury to the optic nerve will obviously produce total blindness in the eye concerned. Damage to the central part of the optic chiasma (e.g., by pressure from an enlarged hypophysis) interrupts the crossing fibres derived from the nasal halves of the two retinae resulting in bitemporal heteronymous hemianopia. It has been claimed that macular fibres are more susceptible to damage by pressure than peripheral fibres and are affected first. When the lateral part of the chiasma is affected a nasal hemianopia results. This may be unilateral or bilateral. Complete destruction of the optic tract, the lateral geniculate body, the optic radiation or the visual cortex of one side, results in loss of the opposite half of the field of vision. A lesion on the right side leads to left homonymous hemianopia. Lesions anterior to the lateral geniculate body also interrupt fibres responsible for the pupillary light reflex (See below).

Oculomotor, Trochlear and Abducent Nerves

These three nerves are responsible for movements of the eyeball. In a routine clinical examination the movements are tested by asking the patient to keep his head fixed and to move his eyes in various directions i.e., upwards, downwards, inwards and outwards. An easy way is to ask the patient to keep his head fixed, and to follow the movements of your finger with his eyes. Such an examination can detect a gross abnormality in movement of the eyes.

Sometimes one of the ocular muscles may not be completely paralysed but may be weak. Two indications of such weakness are as follows.

Diplopia:

This term means that objects are seen double. To understand this phenomenon remember that objects lying in different parts of the visual field produce images over different spots on the retina. The brain judges the position of an object by the position at which its image is formed on the retina. Normally the movements of the right and left eyes are in perfect alignment, and an object casts an image on corresponding spots on the two retinae so that only one image is perceived by the brain. When a muscle of the eyeball is weak, and a movement involving that muscle is performed, the movement of the defective eye is slightly less than that of the normal eye. As a result images of the object on the two retinae are not formed at corresponding points but over two points near each other. The brain therefore 'sees' two images, one from each retina.

To understand the causation of diplopia you can do a little experiment on yourself. Fix your gaze on any object. Place a finger below one eyeball and gently push it upwards. In addition to the normal bright image of the object you will see a second fainter image above the normal image. This illustrates that diplopia will be produced by any factor that distorts the normal alignment of the two eyes relative to each other.

Squint (or strabismus):

This is a condition in which the two eyes do not look in the same direction. The squint becomes obvious when the eye movement involves a muscle that is paralysed or weak, because the weak muscle cannot keep up with the muscle of the normal side.

As explained above squint will be accompanied by diplopia. However, the patient compensates for lack of movement of the eyeball by turning the head in the direction of the object and on doing so the diplopia disappears.

If the normal eye is closed, the patient is unable to judge the position of objects in the field of vision correctly (because the image of the object does not fall on the part of the retina that corresponds to the true position of the object). All the features described above are those of paralytic squint.

There is another type of squint called concomitant squint. This condition is congenital, and manifests itself in early childhood. Squint is present in all positions of the eyeball. There is no muscular weakness and movements are normal in all directions. There is no diplopia.

Paralysis of oculomotor nerve

All movements of the eyeball are lost in the affected eye. When the patient is asked to look directly forwards the affected eye is directed laterally (by the lateral rectus) and downwards (by the superior oblique). There is lateral quint (external strabismus) and diplopia.

As the levator palpebrae superioris is paralysed there is drooping of the upper eyelid (ptosis). As parasympathetic fibres to the sphincter pupillae pass through the oculomotor nerve, the sphincter pupillae is paralysed. Unopposed action of sympathetic nerves produces a fixed and dilated pupil.

Normally the pupil contracts when exposed to light (light reflex). It also contracts when the relaxed eye is made to concentrate on a near object (accommodation reflex). Both these reflexes are lost. The power of accommodation is lost because of paralysis of the ciliaris muscle.

Paralysis of trochlear nerve

The superior oblique muscle (supplied by the trochlear nerve) moves the eyeball downwards and laterally, and the inferior rectus (supplied by the oculomotor nerve) moves it downwards and medially. For direct downward movement synchronized action of both muscles is required. When the superior oblique muscle is paralysed the eyeball deviates medially on trying to look downwards.

Paralysis of abducent nerve

This nerve supplies the lateral rectus muscle which moves the eyeball laterally. In looking forwards the lateral pull of the lateral rectus is counteracted by the medial pull of the medial rectus and so the eye is maintained in the centre. When the lateral rectus is paralysed the affected eye deviates medially (medial squint, or internal strabismus).

Trigeminal nerve

The trigeminal nerve has a wide sensory distribution. It also supplies the muscles of mastication.

The sensation of touch in the area of distribution of the nerve can be tested by touching different areas of skin with a wisp of cotton wool. The sensation of pain can be tested by gentle pressure with a pin.

Motor function is tested by asking the patient to clench his teeth firmly. Contraction of the masseter can be felt by palpation when the teeth are clenched.

Effects of injury or disease

Injury to the trigeminal nerve causes paralysis of the muscles supplied and loss of sensations in the area of supply. Some features of special importance are as follows:

1. Apart from their role in opening and closing the mouth, the muscles of mastication are responsible for side to side movements of the mandible. Contraction of these muscles on one side moves the chin to the opposite side. Normally the chin is maintained in the midline by the balanced tone of the muscles of the right and left sides. In paralysis of the pterygoid muscles of one side the chin is pushed to the paralysed side by muscles of the opposite side.

2. Loss of sensation in the ophthalmic division (specially the nasociliary nerve) is of great importance. Normally the eyelids close as soon as the cornea is touched (corneal reflex). Loss of sensation in the cornea abolishes this reflex leaving the cornea unprotected. This can lead to the formation of ulcers on the cornea which can in turn lead to blindness.

3. Pain arising in a structure supplied by one branch of the nerve may be felt in an area of skin supplied by another branch: this is called referred pain. Some examples are as follows:

(a) Caries of a tooth in the lower jaw (supplied by the inferior alveolar nerve) may cause pain in the ear (auriculotemporal).

(b) If there is an ulcer or cancer on the tongue (lingual nerve) the pain may again be felt over the ear and temple (auriculotemporal).

(c) In frontal sinusitis (sinus supplied by a branch from the supraorbital nerve) the pain is referred to the forehead (skin supplied by supraorbital nerve). In fact headache is a common symptom when any structure supplied by the trigeminal nerve is involved (e.g., eyes, ears, teeth).

4. A source of irritation in the distribution of the nerve may cause severe persistent pain (*trigeminal neuralgia*). Removal of the cause can cure the pain. However, in some cases no cause can be found. In such cases pain can be relieved by injection of alcohol into the trigeminal ganglion, into one of the divisions of the nerve, or into its sensory root. In some cases it may be necessary to cut fibres of the sensory root. In this connection it is important to know that the fibres for the maxillary and mandibular divisions can be cut without destroying those for the ophthalmic division. This is possible as the fibres for the ophthalmic division lie separately in the upper medial part of the sensory root. Finally, it may be noted that trigeminal pain can also be relieved by cutting the spinal tract of the trigeminal nerve: this procedure is useful specially for relieving pain in the distribution of the ophthalmic division as pain can be abolished without loss of the sense of touch and, therefore, without the abolition of the corneal reflex.

5. *Mandibular nerve block*: This is used for anaesthesia of the lower jaw (for extraction of teeth). Palpate the anterior margin of the ramus of the mandible. Just medial to it you will feel the pterygomandibular raphe (ligament). The needle is inserted in the interval between the ramus and the raphe. The tip of the needle is now very near the inferior alveolar nerve, just before it enters the mandibular canal. Anaesthetic injected here blocks the nerve.

6. The lingual nerve lies very close to the medial side of the third molar tooth, just deep to the mucosa. The nerve can be injured in careless extraction of a third molar. In cases of cancer of the tongue, having intractable pain, the lingual can be cut at this site to relieve pain.

Facial nerve

The facial nerve supplies the muscles of the face including the muscles that close the eyelids, and the mouth. The nerve is tested as follows.

1. Ask the patient to close his eyes firmly. In complete paralysis of the facial nerve the patient will not be able to close the eye on the affected side. In partial paralysis the closure is weak and the examiner can easily open the closed eye with his fingers (which is very difficult in a normal person).

2. Ask the person to smile. In smiling the normal mouth is more or less symmetrical, the two angles moving upwards and outwards. In facial paralysis the angle fails to move on the paralysed side.

3. Ask the patient to fill his mouth with air. Press the cheek with your finger and compare the resistance (by the buccinator muscle) on the two sides. The resistance is less on the paralysed side. On pressing the cheek air may leak out of the mouth because the muscles closing the mouth are weak.

4. The sensation of taste should be tested on the anterior two thirds of the tongue (as described under glossopharyngeal nerve).

Paralysis of facial nerve

Paralysis of the facial nerve is fairly common. It can occur due to injury or disease of the facial nucleus (nuclear paralysis) or of the nerve any where along its course (infranuclear paralysis). In the most common type of infranuclear paralysis called *Bell's palsy* the nerve is affected near the stylomastoid foramen. Facial muscles can also be paralysed by interruption of corticonuclear fibres running from the motor cortex to the facial nucleus: this is referred to as supranuclear paralysis.

The effects of paralysis are due to the failure of the muscles concerned to perform their normal actions. Some effects are as follows:

(1) The normal face is more or less symmetrical. When the facial nerve is paralysed on one side the most noticeable feature is the loss of symmetry. (Also see para 4 in this regard).

(2) Normal furrows on the forehead are lost because of paralysis of the occipitofrontalis.

(3) There is drooping of the eyelid and the palpebral fissure is wider on the paralysed side because of paralysis of the orbicularis oculi. The conjunctival reflex is lost for the same reason.

(4) There is marked asymmetry of the mouth because of paralysis of the orbicularis oris and of muscles inserted into the angle of the mouth. This is most obvious when a smile is attempted. As a result of asymmetry the protruded tongue appears to deviate to one side, but is in fact in the midline.

(5) During mastication food tends to accumulate between the cheek and the teeth. (This is normally prevented by the buccinator).

Additional effects are observed in injuries to the facial nerve at levels higher than the stylomastoid foramen, as follows:

(a) If the injury is proximal to the origin of the chorda tympani there is loss of the sensation of taste on the anterior two thirds of the tongue.

(b) The transmission of loud sounds to the internal ear is normally dampened by the stapedius muscle. When the lesion is proximal to the origin of the branch to the stapedius this muscle is paralysed. As a result even normal sounds appear too loud (hyperacusis).

(c) In fractures of the temporal bone, or in lesions near the exit of the nerve from the brain the vestibulocochlear nerve may also be affected (leading to deafness).

(d) In nuclear lesions (within the brainstem) other neighbouring nuclei may be affected leading to lesions of the abducent or trigeminal nerves.

(e) Supranuclear lesions can be distinguished from nuclear or infranuclear lesions because these are usually accompanied by hemiplegia. Movements of the lower part of the face are more affected than those of the upper part: the explanation for this is that the corticonuclear fibres concerned with movements of the upper part of the face are bilateral, whereas those for movements of the lower part of the face are unilateral. Another difference is that while voluntary movements are affected, emotional expressions appear to be normal. It has been suggested that there are separate pathways from the cerebral cortex to the facial nucleus for voluntary and emotional movements; and that usually only the former are involved.

Vestibulocochlear nerve

This nerve is responsible for hearing (cochlear part) and for equilibrium (vestibular part). Normally we test only the cochlear part.

1. The hearing of the patient can be tested by using a watch. First place the watch near one ear so that the patient knows what he is expected to hear. Next ask him to close his eyes and say so when he hears the ticking of the watch. The watch should be held away from the ear and then gradually brought towards it. The distance at which the sounds are first heard should be compared with the other ear.

In doing this test it must be remembered that loss of hearing can occur from various causes such as the presence of wax in the ear, or middle ear disease.

Nerve deafness can be distinguished from deafness due to a conduction defect (as in middle ear disease) by noting the following.

1. Sounds can be transmitted to the internal ear through air (normal way), and can also be transmitted through bone. Normally conduction through air is better than that through bone, but in defects of conduction the sound is better heard through bone.

2. Air conduction and bone conduction can be compared by using a tuning fork. Strike the tuning fork against an object so that it begins to vibrate producing sound. Place the tuning fork near the patients ear and then immediately put the base of the tuning fork on the mastoid process. Ask the patient where he hears the sound better. (This is called **Rinne's test**). In another test the base of a vibrating tuning fork is placed on the forehead. The sound is heard in both ears but is more clear in the ear with a conduction defect (This is **Weber's test**).

Defects in the vestibular apparatus or in the vestibular nerve are difficult to test and such cases need to be examined by a specialist.

Glossopharyngeal nerve

Testing of this nerve is based on the fact that (a) the nerve carries fibres of taste from the posterior one third of the tongue; and (b) that it provides sensory innervation to the pharynx.

1. Sensations of taste can be tested by applying substances that are salty (salt), sweet (sugar), sour (lemon), or bitter (quinine) to the posterior one third of the tongue. The mouth should be rinsed and the tongue dried before the substance is applied.

2. Touching the pharyngeal mucosa causes reflex constriction of pharyngeal muscles. The glossopharyngeal nerve provides the afferent part of the pathway for this reflex.

Vagus nerve (and cranial part of accessory)

This nerve has an extensive distribution but testing is based on its motor supply to the soft palate and to the larynx.

1. Ask the patient to open the mouth wide and say 'aah'. Observe the movement of the soft palate. In a normal person the soft palate is elevated. When one vagus nerve is paralysed the palate is pulled towards the normal side. When the nerve is paralysed on both sides the soft palate does not move at all.

2. In injury to the superior laryngeal nerve the voice is weak due to paralysis of the cricothyroid muscle. At first there is hoarseness but after some time the opposite cricothyroid compensates for the deficit and hoarseness disappears.

3. Injury to the recurrent laryngeal nerve also leads to hoarseness, but this hoarseness is permanent. On examining the larynx through a laryngoscope it is seen that on the affected side the vocal fold does not move. It is fixed in a position midway between adduction and abduction. In cases where the recurrent laryngeal nerve is pressed upon by a tumour it is observed that nerve fibres that supply abductors are lost first.

4. In paralysis of both recurrent laryngeal nerves voice is lost as both vocal folds are immobile.

5. It may be remembered that the left recurrent laryngeal nerve runs part of its course in the thorax. It can be involved in bronchial or oesophageal carcinoma, or by secondary growths in mediastinal lymph nodes.

Accessory nerve (spinal part)

This nerve is tested as follows.

1. Put your hands on the right and left shoulders of the patient and ask him to elevate (shrug) his shoulders. In paralysis the movement will be weak on one side (due to paralysis of the trapezius).

2. Ask the patient to turn his face to the opposite side (against resistance offered by your hand). In paralysis the movement is weak on the affected side (due to paralysis of the sternocleidomastoid muscle).

Hypoglossal nerve

This nerve supplies muscles of the tongue. To test the nerve ask the patient to protrude the tongue. In a normal person the protruded tongue lies in the midline. If the nerve is paralysed the tongue deviates to the paralysed side. The explanation for this is as follows.

Protrusion of the tongue is produced by the pull of the right and left genioglossus muscles. The origin of the right and left genioglossus muscles lies anteriorly (on the hyoid bone), and the insertion lies posteriorly (on to the posterior part of the tongue). Each muscle draws the posterior part of the tongue forwards and medially. Normally, the medial pull of the two muscles cancels out, but when one muscle is paralysed it is this medial pull of the intact muscle that causes the tongue to deviate to the opposite side.

Deviation of the tongue should be assessed with reference to the incisor teeth, and not to the lips. Remember that in facial paralysis the tongue may protrude normally, but may appear to deviate to one side because of asymmetry of the mouth.

11 : Internal Structure of Brainstem

A brief outline of the internal structure of the brainstem has been given in Chapter 6. (This chapter should be revised before proceeding further). We have also considered the cranial nerve nuclei and their connections (Chapter 10), and the tracts passing through the brainstem (Chapter 9). With this background we will now consider the internal structure of the brainstem as seen in transverse sections at various levels.

The Medulla

Section through the medulla at the level of the pyramidal decussation

Some features to be seen at this level have been reviewed on page 66. The pyramids and their decussation, the nucleus gracilis, the nucleus cuneatus, the spinal nucleus of the trigeminal nerve, the central grey matter, the central canal, and the uppermost part of the ventral grey column have been identified (Fig. 6.4). Now note the following additional features (Fig. 11.1).

The ventral grey column is separated from the central grey matter by decussating pyramidal fibres. The neurons in it give origin to the uppermost rootlets of the first cervical nerve, and to some fibres in the spinal root of the accessory nerve. The area between the ventral grey column and the spinal nucleus of the trigeminal nerve is occupied by the lower part of the reticular formation.

The main descending fibres to be seen at this level are the corticospinal fibres that form the pyramids. After crossing the middle line these fibres turn downwards in the region lateral to the central grey matter to form the lateral corticospinal tract. We have already seen that those fibres of the pyramids that do not cross descend into the ventral funiculus of the spinal cord to form the ventral corticospinal tract. Other descending tracts to be seen at this level (in the anterolateral part

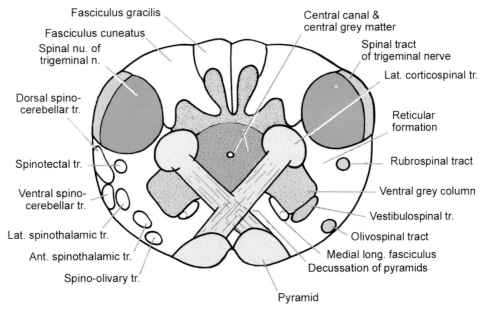

Fig. 11.1. Transverse section through the medulla at the level of the pyramidal decussation.

of the medulla, Fig. 11.1, right half) are the rubrospinal tract, the vestibulospinal tract, the olivospinal tract and the tectospinal tract. The tectospinal tract is incorporated within the medial longitudinal fasciculus. Among descending tracts we may also include the spinal tract of the trigeminal nerve, which forms a layer of fibres superficial to the spinal nucleus of this nerve.

The ascending tracts to be seen at this level include the fasciculus gracilis and fasciculus cuneatus which occupy the areas behind the corresponding nuclei; and the spinothalamic, spinocerebellar, spinotectal and spino-olivary tracts that occupy the anterolateral region.

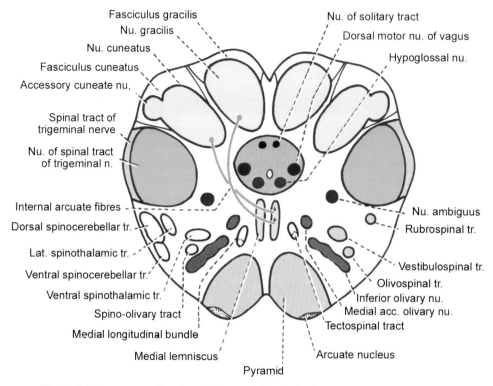

Fig. 11.2. Transverse section through the medulla a little above the pyramidal decussation
(i.e., at the level of the lemniscal decussation).

Section through the medulla at the level of the lemniscal decussation

The level represented by this section lies a little above the level of the pyramidal decussation. Some features of a section at this level have already been seen (page 66, Fig. 6.5). The central canal surrounded by central grey matter, the medial lemniscus, the pyramids, the nucleus gracilis, the nucleus cuneatus, the spinal nucleus of the trigeminal nerve, and the reticular formation have been identified.

The nucleus gracilis and the nucleus cuneatus are much larger than at lower levels (Fig. 11.2). Internal arcuate fibres arising in these nuclei arch forwards and medially around the central grey matter to cross the middle line. These crossing fibres constitute the *lemniscal (or sensory) decussation*. Having crossed the middle line these fibres turn cranially to constitute the *medial lemniscus*. As the fibres from the nucleus gracilis and the nucleus cuneatus pass forwards they cross each other so that the fibres from the nucleus gracilis come to lie ventral to those from the nucleus cuneatus. The most medial fibres (from the legs) come to lie most anteriorly in the medial lemniscus. These are followed by fibres from the trunk and from the upper limb, in that order. Higher up in the brainstem the medial lemniscus changes its orientation, its long axis (as seen in cross section) becoming transverse (Fig. 11.7). The most anterior fibres become lateral, and the posterior fibres become medial. In its course through the medulla the medial lemniscus is joined by the anterior spinothalamic tract.

It has been shown that fibres in the medial lemniscus are arranged in layers corresponding to spinal segments. Fibres from segment C1 are most medial, and those from S4 are most lateral.

The *accessory cuneate nucleus* is placed dorsolateral to the cuneate nucleus. It receives proprioceptive impulses from the upper limb through fibres arising in spinal grey matter of cervical segments of the cord. Efferents of the accessory cuneate nucleus constitute the *posterior external arcuate fibres*. They reach the cerebellum through the inferior cerebellar peduncle of the same side.

A number of cranial nerve nuclei can be identified at this level. Several of these are present in relation to the central grey matter. The hypoglossal nucleus is located ventral to the central canal just lateral to the middle line. The dorsal vagal nucleus lies dorsolateral to the hypoglossal nucleus. The nucleus of the solitary tract is seen dorsal to the central canal near the middle line. The lower ends of these nuclei of the two sides become continuous with each other to form the commissural nucleus of the vagus. The nucleus ambiguus lies in the reticular formation medial to the spinal nucleus of the trigeminal nerve.

Other masses of grey matter that may be recognised at this level are:

  (a) the lowest part of the *inferior olivary nucleus* (page 61);

  (b) the *medial accessory olivary nucleus* which lies dorsal to the medial part of the inferior olivary nucleus (see below);

  (c) the *lateral reticular nucleus* lying in the lateral part of the reticular formation; and

  (d) *arcuate nuclei* lying on the anterior aspect of the pyramids.

The gracile and cuneate fasciculi are much smaller than at lower levels as the fibres of these tracts progressively terminate in the gracile and cuneate nuclei. Other ascending tracts to be seen at this level are the spinothalamic, spinocerebellar, spinotectal and spino-olivary tracts all of which lie in the anterolateral region (Fig. 11.2, left half).

The descending tracts present are (Fig. 11.2, right half) the pyramids, the rubrospinal, vestibulospinal and olivospinal tracts, and the medial longitudinal fasciculus which includes the tectospinal tract.

Section through the medulla at the level of the olive

Some features of a transverse section at this level have been introduced on page 67(Fig. 6.6). The floor of the fourth ventricle lined by grey matter, the reticular formation, the spinal nucleus and tract of the trigeminal nerve, the inferior cerebellar peduncle, the inferior olivary nucleus, the medial lemniscus and the pyramids have been briefly considered.

Several cranial nerve nuclei can be recognised in relation to the floor of the fourth ventricle (Fig. 11.3). From medial to lateral side these are the hypoglossal nucleus, the dorsal vagal nucleus, and the vestibular nuclei. The solitary tract and its nucleus lie ventrolateral to the dorsal vagal nucleus. The nucleus ambiguus lies much more ventrally within the reticular formation.

The dorsal and ventral cochlear nuclei can be seen in relation to the inferior cerebellar peduncle. (They are shown schematically in Fig. 11.3. They are actually seen at higher levels of the medulla, near its junction with the pons).

Other masses of grey matter present are the medial and dorsal accessory olivary nuclei (lying medial and dorsal, respectively, to the inferior olivary nucleus), and the lateral reticular nucleus and arcuate nuclei which occupy the same relative positions as at lower levels. The pontobulbar body lies on the dorsolateral aspect of the inferior cerebellar peduncle (Fig. 11.3, right).

BASIC

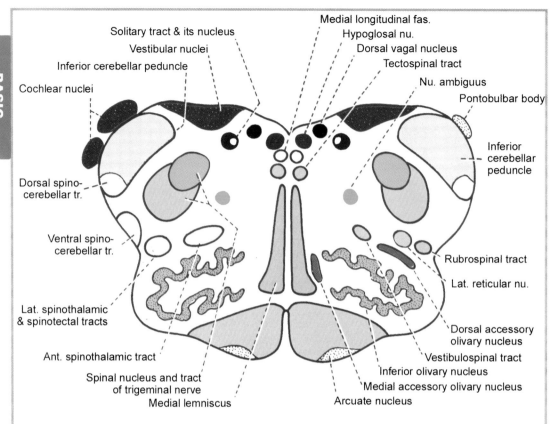

Fig. 11.3. Transverse section through the medulla at the level of the olive.

The descending tracts to be seen at this level (Fig. 11.3, right half) are the pyramids, the tectospinal, vestibulospinal, and rubrospinal tracts; and the spinal tract of the trigeminal nerve.

The ascending tracts are the medial lemniscus forming an anteroposterior L-shaped band lying next to the middle line; the spinothalamic, spinocerebellar and spino-tectal tracts. At this level the dorsal spino-cerebellar tract lies within the inferior cerebellar peduncle. The ventral spino-cerebellar tract lies more anteriorly near the surface of the medulla. The spinothalamic tracts lie dorsolateral to the inferior olivary nucleus. The medial longitudinal fasciculus lies dorsal to the medial lemniscus.

The connections of the cranial nerve nuclei of the medulla have been described in Chapter 10. The reticular formation is considered on page 151. Some details about other masses of grey matter to be seen in the medulla are considered below.

Gracile and Cuneate nuclei

ADVANCED

We have seen that the gracile and cuneate nuclei receive fibres of the fasciculus gracilis and fasciculus cuneatus respectively; and give origin to the internal arcuate fibres which form the medial lemniscus, ultimately reaching the thalamus. However, the gracile and cuneate nuclei are not to be regarded as simple relay stations. The neurons in them are of various types. In both nuclei an upper *reticular region* can be distinguished. Apart from receiving fibres derived from the dorsal nerve roots of spinal nerves, this region receives fibres originating in spinal grey matter. It also receives fibres descending from the sensory cortex: these could presumably inhibit or facilitate conduction through the gracile and cuneate nuclei. Some fibres from these nuclei descend to the spinal grey matter (constituting a feedback circuit).

The arrangement of neurons in the gracile and cuneate nuclei is somatotropic. The upper (reticular) parts of the nuclei receive proprioceptive inputs. The lower parts of the nuclei receive impulses arising (mainly) in skin.

In the cuneate nucleus there is a middle zone called **the pars rotunda**. Within the pars rotunda distinct areas which receive impulses from individual digits, palm and dorsum of the hand, and from the forearm can be distinguished.

Connections of the Inferior Olivary Complex

The main afferents of the inferior olivary nucleus are from the cerebral cortex and from the spinal cord (Fig. 11.4). The main efferents are to the cerebellar cortex. Details of olivocerebellar connections are considered on page 174. An olivospinal tract is traditionally described, but some authorities hold that the inferior olivary nuclei do not send any fibres to the spinal cord. The nucleus may be regarded as a relay station on the cortico-olivo-cerebellar and spino-olivo-cerebellar pathways. Other connections of the nucleus are shown in Fig. 11.4.

The **accessory olivary nuclei** are connected to the cerebellum by **parolivo-cerebellar fibres**.

Connections of arcuate nuclei and pontobulbar body

The **arcuate nuclei** are generally regarded as displaced pontine nuclei. Cortical fibres reach them through the pyramids. These are relayed to the cerebellum by fibres which follow two separate pathways. Some of them wind round the anterior and lateral aspect of the medulla as **anterior external arcuate fibres** to reach the inferior cerebellar peduncle of the opposite side. Other fibres pass dorsally through the substance of the medulla to reach the floor of the fourth ventricle. Here they run under the ependyma to the inferior cerebellar peduncle of the opposite side as fibres of the **striae medullares**. Fibres from the arcuate nuclei probably end in the flocculus of the cerebellum.

Students must distinguish carefully between the stria medullares described above and the stria medullaris thalami present in relation to the wall of the third ventricle.

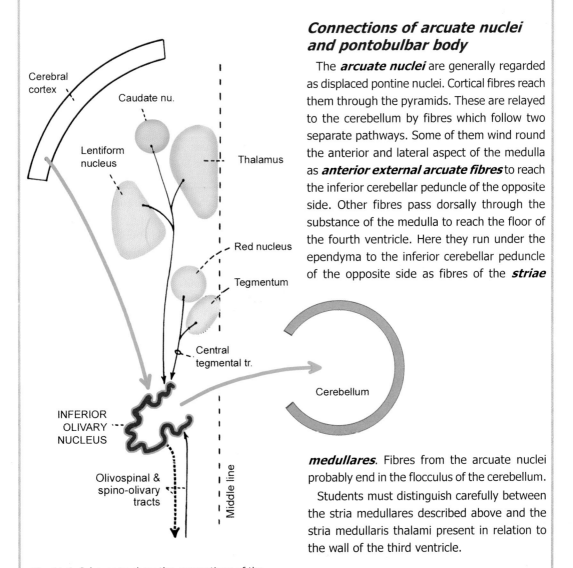

Fig. 11.4. Scheme to show the connections of the inferior olivary nucleus.

Like the arcuate nuclei, the **pontobulbar body** is made up of neurons that represent displaced pontine nuclei. Fibres arising in this body form the **circumolivary bundle**. These fibres join those from the arcuate nuclei to reach the inferior cerebellar peduncle of the opposite side. Some of them possibly pass through the striae medullares.

The Pons

Transverse sections through the lower and upper parts of the pons are illustrated in Figs. 11.5 and 11.7. Some features common to both these levels have been already considered (page 68, Fig. 6.7). The subdivision of the pons into dorsal and ventral parts and its relationship to the superior, middle and inferior cerebellar peduncles has been noted.

We have seen that the **ventral part of the pons** contains: **(a)** the pontine nuclei, **(b)** vertically running corticospinal and corticopontine fibres, and **(c)** transversely running fibres arising in the pontine nuclei and projecting to the opposite half of the cerebellum through the middle cerebellar peduncle.

The **pontine nuclei** (or **nuclei pontis**) receive corticopontine fibres from the frontal, temporal, parietal and occipital lobes of the cerebrum. Their efferents form the transverse fibres of the pons. We have seen that most of these fibres cross to the opposite side, but some may end ipsilaterally.

The pontine nuclei also receive fibres from various other sources including the tectum (superior colliculus), the mamillary body, the lateral geniculate body, the nuclei gracilis and cuneatus, trigeminal nuclei, hypothalamus, cerebellar nuclei and reticular formation.

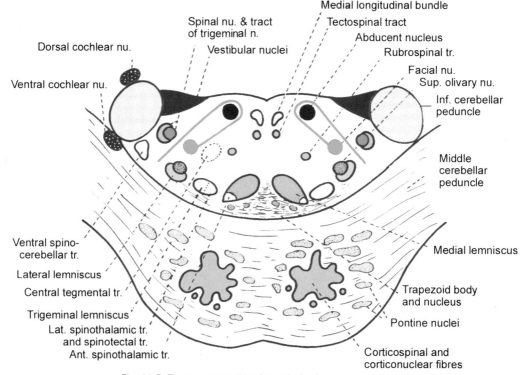

Fig. 11.5. Transverse section through the lower part of the pons.

It has been estimated that there are about twenty million neurons in pontine nuclei. Most of them are glutaminergic. About 5% are GABAergic and are inhibitory.

The **dorsal part of the pons** is occupied, predominantly, by the reticular formation. Its posterior surface helps to form the floor of the fourth ventricle. This surface is lined by grey matter and is related to some cranial nerve

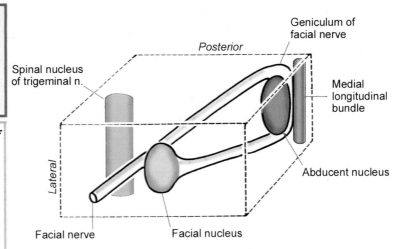

Fig. 11.6. Scheme to show the course of the fibres of the facial nerve through the pons, and the formation of the facial colliculus.

nuclei. The dorsal part is bounded laterally by the inferior cerebellar peduncle in the lower part of the pons, and by the superior cerebellar peduncle in the upper part. The region adjoining the ventral part (of the pons) is occupied by important ascending tracts. The medial lemniscus occupies a transversely elongated oval area next to the middle line. Lateral to this are the trigeminal lemniscus and the spinal lemniscus (lateral spinothalamic tract). The fibres of the spinotectal tract run along with the spinal lemniscus, while those of the ventral spinothalamic tract lie within the medial lemniscus. Still more laterally, there is the lateral lemniscus. Ventral to these lemnisci there are conspicuous transversely running fibres that form the **trapezoid body**. The ventral spinocerebellar tract lies ventromedial to the inferior cerebellar peduncle in the lower part of the pons (Fig. 11.5). In the upper part of the pons

BASIC

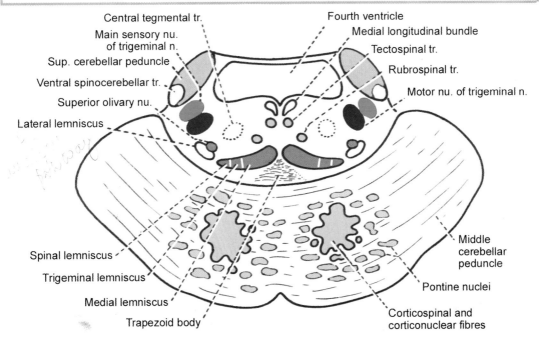

Fig. 11.7. Transverse section through the upper part of the pons.

it is seen within the superior cerebellar peduncle (Fig. 11.7). Descending tracts passing through the dorsal part of the pons are the tectospinal tract and the rubrospinal tract. The medial longitudinal fasciculus lies dorsally near the middle line.

In the preceding paragraphs we have studied those features of the pons that are common to upper and lower levels. We will now consider those features that are different in the upper and lower parts.

Section through the lower part of the pons

This secton (Fig. 11.5) shows two cranial nerve nuclei that are closely related to the floor of the fourth ventricle. These are the abducent nucleus lying medially and the vestibular nuclei that lie laterally. At a deeper level in the lateral part of the reticular formation two additional nuclei are seen. These are the spinal nucleus of the trigeminal nerve (along with its tract) lying laterally, and the facial nucleus lying medially. The dorsal and ventral cochlear nuclei lie dorsal and ventral, respectively, to the inferior cerebellar peduncle.

The fibres arising from the facial nucleus follow an unusual course (Fig. 11.6). They first run backwards and medially to reach the lower pole of the abducent nucleus. They then ascend on the medial side of that nucleus. Here the fibres are closely related to the medial longitudinal fasciculus. Finally, the fibres of the facial nerve turn forwards and laterally passing above the upper pole of the abducent nucleus. As they pass forwards the fibres lie between the facial nucleus medially, and the spinal nucleus of the trigeminal nerve laterally . The abducent nucleus and the facial nerve fibres looping around it together form a surface elevation, the *facial colliculus,* in the floor of the fourth ventricle (Fig. 20.12).

The vestibular nuclei occupy the vestibular area in the lateral part of the floor of the fourth ventricle. These nuclei are to be seen in the lower part of the pons and in the upper part of the medulla

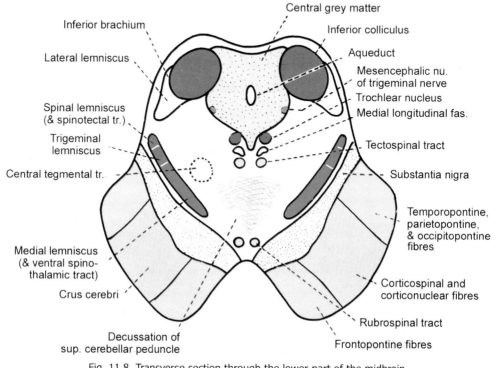

Fig. 11.8. Transverse section through the lower part of the midbrain.

(Figs. 11.3, 11.5). Their subdivisions are described on page 121, and their connections on page 125 (Fig. 10.8).

Other masses of grey matter to be seen in the lower part of the pons are the **superior olivary complex** (made up of several nuclei) which lies dorsomedial to the lateral lemniscus, and the nuclei of the trapezoid body which consist of scattered cells lying within this body. The significance of these nuclei has been considered on page 123.

Section through the upper part of the pons

At this level (Fig. 11.7) the dorsal part is bounded laterally by the superior cerebellar peduncles. Medial to each peduncle there is the main sensory nucleus of the trigeminal nerve, and further medially there is the motor nucleus of the same nerve. The superior olivary nucleus extends to this level, but is less prominent; while the lateral lemniscus forms a more conspicuous bundle. Some fibres of the trapezoid body can be seen ventral to the medial lemniscus.

The reticular formation of the pons is described on page 151.

The Midbrain

Some features of the internal structure of the midbrain have been considered on page 69 (Fig. 6.9). The subdivision of the midbrain into the tectum, the tegmentum, the substantia nigra, and the crus cerebri (or basis pedunculi) has been noted. The superior and inferior colliculi, the red nucleus and the reticular formation have been identified.

Transverse sections through the midbrain

A transverse section through the midbrain at the level of the inferior colliculus is shown in Fig. 11.8 and a section at the level of the superior colliculus in Fig. 11.9. We will first consider those features that are common to both these levels.

The **crus cerebri** (or **basis pedunculi**) consists of fibres descending from the cerebral cortex. Its medial one-sixth is occupied by corticopontine fibres descending from the frontal lobe; and the lateral one-sixth is occupied by similar fibres from the temporal, occipital and parietal lobes. The intermediate two-thirds of the crus cerebri are occupied by corticospinal and corticonuclear fibres. The fibres for the leg are most lateral and those for the head are most medial.

The **substantia nigra** lies immediately behind and medial to the basis pedunculi. It appears dark in unstained sections as neurons within it contain pigment (neuromelanin).

The substantia nigra is divisible into a dorsal part, the **pars compacta**; and a ventral part, the **pars reticularis**. The pars compacta contains dopaminergic and cholinergic neurons. Most of the neurons in the pars reticularis are GABAergic. Superiorly, the pars reticularis becomes continuous with the globus pallidus. The connections of the substantia nigra are considered on page 151 and are shown in Fig. 11.13. The substantia nigra is closely connected, functionally, with the corpus striatum (and in causation of Parkinsonism, page 151).

The midbrain is traversed by the cerebral aqueduct which is surrounded by central grey matter. Ventrally, the central grey matter is related to cranial nerve nuclei (oculomotor and trochlear). The region between the substantia nigra and the central grey matter is occupied by the reticular formation.

Section through midbrain at level of inferior colliculus

A section through the midbrain at the level of the inferior colliculus shows the following additional features (Fig. 11.8).

The *inferior colliculus* is a large mass of grey matter lying in the tectum. It forms a cell station in the auditory pathway and is probably concerned with reflexes involving auditory stimuli. Its connections are considered on page 148 and are shown in Fig. 11.11.

The *trochlear nucleus* lies in the ventral part of the central grey matter. Fibres arising in this nucleus follow an unusual course. They run dorsally and decussate (in the superior medullary velum) before emerging on the dorsal aspect of the brainstem. The *mesencephalic nucleus of the trigeminal nerve* lies in the lateral part of the central grey matter.

A compact bundle of fibres lies in the tegmentum dorsomedial to the substantia nigra. It consists of the medial lemniscus, the trigeminal lemniscus and the spinal lemniscus in that order from medial to lateral side. The medial lemniscus includes fibres of the ventral spinothalamic tract while the spinal lemniscus (made up mainly of the lateral spinothalamic tract) includes fibres of the spinotectal tract. More dorsally, the lateral lemniscus forms a bundle ventrolateral to the inferior colliculus (in which most of its fibres end). Important fibre bundles are also located near the middle line of the tegmentum. The medial longitudinal fasciculus lies ventral to the trochlear nucleus; and ventral to the fasciculus there is the tectospinal tract. The region ventral to the tectospinal tracts is occupied by decussating fibres of the superior cerebellar peduncle. These fibres have their origin in the dentate nucleus of the cerebellum. They cross the middle line in the lower part of the tegmentum. Some of these fibres end in the red nucleus while others ascend to the thalamus. The part of the tegmentum ventral to the decussation of the superior cerebellar peduncle is occupied by the rubrospinal tracts.

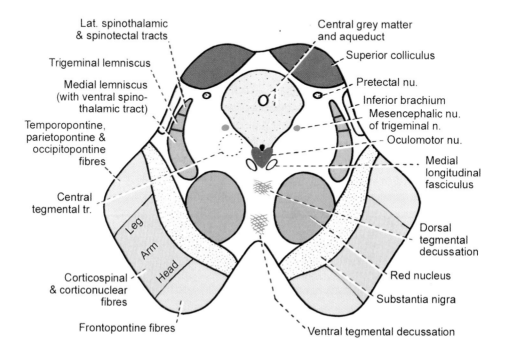

Fig. 11.9. Transverse section through the upper part of the midbrain.

Section through midbrain at level of superior colliculus

A section through the upper part of the midbrain (Fig. 11.9) shows two large masses of grey matter not seen at lower levels. These are the **superior colliculus** in the tectum, and the **red nucleus** in the tegmentum. The superior colliculus is a centre concerned with visual reflexes. Its connections are considered on page 150 and are shown in Fig. 11.12.

The red nucleus lies in the anterior part of the tegmentum dorsomedial to the substantia nigra. It is so called because of a reddish colour in fresh material. The colour is produced by the presence of an iron pigment in its neurons. The connections of the red nucleus are considered below and are shown in Fig. 11.10.

The **oculomotor nucleus** lies in relation to the ventral part of the central grey matter. The nuclei of the two sides lie close together forming a single complex. The **Edinger Westphal nucleus** (which supplies the sphincter pupillae and ciliaris muscle) forms part of the oculomotor complex. The oculomotor complex is related ventrally to the medial longitudinal fasciculus.

Closely related to the cranial part of the superior colliculus there is a small collection of neurons that constitute the **pretectal nucleus**. This nucleus is concerned with the pathway for the pupillary light reflex.

BASIC

> The pretectal nucleus extends cranially to the junction of the midbrain with the diencephalon. It receives retinal fibres through the optic tract. It also receives some fibres from the superior colliculus and from the visual cortex. The main efferents of the nucleus reach the oculomotor nuclei (of both sides). Some efferents reach the superior colliculus and the pulvinar.

ADVANCED

The bundle of ascending fibres consisting of the medial lemniscus, the trigeminal lemniscus and the spinal lemniscus lies more dorsally than at lower levels (because of the presence of the red nucleus). The lateral lemniscus is not seen at this level as its fibres end in the inferior colliculus. However, the **inferior brachium** that conveys auditory fibres to the medial geniculate body can be seen near the surface of the tegmentum. The region of the tegmentum near the middle line shows two groups of decussating fibres.

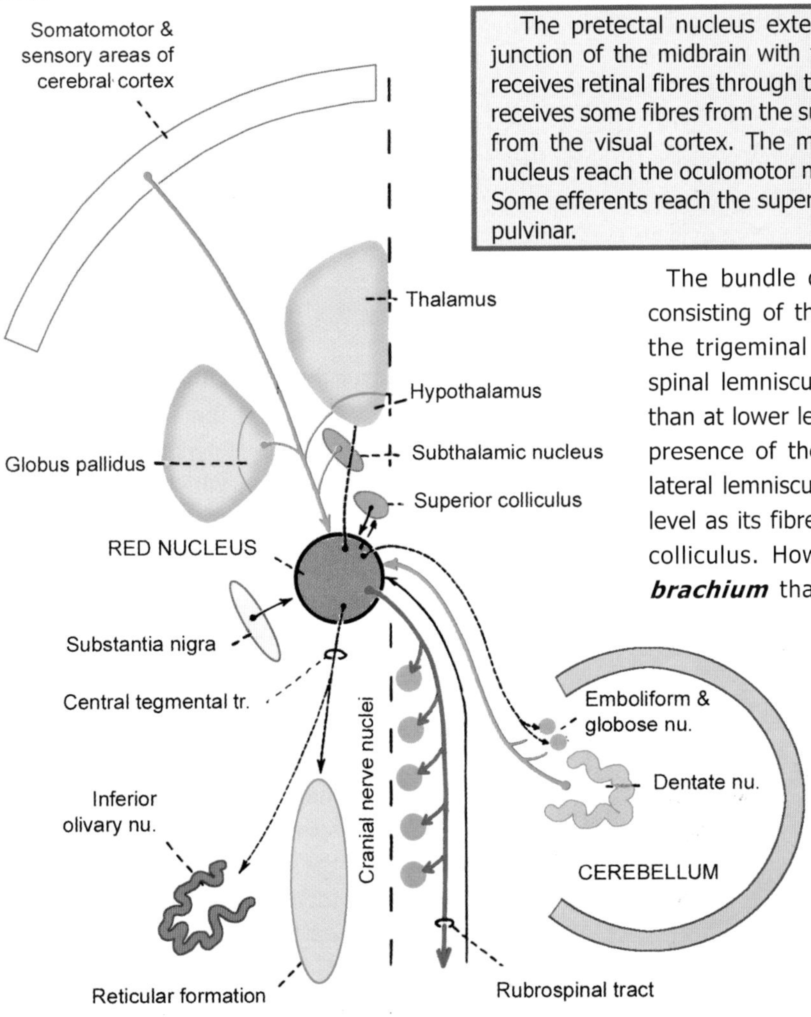

Fig. 11.10. Scheme to show the connections of the red nucleus.

The ***dorsal tegmental decussation*** consists of fibres that have their origin in the superior colliculus and cross to the opposite side to descend as the tectospinal tract. The ***ventral tegmental decussation*** consists of fibres that originate in the red nucleus and decussate to form the rubrospinal tracts.

Connections of the red nucleus

The red nucleus consists of a cranial ***parvicellular part*** and a caudal ***magnocellular part***. The magnocellular part is prominent in lower species, but in man it is much reduced and is distinctly smaller than the parvicellular part.

The red nucleus receives its main afferents from:

(a) the cerebral cortex (directly, and as collaterals from the corticospinal tract); and

(b) the cerebellum (dentate, emboliform and globose nuclei).

The efferents of the nucleus are as follows. The magnocellular part projects to the spinal cord through the rubrospinal tract; and to motor cranial nerve nuclei (III, IV, V, VI, VII) through the rubrobulbar tract. Some fibres reach the reticular formation. The parvicellular part of the nucleus gives origin to fibres that descend through the ***central tegmental fasciculus*** to reach the inferior olivary nucleus. Some fibres reach the reticular formation.

Other connections of the red nucleus are shown in Fig. 11.10.

Inferior Colliculus

The inferior colliculus is an important relay centre in the acoustic (auditory) pathway. It receives fibres of the lateral lemniscus arising in the superior olivary complex. Each colliculus receives auditory impulses from both ears. These impulses are relayed to the medial geniculate body (the fibres passing through the inferior brachium) and from there to the acoustic (auditory) area of the cerebral cortex. Other connections of the inferior colliculus are shown in Fig. 11.11 which illustrates the complete auditory pathway. Note that the inferior colliculus can influence motor neurons in the spinal cord and brainstem through the superior colliculus and the tectospinal and tectotegmental tracts.

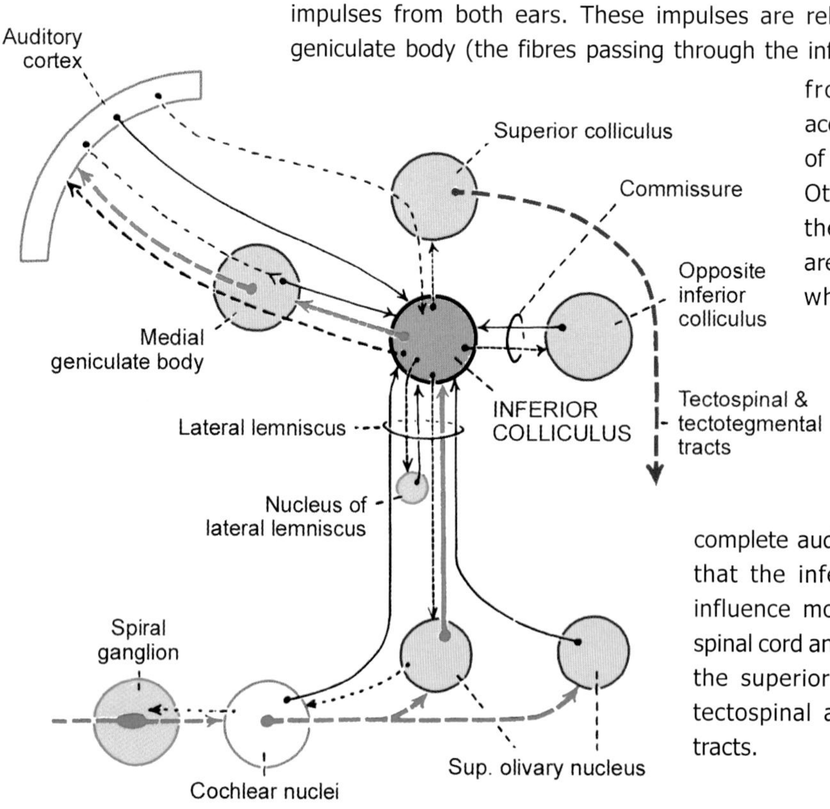

Fig. 11.11. Scheme to show the connections of the inferior colliculus.

Traditionally, the inferior colliculi have been regarded as reflex centres for responses to auditory stimuli. The colliculi are important in differentiating sounds received by the two ears, and thus, in locating the source of sound.

Each inferior colliculus has a main nucleus (placed centrally). This nucleus is divisible into dorsomedial and ventrolateral zones. More superficially, in the colliculus, there is a dorsal cortex which is divided into four laminae. The neurons of the inferior colliculus are arranged in groups responding to

ADVANCED

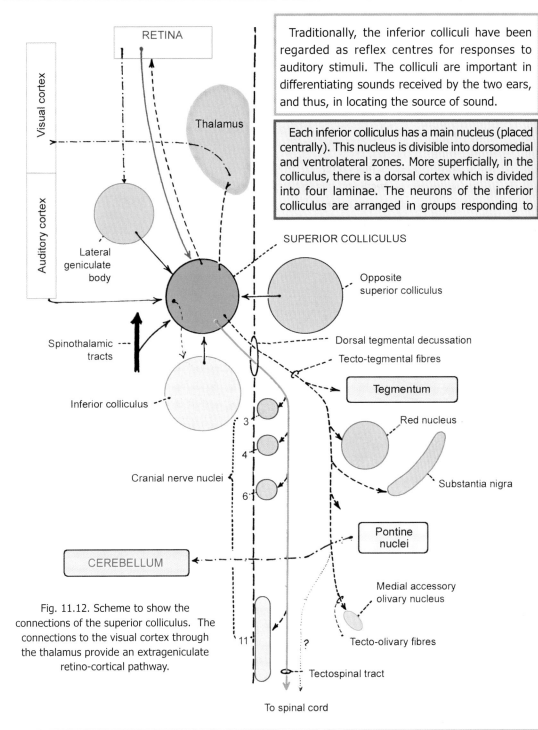

Fig. 11.12. Scheme to show the connections of the superior colliculus. The connections to the visual cortex through the thalamus provide an extrageniculate retino-cortical pathway.

different frequencies of sound. Those in the dorsal part of the central nucleus respond to low frequencies, while ventrally placed cells respond to higher frequencies. Recent studies suggest that a similar arrangement probably exists at all levels of the auditory pathway.

Lesions of the inferior colliculus produce defects in appreciation of tones, of localisation of sound, and of reflex movements in response to sound.

In Fig. 11.11 note that the various auditory centres are also interconnected by fibres running in a direction opposite to that of the main auditory pathway. These ***descending auditory fibres*** probably have a regulatory role on conduction through the pathway.

Connections of the Superior Colliculus

The superior colliculus has a complex laminar structure, being made up of seven layers. Its connections are shown in Fig. 11.12. Its most important afferents are those that bring visual impulses from the retina. The major efferents are the tectospinal tract, and tectonuclear fibres to the nuclei of cranial nerves responsible for moving the eyes and head. Some efferents also reach the retina. The colliculus has, therefore, been regarded as a centre for reflex movements of the head and eyes in response to visual stimuli.

However, recent work has shown that the functions of the superior colliculi may be much more complex. In addition to visual impulses the superior colliculi receive auditory impulses (through the inferior colliculi), and somatic impulses (touch, pain, temperature) through collaterals of spinothalamic tracts. They also receive fibres from the temporal and occipital cerebral cortex. The colliculi send efferents to various centres in the brainstem (red nucleus, substantia nigra, reticular formation) and can influence the cerebellum through the pontine nuclei. The fibres to the reticular formation reach reticular nuclei in the midbrain, pons and medulla.

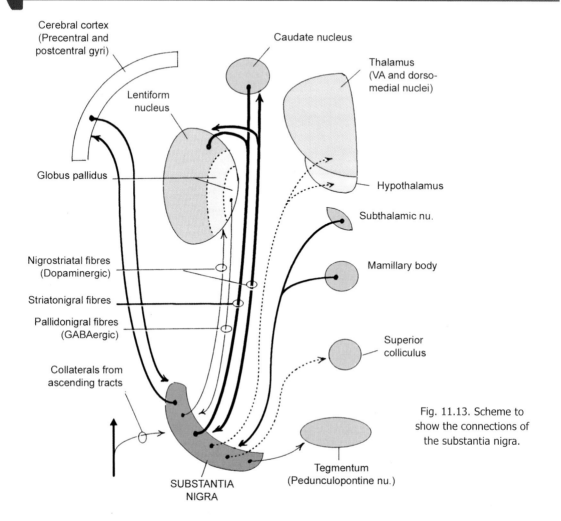

Fig. 11.13. Scheme to show the connections of the substantia nigra.

From these connections it appears likely that the superior colliculi are concerned with complex interactions between visual inputs and various activities of the body. Some fibres descend to the superior colliculus from the auditory cortex, and may be involved in integration of visual and auditory behaviour.

For role of the superior colliculus in control of eye movements see page 159.

Connections of the Substantia Nigra

The main connections (both afferent and efferent) are with the striatum (i.e., caudate nucleus and putamen). Dopamine produced by neurons in the substantia nigra (pars compacta) passes along their axons to the striatum (*mesostriatal dopamine system*). Dopamine is much reduced in patients with a disease called *Parkinsonism* in which there is a degeneration of the striatum.

Other connections of the substantia nigra are shown in Figs. 11.13, 11.14. The functional relationships of the substantia nigra with the basal nuclei are considered further in Chapter 14.

Along with other groups of dopaminergic neurons present in the ventral part of the tegmentum, the substantia nigra is believed to be a neural centre for "adaptive behaviour". Efferents of this system are widely distributed.

Some fibre bundles seen in the brainstem

In addition to the various ascending and descending tracts described in Chapter 9, there are a number of fibre bundles to be seen in the brainstem. These include:

1. The medial longitudinal fasciculus (or bundle)
2. The central tegmental tract.
3. The dorsal longitudinal fasciculus.

Parts of the medial forebrain bundle, and of the mamillary peduncle are also seen.

Reticular Formation of the Brainstem

The term reticular formation was originally used to designate areas of the central nervous system which were not occupied by well defined nuclei or fibre bundles, but consisted of a network of fibres within which scattered neurons were situated. Such areas are to be found at all levels in the nervous system. In the spinal cord there is an intermingling of grey and white matter on the lateral side of the neck of the dorsal grey column. This area is sometimes referred to as the reticular formation of the spinal cord. The reticular formation is, however, best defined in the brainstem where it is now recognised as an area of considerable importance. Some centres in the cerebrum and cerebellum are regarded by some authorities to be closely related, functionally, to this region.

The reticular formation extends throughout the length of the brainstem. In the medulla it occupies the region dorsal to the inferior olivary nucleus. In the pons it lies in the dorsal part, while in the midbrain it lies in the tegmentum.

The neurons to be seen in the reticular formation vary considerably in the size of their cell bodies, the length and ramifications of their axons, and the behaviour of their dendrites. Many neurons have extensive dendritic trees and their ramifications may cover a wide extent both vertically and transversely. The connections of individual neurons are difficult to determine as many of the pathways concerned are polysynaptic.

ADVANCED

CLINICAL

BASIC

Fig. 11.14. Nuclei in the reticular formation of the brainstem. Also see Fig. 11.15

	MEDIAN COLUMN (Nuclei of Raphe)	MEDIAL COLUMN (Magnocellular)	LATERAL COLUMN (Magnocellular)
MID BRAIN	Nu raphes dorsalis	Circumaqueductal grey Deep tegmental nucleus Dorsal tegmental nucleus Nu. subcuneiformis Nu. cuneiformis	Nu. pedunculopontis Lat. partabrachial nucleus Med. parabrachial nucleus
PONS	Nu. raphes centralis superior Nu. raphes pontis Nu raphes magnus	Nu. coeruleus Nu. reticularis pontis oralis Nu. reticularis tegmenti pontis Nu. reticularis pontis caudalis Gigantocellular nucleus (Pontine part)	Central nucleus of pons
MEDULLA	Nu. raphes obscurus Nu. raphes pallidus	Gigantocellular nucleus (Medullary part)	Central nucleus of medulla Lateral reticular nucleus Ventral reticular nucleus

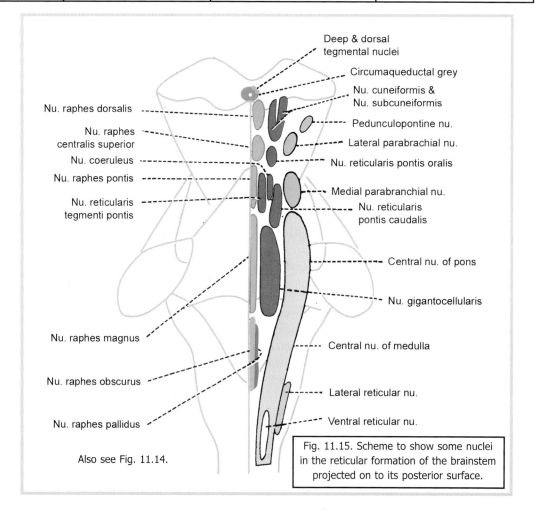

Fig. 11.15. Scheme to show some nuclei in the reticular formation of the brainstem projected on to its posterior surface.

A number of reticular nuclei have been described. The limits of such nuclei are ill defined, and their functional significance is often obscure. The following scheme includes the better known nuclei of the reticular formation.

Nuclei of the reticular formation of the brainstem

These can be divided into three longitudinal columns (in each half of the brainstem).

(a) The *median column* lies next to the middle line. The nuclei in it are called the *nuclei of the raphe,* or *paramedian nuclei.*

(b) The *medial column* (or *magnocellular* column) consists of nuclei having neurons of large or medium size.

(c) The nuclei of the *lateral column* are made up of small neurons. Because of this the lateral column is also referred to as the *parvocellular column.* The nuclei to be seen in each of these columns are named in Fig. 11.14 and are shown in Fig. 11.15.

Chemoarchitectonics of reticular formation

With the development of immuno-fluorescence techniques a number of neuromediators have been demonstrated in the reticular formation. These include acetylcholine, noradrenaline, adrenaline, dopamine (confined to the midbrain), and serotonin. New maps of the reticular formation, based on the distribution of such neuromediators, are now being drawn up (as for other regions of the nervous system). Such studies have created a new interesting science of *chemoarchitectonics*. It appears logical to assume that grouping of areas in this way may be of greater functional relevance than the division into ill defined nuclei.

Many neurons in the raphe nuclei are serotoninergic and constitute part of a system that ramifies into the entire central nervous system. This serotoninergic system is considered on page 157.

Connections of Reticular Formation

The reticular formation has numerous connections. Directly, or indirectly, it is connected to almost all parts of the nervous system. The better established afferents are shown in Fig. 11.16; and the efferents in Fig. 11.17.

The pathways involved are both ascending and descending; crossed and uncrossed; somatic and visceral. In the description that follows, the major pathways involving the reticular formation are taken up one by one. It must be emphasised, however, that the reticular formation is not to be regarded merely as a relay station on these pathways. It has an important regulatory role, both facilitatory and inhibitory.

Cortico-reticulo-spinal pathways

The reticular formation receives impulses from the motor and other areas of the cerebral cortex and relays them to the spinal cord through the medial and lateral reticulospinal tracts. The corticoreticular fibres descend along with corticospinal fibres. They terminate mainly in relation to the oral and caudal reticular nuclei of the pons, and the gigantocellular nucleus of the medulla. Fibres arising in the oral and caudal nuclei of the pons form the pontine (or medial) reticulospinal tract, while fibres arising in the gigantocellular nucleus form the medullary (or lateral) reticulospinal tract. Apart from these relatively better defined tracts reticulospinal fibres are widely scattered in the anterior and lateral funiculi of the spinal cord; and some descend through the intersegmental tracts. Apart from the nuclei mentioned above reticulospinal fibres may arise from other nuclei including the central nucleus of the medulla. The reticulospinal tracts are described on page 100.

The reticular formation also establishes connections with motor cranial nerve nuclei.

Cerebelloreticular connections

The following nuclei of the reticular formation have reciprocal connections with the cerebellum (Fig. 11.18).

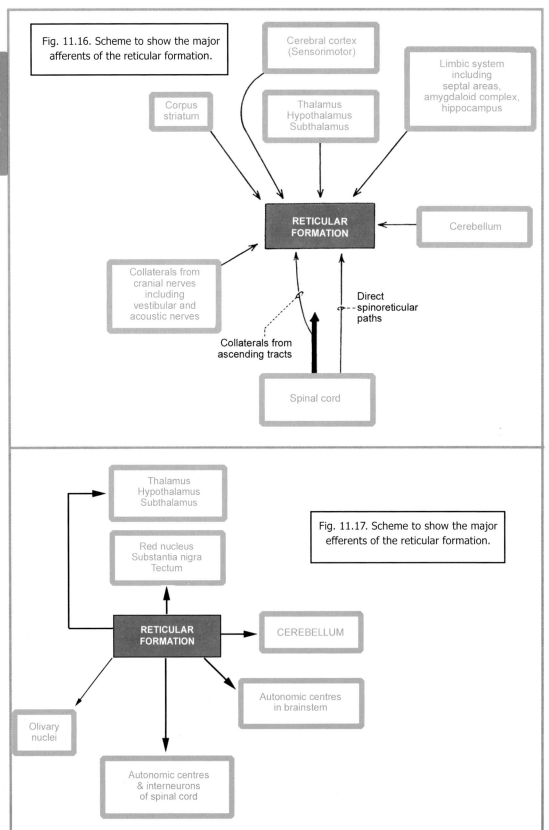

Fig. 11.16. Scheme to show the major afferents of the reticular formation.

Cerebral cortex (Sensorimotor)

Limbic system including septal areas, amygdaloid complex, hippocampus

Corpus striatum

Thalamus Hypothalamus Subthalamus

RETICULAR FORMATION

Cerebellum

Collaterals from cranial nerves including vestibular and acoustic nerves

Collaterals from ascending tracts

Direct spinoreticular paths

Spinal cord

Thalamus Hypothalamus Subthalamus

Red nucleus Substantia nigra Tectum

Fig. 11.17. Scheme to show the major efferents of the reticular formation.

RETICULAR FORMATION

CEREBELLUM

Autonomic centres in brainstem

Olivary nuclei

Autonomic centres & interneurons of spinal cord

ADVANCED

(1) Lateral reticular nucleus

(2) Paramedian reticular nucleus. (This nucleus is not included in the list given in Fig. 11.14. It is located in the medulla within the medial longitudinal fasciculus).

(3) Pontine tegmental reticular nucleus.

Through these connections the reticular formation connects the cerebral cortex, and the spinal cord, to the cerebellar cortex. For further details of reticulo-cerebellar connections see Chapter 12.

Ascending reticular activating system

It has been seen that many ascending tracts passing through the brainstem are intimately related to the reticular formation. Many of the fibres in these tracts give off collaterals to it. These come from the spinothalamic tracts, from secondary trigeminal pathways and from auditory pathways. These collaterals terminate predominantly in the lateral part of the reticular formation. Fibres arising here project to the intralaminar and reticular nuclei of the thalamus. These nuclei in turn project to widespread areas of the cerebral cortex. These pathways form part of the ***ascending reticular activating system*** (ARAS) which is believed to be responsible for maintaining a state of alertness.

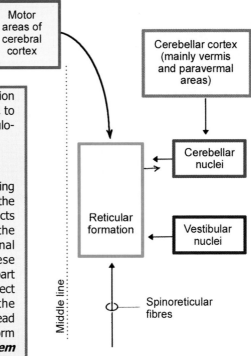

Fig. 11.18. Cerebello-reticular connections.

Summary of Functions of the Reticular Formation

Because of its diverse connections the reticular formation is believed to have a controlling or modifying influence on many functions. Some of them are as follows.

BASIC

A. Somatomotor control

Through its direct connections with the spinal cord; and indirectly through the corpus striatum, the cerebral cortex and the cerebellum, the reticular formation has an influence on fine control of movements including those involved in postural adjustments, locomotion, skilled use of the hands, speech etc.

B. Somatosensory control

The reticular formation influences conduction through somatosensory pathways. Similar effects may also be exerted on visual and auditory pathways.

C. Visceral control

Physiological studies have shown that stimulation of certain areas in the reticular formation of the medulla has great influence on respiratory and cardiovascular function. The region influencing respiratory activity corresponds approximately to the giganto-cellular nucleus and parvocellular nucleus. Stimulation of the gigantocellular nucleus and the upper part of the ventral reticular nucleus causes depression of vasomotor activity while stimulation of other areas has a pressor effect. These effects are through connections between the reticular formation and autonomic centres in the brainstem and spinal cord, but the pathways concerned are not well defined.

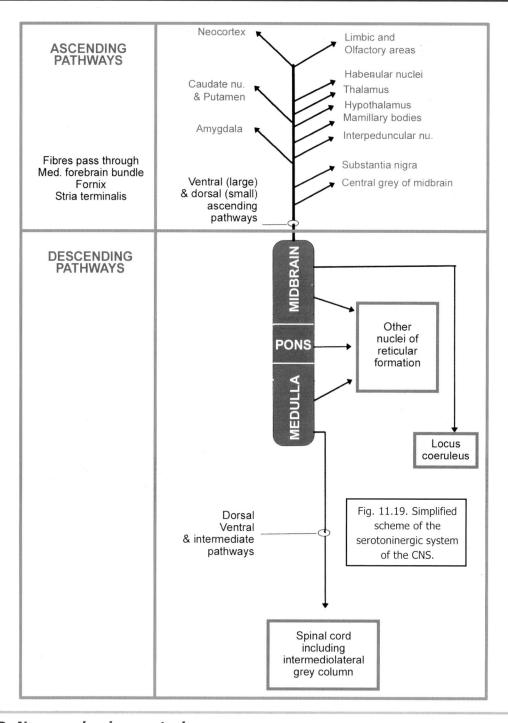

Fig. 11.19. Simplified scheme of the serotoninergic system of the CNS.

D. Neuroendocrine control

Through its connections with the hypothalamus, the reticular formation influences activity of the adenohypophysis and of the neurohypophysis.

A similar influence is also exerted on the pineal body.

E. The reticular formation also influences other hypothalamic functions. These include a possible effect on circadian rhythms.

BASIC

F. The significance of the reticular formation in controlling arousal and the state of consciousness through the ascending reticular activating system has been mentioned above.

The summary of the functions of the reticular formation given in the preceding paragraphs is based on traditional teaching. In the sections that follow some newer insights into the functional significance of the reticular formation are presented.

Serotoninergic Raphe System

The nuclei of the raphe (or raphe nuclei) have been described on page 153. They are also referred to as the paramedian reticular nuclei. Special interest in the raphe nuclei has ensued after the demonstration that they are the central part of an extensive serotoninergic system that permeates the entire nervous system as summarised below (Fig. 11.19).

1. Serotoninergic fibres descending from the raphe nuclei (mainly of the medulla) reach all levels of the spinal cord. Dorsal (or lateral) and ventral pathways are described. Many of the fibres end in relation to neurons of the intermediolateral grey column.

2. Descending fibres (from raphe nuclei in the midbrain, pons and medulla) also reach other nuclei of the reticular formation (dorsal tegmental nucleus in the midbrain, and other nuclei in the pons and medulla).

3. Fibres from the dorsal raphe nucleus (midbrain) descend to the locus coeruleus.

4. The nucleus raphe magnus projects to the caudal part of the spinal nucleus of the trigeminal nerve and influences perception of pain through the nucleus.

5. Ascending serotoninergic fibres take origin mainly from the dorsal raphe nucleus, and from the superior central nucleus. The fibres ascend as a large ventral bundle, and a much smaller dorsal bundle. On their journey upwards many of the fibres pass through the medial forebrain bundle. Some traverse the fornix, and the stria terminalis. The centres these fibres reach include the following.

Midbrain: Substantia nigra, central grey matter.

Diencephalon: Hypothalamus and mamillary body, thalamus, habenular nuclei.

Basal nuclei: Caudate nucleus, putamen, amygdala.

Cerebral cortex: Limbic, septal and olfactory areas; parts of neocortex.

The functions attributed to the serotoninergic system include the following.

(a) Fibres descending dorsally in the spinal cord may form part of a pain controlling pathway. They terminate mainly in the posterior grey column. Cranially, this pathway connects to some centres in the midbrain that constitute a pain control centre (periaqueductal grey, dorsal raphe nucleus and cuneiform nuclei).

(b) The 'intermediate' fibres descending into the spinal cord influence sympathetic control of the cardiovascular system.

(c) Ventrally descending fibres influence ventral horn cells to which they are facilitatory.

(d) Ascending serotoninergic fibres influence the activities of the areas to which they project, mainly those of the limbic and related areas.

Locus Coeruleus and Noradrenergic System

The locus coeruleus is an area in the floor of the fourth ventricle, at the upper end of the sulcus limitans. The area has a bluish colour caused by the presence of pigment in the underlying neurons. These neurons constitute the nucleus coeruleus.

With the development of techniques for localisation of neuropeptides in neurons and their processes it has been found that the locus coeruleus contains noradrenergic neurons. It lies at the heart of an extensive system of noradrenergic fibres permeating the brain. Apart from the locus coeruleus noradrenergic neurons are located in the nuclei forming the lateral column of the reticular formation; in the median eminence; and in some other situations. The fibres of the noradrenergic system are ascending and descending.

ADVANCED

Descending fibres:

Descending fibres travel to the pontine nuclei, reticular formation of the medulla, and several cranial nerve nuclei (cochlear nuclei, nucleus of tractus solitarius, spinal nucleus of trigeminal nerve, dorsal nucleus of vagus). Fibres descend into the spinal cord in the anterior and lateral funiculi. These fibres terminate in both the dorsal and ventral grey columns, and specially in relation to neurons giving origin to the sacral parasympathetic outflow.

Ascending fibres

Ascending noradrenergic fibres permeate into many parts of the brain. Within the midbrain they reach the colliculi and the central grey matter. Some fibres reach the cerebellum (cortex as well as cerebellar nuclei).

Fibres ascending into the cerebral hemisphere travel through many fibre bundles mentioned elsewhere. They include the central tegmental tract, medial and lateral longitudinal striae, stria terminalis, fornix, mammilothalamic tract and the diagonal band. The areas receiving the noradrenergic fibres include the following.

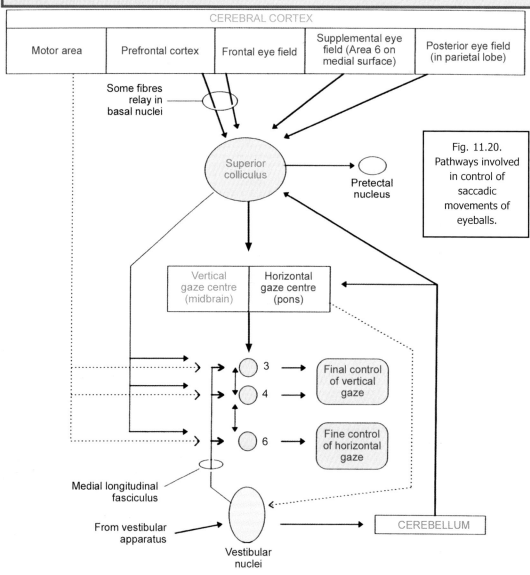

Fig. 11.20. Pathways involved in control of saccadic movements of eyeballs.

In the diencephalon: Thalamus, hypothalamus, habenular nuclei, interpeduncular nucleus.

In the telencephalon: Parts of neocortex; limbic cortex including the cingulate gyrus, the parahippocampal gyrus and the hippocampus; septal areas, anterior perforated substance, olfactory bulb and anterior olfactory nucleus.

The functions of the noradrenergic system are not well understood. The system probably plays a role in control of cardiovascular, respiratory and gastrointestinal functions. It may have a role in circadian rhythms (including the sleep-waking cycle).

Control of Eye Movements

The cranial nerve nuclei that innervate the muscles that move the eyeballs are under the influence of a complex network involving the cerebral cortex, the cerebellum, the superior colliculus, the vestibular nuclei and other centres (Figs. 11.20, 11.21). As many of the centres involved lie in the brainstem it is convenient to consider the entire system here.

The gross control of ocular movements is similar to that for other movements. The motor area of the cerebral cortex projects to the cranial nerve nuclei concerned through corticonuclear fibres. The nuclei are also influenced by other centres. In this section we will consider some aspects of the control of fine movements of the eyeballs.

When the gaze is shifted from one object to another the eyes undergo sharp movements called *saccades*. The controlling centres determine the velocity and extent of a saccade. A different kind of control is required when the eyes follow a moving object (*pursuit movement*).

A. The areas of cerebral cortex involved in programming and co-ordination of all eye movements are:

(a) the frontal eye field (area 8);

(b) the supplemental eye field located on the medial surface of the hemisphere (area 6).

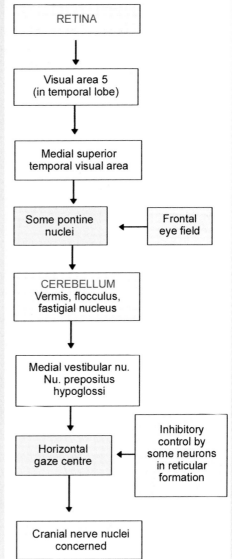

Fig. 11.21. Scheme to show control of smooth pursuit eye movements.

(c) the prefrontal cortex (anterior to the frontal eye field); and

(d) the posterior eye field (in the parietal lobe).

B. The areas of cerebral cortex listed above project to the superior colliculus (some of them passing via the basal nuclei). The superior colliculus also receives fibres from the retinae, from pretectal nuclei, and from the cerebellum.

C. The superior colliculus projects to two important centres which are as follows.

(1) The *vertical gaze centre* lies in the midbrain. It is located in the rostral interstitial nucleus (a collection of neurons within the medial longitudinal fasciculus), and in the interstitial nucleus of Cajal. This centre controls vertical eye movements.

(2) The ***horizontal gaze centre*** lies in the pons, in the paramedian reticular formation. The centre controls horizontal eye movements.

In addition to the afferents from the superior colliculus, these centres also receive:

(a) some direct cortical fibres; and

(b) fibres from the cerebellum.

Efferents from the vertical and horizontal gaze centres project to the oculomotor, trochlear and abducent nuclei.

D. The cranial nerve nuclei supplying muscles of the eyeball receive the following afferents.

(a) Corticonuclear fibres.

(b) Fibres from the vertical and horizontal gaze centres described above.

(c) Direct fibres from the superior colliculus and from pretectal nuclei.

(d) Fibres from vestibular nuclei. These travel through the medial longitudinal fasciculus. They provide information about movements of the head and neck (from the vestibular apparatus). Through the vestibular nuclei, the oculomotor trochlear and abducent nuclei are brought under cerebellar control.

E. The final control of vertical gaze is by fibres passing from the oculomotor and trochlear nuclei (to reach muscles producing upward and downward movements of the eyeballs). The final control of horizontal gaze is mainly by the abducent nerve (lateral rectus), but is also influenced by the oculomotor nerve (medial rectus).

The horizontal gaze centre is also involved in control of eye movements when the gaze follows a moving object. These are called 'pursuit movements'. The control of these movements is complex and is summarised in Fig. 11.21.

Injury to the medulla is usually fatal because vital centres controlling the heart and respiration are located here. As tracts are closely packed as they pass through the brainstem lesions produce widespread effect. Paralysis due to a lesion in the medulla is called ***bulbar palsy***. In this condition the 9th, 10th, 11th and 12th cranial nerves are affected.

Damage to corticospinal tracts in the brainstem roduces various syndromes. See ***Weber's syndrome***, ***Raymond's syndrome*** and ***Millard Gubler syndrome*** (all on page 104).

The blood supply of the medulla is described in Chapter 21. See ***pontine haemorrhage, lateral medullary syndrome*** and ***medial medullary syndrome*** in thiat chapter.

Abnormality in upward gaze can occur in tumours of the pineal body. This is called ***Parinaud's syndrome***.

DEVELOPMENT OF THE MEDULLA OBLONGATA

The medulla oblongata develops from the myelencephalon. The early development of the medulla is similar to that of the spinal cord. The appearance of the sulcus limitans divides each lateral wall into a dorsal or alar lamina, and a ventral or basal lamina. Subsequently, the thin ***roof plate*** becomes greatly widened as a result of which the alar laminae come to lie dorso-lateral to the basal laminae. Thus, both these laminae are now in the floor of the developing fourth ventricle.

Cells developing in the lateral part of each alar lamina migrate ventrally, and reach the marginal layer overlying the ventrolateral aspect of the basal lamina. These cells constitute the caudal part of the ***bulbo-pontine extension***, and develop into the ***olivary nuclei***. The remaining cells of the alar lamina develop into the sensory nuclei of the cranial nerves related to the medulla. The motor nuclei of these nerves are derived from the basal lamina as described in Chapter 10.

The ***gracile and cuneate nuclei*** are derived from the lowermost part of the somatic afferent column.

The *white matter* of the medulla is predominantly extraneous in origin, being composed of fibres constituting the ascending and descending tracts that pass through the medulla.

DEVELOPMENT OF PONS

The pons arises from the ventral part of the metencephalon. It also receives a contribution from the alar lamina of the myelencephalon, in the form of the cranial part of the bulbopontine extension. This extension comes to lie ventral to the metencephalon, and gives rise to the *pontine nuclei*. Axons of cells in these nuclei grow transversely to form the *middle cerebellar peduncle*.

As in the myelencephalon, the roof of the metencephalon becomes thin and broad. The alar and basal laminae are thus orientated as in the medulla.

The lateral part of each alar lamina (often called the *rhombic lip*) becomes specialised to form the cerebellum. The ventral part of the alar lamina gives origin to the sensory cranial nerve nuclei, and the basal lamina to the motor cranial nerve nuclei, of the pons as described in Chapter 10..

The nuclei derived from the basal, and alar, laminae lie in the dorsal or tegmental part of the pons. The ventral part of the pons is constituted by:

(a) Cells of the bulbopontine extension (derived from the alar lamina of the myelencephalon), form the pontine nuclei. Axons of the cells in these nuclei grow transversely and form the *middle cerebellar peduncle*.

(b) Corticospinal and corticobulbar fibres that descend from the cerebral cortex, and pass through this region on their way to the medulla and spinal cord. Some fibres from the cerebral cortex terminate in relation to the pontine nuclei. These are the corticopontine fibres.

DEVELOPMENT OF THE MIDBRAIN

The midbrain is developed from the mesencephalon. The cavity of the mesencephalon remains narrow and forms the aqueduct. As described in the case of the spinal cord, the mantle layer becomes subdivided into a dorsal or alar lamina and a ventral or basal lamina by the appearance of the sulcus limitans. The nuclei which develop from the basal lamina are: (1) the oculomotor nerve nucleus, (2) the trochlear nerve nucleus, and (3) the Edinger Westphal nucleus (GVE).

The alar lamina gives rise to the cells of the colliculi. At first, these form one mass which later becomes subdivided by a transverse fissure. Some cells of the alar lamina migrate ventrally to form the *red nucleus* and the *substantia nigra*.

The marginal layer of the ventral part of the mesencephalon is invaded by downward growing fibres of the corticospinal, corticobulbar and corticopontine pathways. This region, thus, becomes greatly expanded, and forms the *basis pedunculi* (crus cerebri).

RELATED TOPICS IN OTHER CHAPTERS

12 : Internal Structure of Cerebellum

PART 1 : BASIC FACTS ABOUT CEREBELLAR STRUCTURE

The gross anatomy of the cerebellum has been described on page 73. It has been noted that the grey matter of the cerebellum consists of the cerebellar cortex and of the cerebellar nuclei: dentate, emboliform, globose and fastigial (Fig. 7.4). The structure of the cerebellar cortex and the connections of the cerebellum are considered in this chapter. As this chapter contains many details (that the average undergraduate does not need to know) the chapter is divided into two parts. Part 1 gives essential facts only, while details are given in Part 2.

Basic Structure of the Cerebellar Cortex

In striking contrast to the cortex of the cerebral hemispheres, the cerebellar cortex has a uniform structure in all parts of the cerebellum. It may be divided into three layers (Fig. 12.1) as follows.

(a) **Molecular layer** (most superficial).

(b) **Purkinje cell layer**. (The Purkinje cell layer is often described as part of the molecular layer).

(c) **Granular layer**, which rests on white matter.

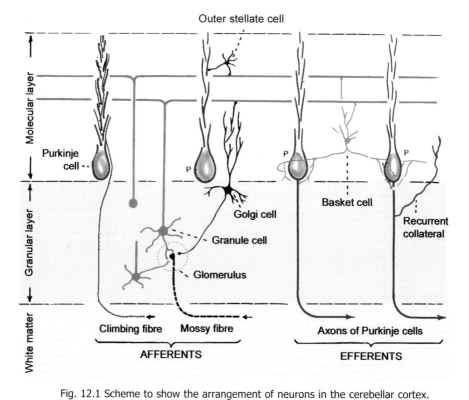

Fig. 12.1 Scheme to show the arrangement of neurons in the cerebellar cortex.

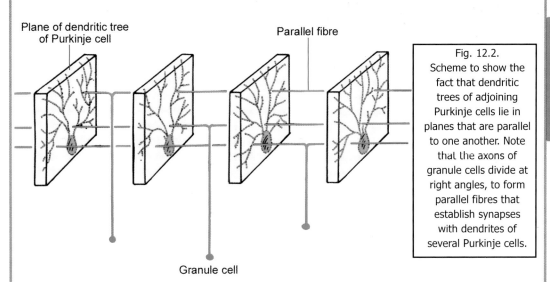

Plane of dendritic tree of Purkinje cell

Parallel fibre

Granule cell

Fig. 12.2. Scheme to show the fact that dendritic trees of adjoining Purkinje cells lie in planes that are parallel to one another. Note that the axons of granule cells divide at right angles, to form parallel fibres that establish synapses with dendrites of several Purkinje cells.

The neurons of the cerebellar cortex are of five main types.

(a) *Purkinje cells*, forming the layer named after them.

(b) *Granule cells*, forming the granular layer.

(c) *Outer (external) stellate cells;* and

(d) *Basket cells*, lying in the molecular layer.

(e) *Golgi cells*, present in the granular layer.

(f) *Brush cells* present in the granular layer.

The processes of these neurons have a definite orientation in relation to cerebellar folia. The main relationships are illustrated in Figs 12.1 and 12.2. The neurons in the molecular layer are supported by large neuroglial cells.

Purkinje cells

The Purkinje cell layer is unusual in that it contains only one layer of neurons. The cell bodies of these neurons are large and flask-shaped. The cells are evenly spaced. A dendrite arises from the 'neck' of the 'flask' and passes 'upwards' into the molecular layer. Here it divides and subdivides to form an elaborate dendritic tree. The branches of this 'tree' all lie in one plane (like the fins of a fan; or like a vine branching against a wall, Fig. 12.2). This plane is transverse to the long axis of the folium. As a result of this arrangement the dendritic trees of adjoining Purkinje cells lie in planes more or less parallel to one another.

The axon of each Purkinje cell passes 'downwards' through the granular layer to enter the white matter. As described later these axons constitute the only efferents of the cerebellar cortex. They end, predominantly, by synapsing with neurons in cerebellar nuclei. They are inhibitory to these neurons.

Further facts about these cells are given on page 169.

Granule cells

These are very small, numerous, spherical neurons that occupy the greater part of the granular layer. The spaces not occupied by them are called *cerebellar islands*. These islands are occupied by special synaptic structures called *glomeruli*.

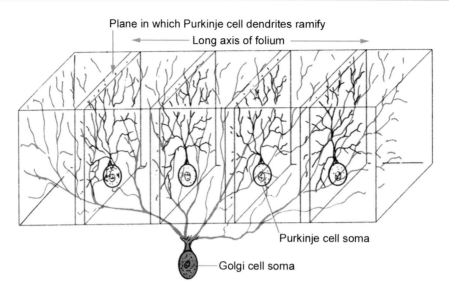

Fig. 12.3. Diagram showing relationship of dendrites of one Golgi neuron to those of Purkinje cells.

Each granule cell gives off three to five short dendrites. These end in claw-like endings which enter the glomeruli where they synapse with the terminals of mossy fibres (see below). The axon of each granule cell enters the molecular layer. Here it divides into two subdivisions each of which is at right angles to the parent axon (forming a T-junction). These axonal branches of granule cells are called **parallel fibres**. The granule cells being extremely numerous, the parallel fibres are also abundant and almost fill the molecular layer. The parallel fibres run at right angles to the planes of the dendritic trees of Purkinje cells. As a result each parallel fibre comes into contact, and synapses, with the dendrites of numerous Purkinje cells. Parallel fibres also synapse with Golgi cells, basket cells and stellate cells.

Golgi neurons

These are large, stellate cells lying in the granular layer (Fig. 12.2, 12.3), just deep to the Purkinje cells. They are GABAergic inhibitory neurons. Their dendrites enter the molecular layer, where they branch profusely, and synapse with the parallel fibres. Some dendrites ramify in the granular layer. The axons of these neurons also branch profusely. These branches permeate the whole thickness of the granular layer. They take part in the formation of glomeruli. Some dendritic branches also reach the glomeruli. For some details see page 170

Other cells of the cerebellar cortex are described on page 170.

Afferent Fibres entering the Cerebellar Cortex

In addition to the dendrites and axons of the cells described listed on page 163, the cerebellar cortex contains fibres that are terminations of cerebellar afferents. Histologically, these are of two distinct types.

(a) Mossy fibres:

Some fibres terminate in the granular layer of the cortex, within glomeruli. These are called mossy fibres. They branch profusely within the granular layer, each branch ending in an expanded terminal called a **rosette** (See below).

All fibres entering the cerebellum, other than olivocerebellar, end as mossy fibres. As explained below, afferent inputs through mossy fibres pass through granule cells to reach Purkinje cells.

(b) Climbing fibres:

These fibres represent terminations of axons reaching the cerebellum from the inferior olivary complex (Fig. 12.4). They pass through the granular layer, and the Purkinje cell layer, to reach the molecular layer. Each climbing fibre become intimately associated with the proximal part of the dendritic tree of one Purkinje cell, and establishes numerous synapses on them. (These are called climbing fibres as they appear to **climb up** along the Purkinje cell dendrites).

There has been considerable doubt regarding the source of mossy fibres and of climbing fibres.

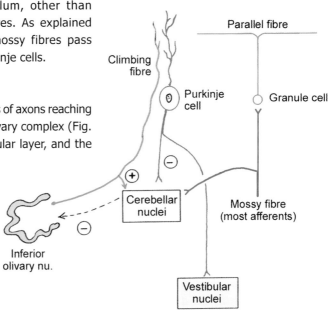

Fig. 12.4. Basic arrangement of connections within the cerebellar cortex.

It is now established that olivo-cerebellar fibres end predominantly as climbing fibres, while all other afferents end predominantly as mossy fibres. Both mossy fibres and climbing fibres are excitatory.

Main Connections of the Cerebellum

The fundamental points to be appreciated in considering the connections of the cerebellum are that, as a rule (Fig. 12.5):

(a) afferent fibres terminate in the cortex;

(b) efferent fibres arising in the cortex end in cerebellar nuclei; and

(c) fibres arising in the nuclei project to centres outside the cerebellum.

There are, however, important exceptions to these rules. Some fibres (notably vestibular) project directly to the cerebellar nuclei. Some parts of the cortex give off efferents that bypass the nuclei to reach centres outside the cerebellum.

The cerebellum receives direct afferents from the spinal cord and from various centres in the brainstem. The main afferents are (Fig. 12.6):

(1) *Spinocerebellar*. These terminate predominantly in the paleocerebellum.

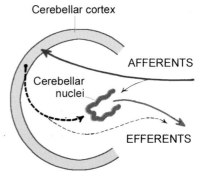

Fig. 12.5. Scheme to show the fundamental arrangement of cerebellar afferents and efferents.

(2) *Pontocerebellar*. These are part of the cortico-ponto-cerebellar pathway. They end predominantly in the neocerebellum.

(3) *Olivocerebellar*. These end mainly in the neocerebellum and partly in the paleocerebellum.

(4) *Vestibulocerebellar*, from the vestibular nuclei, and also direct fibres of the vestibular nerve.

(5) *Reticulocerebellar* fibres from the reticular formation of the pons and of the medulla.

The cerebellum also receives fibres from the tectum, the arcuate nuclei, the accessory cuneate nucleus, and from the sensory nuclei of the trigeminal nerve.

The main efferents of the cerebellum are (Fig. 12.6):

(1) *Cerebellorubral*, to the red nucleus of the opposite side.

(2) *Cerebellothalamic*, to the thalamus of the opposite side.

(3) *Cerebellovestibular*, to the vestibular nuclei.

(4) *Cerebelloreticular*, to the reticular formation.

Some fibres from the cerebellum also reach the inferior olivary nucleus, the nucleus of the oculomotor nerve, and the tectum.

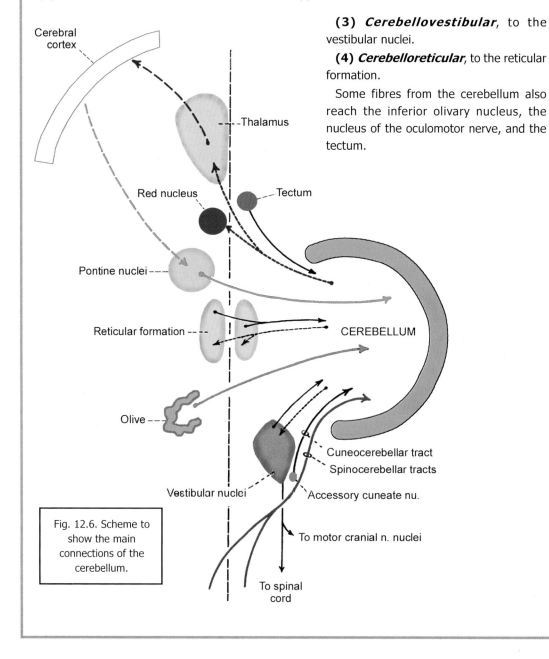

Fig. 12.6. Scheme to show the main connections of the cerebellum.

Cerebellar peduncles

Some features of cerebellar peduncles have been described on page 76. The various fibres entering or leaving the cerebellum pass through the superior, middle and inferior cerebellar peduncles. These connect the cerebellum to the midbrain, the pons and the medulla respectively The fibres composing each peduncle are enumerated below.

BASIC

SUPERIOR CEREBELLAR PEDUNCLE

A. Fibres entering the cerebellum
1. Ventral spino-cerebellar tract. **2**. Rostral (or superior) spino-cerebellar tract.
3. Tecto-cerebellar fibres. **4**. Rubro-cerebellar fibres.
5. Trigemino-cerebellar fibres, from mesencephalic nucleus.
6. Hypothalamo-cerebellar fibres.
7. Coerulo-cerebellar fibres. These are noradrenergic fibres from the nucleus coeruleus.

B. Fibres leaving the cerebellum
1. Cerebello-rubral fibres. **2**. Cerebello-thalamic fibres. Cerebellorubral and cerebellothalamic fibres arise from the dentate, emboliform and globose nuclei.
3. Cerebello-reticular fibres (from dentate nucleus, some from the fastigial nucleus).
4. Cerebello-olivary fibres (from dentate, emboliform and globose nuclei).
5. Cerebello-nuclear fibres. These enter the medial longitudinal fasciculus to reach motor nuclei of nerves supplying the muscles of the eyeball.
6. Some fibres to the hypothalamus and subthalamus.

MIDDLE CEREBELLAR PEDUNCLE

This is made up of ponto-cerebellar fibres. Some serotoninergic fibres from the reticular formation of the pons also pass through it.

INFERIOR CEREBELLAR PEDUNCLE

A. Fibres entering the cerebellum
1. Posterior spino-cerebellar tract. **2**. Cuneo-cerebellar tract (posterior external arcuate fibres).
3. Olivo-cerebellar fibres from the inferior olivary complex (including parolivocerebellar fibres from accessory olivary nuclei). **4**. Reticulo-cerebellar fibres.   **5**. Vestibulo-cerebellar fibres.
6. Anterior external arcuate fibres from arcuate nuclei. **7**. Fibres of striae medullares.
8. Trigemino-cerebellar fibres, from main sensory and spinal nuclei.

B. Fibres leaving the cerebellum
1. Cerebello-olivary fibres. **2**. Cerebello-vestibular fibres. **3**. Cerebello-reticular fibres (from fastigial nucleus). **4**. Some cerebello-spinal and cerebello-nuclear fibres are also present.

Connections between Cerebellum and Spinal Cord

From a clinical point of view the most important connections of the cerebellum are with the spinal cord, and with the cerebral cortex. These connections are through various pathways that are summarised below.

Spinocerebellar pathways convey to the cerebellum proprioceptive information necessary for controlling muscle tone and for maintaining body posture. These pathways also carry exteroceptive impulses.

(a) Direct pathways from spinal cord to cerebellum

These are the ventral spinocerebellar tract, and the dorsal spinocerebellar tract which convey information from the hind limb. Information from the forelimb is probably conveyed by the rostral spinocerebellar tract and the cuneocerebellar tract (page 112). The cuneocerebellar tract begins in the medulla, but is included here as it is functionally equivalent to spinocerebellar tracts.

(b) Indirect pathways from spinal cord to cerebellum

These are:

(a) Spino-olivo-cerebellar; (b) Spino-reticulo-cerebellar; (c) Spino-vestibulo-cerebellar; and (d) Spino-tecto-cerebellar pathways.

Although these are not concerned with the spinal cord it is useful to consider here the pathways that carry impulses from tissues in the head to the cerebellum. Exteroceptive impulses from the head (and parts of the neck) reach the cerebellum through trigemino-cerebellar fibres arising in the main sensory and spinal nuclei of this nerve. Fibres from the mesencephalic nucleus convey proprioceptive information from the muscles of mastication to the cerebellum. (Also see page 120).

(c) Cerebello-spinal pathways

Although the presence of some direct cerebellospinal fibres has been claimed, their existence is not established. The cerebellum can, however, influence the spinal cord through the following pathways:

(a) Cerebello-rubro-spinal; (b) Cerebello-vestibulo-spinal; (c) Cerebello-reticulo-spinal; (d) Cerebello-tecto-spinal; and (e) Cerebello-thalamo-cortico-spinal.

Connections between Cerebellum and Cerebral Cortex

The connections between the cerebellum and the cerebral cortex are all indirect.

Cortico-cerebellar pathways

The cerebral cortex influences the cerebellum through various centres in the brainstem (and possibly even through the spinal cord) through the following pathways.

(a) The most important of these is the cortico-ponto-cerebellar pathway considered on page 102. The arcuate nuclei and the pontobulbar body represent displaced pontine nuclei. The cortico-arcuato-cerebellar, and the cortico-pontobulbar-cerebellar pathways are, functionally, equivalent to the cortico-ponto-cerebellar pathway.

Other pathways connecting the cerebral cortex to the cerebellum are as follows.

(b) Cortico-olivo-cerebellar; (c) Cortico-reticulo-cerebellar; (d) Cortico-rubro-cerebellar; (e) Cortico-tecto-cerebellar; and (f) Cortico-spino-cerebellar.

Some of the impulses may reach these intermediary centres through the corpus striatum.

Cerebello-cortical pathways

We have seen that the cerebellum projects upon the cerebellar nuclei from where fresh fibres relay to the thalamus. Thalamocortical fibres carry these impulses to the cerebral cortex. Cerebellar impulses can also reach the cerebral cortex through a cerebello-reticulo-thalamo-cortical pathway.

Functions of the Cerebellum

BASIC

The cerebellum plays an essential role in the control of movement. It is responsible for ensuring that movement takes place smoothly, in the right direction, and to the right extent. Cerebellar stimulation modifies movements produced by stimulation of motor areas of the cerebral cortex. The cerebellar cortex is also important for learning of movements (e.g., in learning to write).

Through its vestibular and spinal connections the cerebellum is responsible for maintaining the equilibrium of the body.

These functions are possible because the cerebellum receives constant information regarding the state of contraction of muscles, and of the position of various joints. It also receives information from the eyes, the ears, the vestibular apparatus, the reticular formation and the cerebral cortex. All this information is integrated, and is used to influence movement through motor centres in the brainstem and spinal cord, and also through the cerebral cortex.

Recent studies have shown that the importance of the cerebellum may extend beyond control of motor activity. It has been postulated that the cerebellum may influence autonomic functions; that through the reticular formation and the thalamus it may influence conduction in ascending sensory pathways; and that the cerebral cortex and cerebellar cortex may cooperate in other complex ways. The role of the cerebellum in the control of complex eye movements is discussed on page 181.

Some effects of cerebellar dysfunction see page 181.

PART 2: FURTHER DETAILS ABOUT CEREBELLAR STRUCTURE

Further Details about the Cerebellar Cortex

ADVANCED

Some details about Purkinje cells

First see page 163. With the EM the dendrites of these cells can be seen to be studded with numerous spines. Some synapses occur on these spines, and others on the 'smooth' parts of dendrites between the spines. The dendrites of Purkinje cells synapse with axons of granule cells (parallel fibres), outer stellate cells, and basket cells (see below); and with climbing fibres (representing olivocerebellar afferents). Climbing fibres synapse with the proximal parts of dendrites while parallel fibres synapse on the distal parts.

The axons give off collaterals that remain within the cortex and synapse with Golgi cells. Some collaterals enter the molecular layer. The part of the Purkinje cell axon next to the cell body resembles the cell body in structure and is called the preaxon.

Purkinje cell zones

From the point of view of its connections the cerebellar cortex can be divided into vermal, paravermal and lateral zones. The paravermal zone is also called the pars intermedia. On the basis of recent studies a more detailed map of parasagittal zones (called Purkinje cell zones) has been described (Fig. 12.4). The zones (in each half of the cerebellar cortex) are designated A to D (in medial to lateral sequence). Zones A and B lie in the vermis, zone C in the pars intermedia, and zone D in the lateral area.

Zone A lies immediately lateral to the middle line and includes the whole of the vermis except a strip occupied by zone B (see below).

Zone B occupies the lateral and anterior part of the vermis. It includes the lateral parts of the lingula, central lobule, culmen and declive.

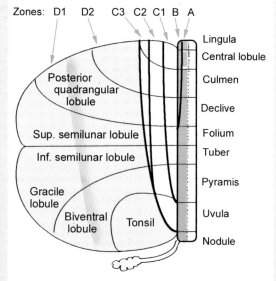

Fig. 12.7. Diagram showing Purkinje cell zones.

Zone C occupies the pars intermedia. It is divided into three strips C1, C2 and C3 (medial to lateral). Strips C1 and C3 extend caudally up to the level of the pyramis. Strip C2 (lying between C1 and C3) extends further caudally into the medial part of the tonsil.

Zone D is constituted by the part of the cerebellar hemisphere not occupied by zone C. It occupies the greater part of the hemisphere. It is sometimes divided into a medial part zone D1, and a lateral part zone D2.

Some details about Golgi neurons

First see page 164. Each Golgi neuron occupies a definite area there being no overlap between the territories of neighbouring Golgi cells. It is interesting to note that the territory of each Golgi cell corresponds to that of about ten Purkinje cells.

The outer stellate cells, the basket cells, and the Golgi cells are inhibitory neurons. Golgi cells are responsible for feedback inhibition of granule cells.

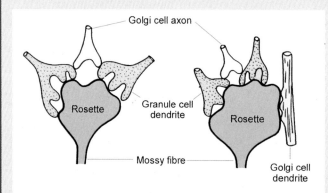

Fig. 12.8. Structure of cerebellar glomeruli.
The outer capsule is not shown.

Outer Stellate cells

These cells and their processes are confined to the molecular layer of the cerebellar cortex. Their dendrites (which are few) synapse with parallel fibres (of granule cells) while their axons synapse with dendrites of Purkinje cells (near their origin).

Basket cells

These cell lie in the deeper part of the molecular layer of the cerebellar cortex. Their dendrites that are few ramify in the molecular layer and are intersected by parallel fibres with which they synapse. They also receive recurrent collaterals from

Purkinje cells, climbing fibres, and mossy fibres. The axons of these cells branch, and form networks (or baskets) around the cell bodies of Purkinje cells. Their terminations synapse with Purkinje cells at the junction of cell body and axon (preaxon). Each basket cell may synapse with about 70 Purkinje neurons. Basket cells and stellate cells are GABAergic. They are inhibitory to Purkinje cells.

Brush cells (or monodendritic cells)

These are small cells present in the granular layer. Each cell gives off a single dendrite the branches of which give a brush-like appearance. The dendrite synapses with mossy fibres. The axon of the cell is thin and its connections are unknown.

Structure of Glomeruli

The glomeruli (referred to on page 163) are complex synaptic structures. The core of each glomerulus is formed by the expanded termination of a mossy fibre (Fig. 12.8). This termination is called a *rosette*. Numerous (up to 20) dendrites of granule cells synapse with the rosette. These synapses are axodendritic and excitatory.

The glomerulus also receives axon terminals of Golgi cells. These also synapse with granule cell dendrites. These synapses are inhibitory. Occasionally, a Golgi cell dendrite may enter a glomerulus and synapse directly with the rosette. The entire glomerulus (which is about 10 μm in diameter) is surrounded by a neuroglial capsule.

Some quantitative data regarding the Cerebellar Cortex

Extensive researches have revealed interesting quantitative data about the cerebellar cortex as follows.

1. The cerebellar cortex has a total surface area of approximately 200,000 square millimeters.
2. The cortex underlying each square millimetre of surface area contains:
(a) about 500 Purkinje neurons;
(b) about 600 basket cells;
(c) about 50 Golgi neurons;
(d) about 3,000,000 granule cells; and
(e) about 600,000 glomeruli.
3. Each axon reaching the cerebellar cortex from the olive divides into about ten climbing fibres. Each olivary neuron, therefore, establishes connections with about ten Purkinje cells.
4. Each mossy fibre synapses with about 400 granule cells. The axons of each granule cell synapse with about 300 to 450 Purkinje neurons.
5. Each Purkinje neuron may bear up to 80,000 synapses with different parallel fibres. The dendritic tree of a single Purkinje cell may be crossed by about 250,000 parallel fibres.

Neurochemistry of the Cerebellum

Recent researches have revealed the presence of several neuroactive substances, and receptors for them, in the cerebellum. Details of these are beyond the scope of this book. Some facts are as follows.

1. Neuroactive substances present in the cerebellum include L-glutamate, aspartate, GABA, serotonin, noradrenalin, acetyl choline, enkephalin and somatostatin.
2. The main neurotransmitter in the cerebellum is L-glutamate. Afferents reaching Purkinje cells through climbing fibres and through the mossy fibre — granule cell — parallel fibre system are glutamatergic. They are excitatory. Some mossy fibres arising in vestibular nuclei are cholinergic. Some reticulocerebellar fibres are serotoninergic, while coeruleo-cerebellar fibres are noradrenergic. Some dopaminergic and cholinergic fibres are also present.
3. Purkinje cells themselves are GABAergic and are inhibitory to cerebellar (and vestibular) nuclei. Some Purkinje cells contain a class of proteins called zebrins. Zebrin containing and non-zebrin containing Purkinje cells may occupy alternating bands of cortex.

ADVANCED

Golgi cells, stellate cells and basket cells are GABAergic. Some basket cells, and some granule cells, show the presence of nitrous oxide (NO) which may be a neurotransmitter.

4. Neurons in cerebellar nuclei are glutamatergic (excitatory), or GABAergic (inhibitory). The latter project to olivary nuclei. Some neurons in cerebellar nuclei are glycinergic. These are interneurons and may contain GABA in addition to glycine.

Apart from the neurotransmitters associated with them, cerebellar nerve fibres show the presence of various other neuroactive substances. These include enkephalin, somatostatin, aspartate, and corticotropin releasing factor.

Cerebellar neurons show interesting specialisations of their enzyme systems.

Receptors for neurotransmitters have been demonstrated in cerebellar neurons. Several types of glutamate receptors and GABA receptors can be distinguished. The receptors may be ionotropic (coupled to ion channels) or metabotropic (coupled to other messengers). Some are voltage dependent and cause opening of Ca^{++} channels in postsynaptic neurons.

Further Details of Cerebellar Connections

Intracortical connections

Within the cerebellum the Purkinje cell axons are the only ones that enter the white matter from the cortex. Hence all afferent impulses (brought by climbing fibres and mossy fibres must ultimately reach Purkinje cells. We have seen that climbing fibres synapse directly with Purkinje cells. Mossy fibres, however, influence Purkinje cells through granule cells. Another important difference between the climbing and mossy fibres is that whereas one climbing fibre specifically influences one Purkinje cell, the influence of a mossy fibre is far more diffuse. This is so because, firstly, one mossy fibre synapses with several granule cells; and secondly, each granule cell synapses with numerous Purkinje cells through parallel fibres (See page 164). Both these influences (i.e., of climbing fibres, and of mossy fibres through granule cells) are excitatory to Purkinje cells.

We have seen that parallel fibres (carrying impulses from mossy fibres relayed by granule cells) synapse with dendrites of basket cells, stellate cells and Golgi cells. The axons of stellate and basket cells end in direct relation to Purkinje cells. They are inhibitory to the Purkinje cells. The axons of Golgi cells (terminating in relation to glomeruli) are believed to exert an inhibiting influence on the synapses between mossy fibres and granule cell dendrites.

Purkinje cell activity occurs as a result of all these influences. We have seen that Purkinje cells project to cerebellar nuclei. Physiological

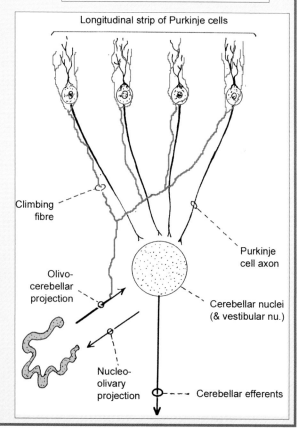

Fig. 12.9. Scheme to illustrate the concept of cerebellar modules

Longitudinal strip of Purkinje cells

Climbing fibre

Olivo-cerebellar projection

Nucleo-olivary projection

Purkinje cell axon

Cerebellar nuclei (& vestibular nu.)

Cerebellar efferents

evidence suggests that this influence is inhibitory to these nuclei. Excitatory influences probably reach these nuclei through collaterals from various cerebellar afferents.

Cerebellar modules

Recently it has been proposed that the cerebellum is divisible into a large number of discrete 'modules' each consisting of a group of Purkinje cells, their axons, and groups of cells in cerebellar nuclei in which they end (Fig. 12.9). Climbing fibres are also included in this modular concept which has been described as 'modular organisation of cerebellar output'.

Functional localisation in the cerebellum

In the cerebellar cortex it is possible to localise areas that receive afferents from different parts of the body. There is a double representation on the superior and inferior surfaces of the cerebellum. Representation on the superior surface is ipsilateral; and that on the inferior surface is bilateral. On either surface the anteroposterior sequence of parts represented is leg, trunk, arm and head. These area are located in vermal and paravermal areas (paleocerebellum) and correspond to areas that receive fibres from the spinal cord. Stimulation of these areas produces movements in parts of the body that correspond roughly to those from which sensory impulses are received.

In addition to proprioceptive impulses the cerebellum receives visual impulses which reach the folium and tuber. A second visual area is located in the biventral lobule and tonsil. These visual areas also receive auditory impulses. Vestibular impulses are received mainly by the nodule and flocculus.

The regions of cerebellar cortex from which efferent projections pass to the cerebellar nuclei are arranged in a medio-lateral sequence corresponding to the position of the nuclei. The fastigial nucleus receives fibres from the vermis, the globose and emboliform nuclei from paravermal regions, and the dentate nucleus from the lateral region. Further details are given on page 177.

Cerebello vestibular connections

The vestibular nuclei receive direct projections from the cerebellar cortex (Fig. 12.10). They are, therefore, regarded as displaced cerebellar nuclei.

At the outset it is necessary to emphasise that, as far as cerebellar connections are concerned, the lateral vestibular nucleus (Dieter's nucleus) is distinct from other vestibular nuclei.

Connections of vestibular nuclei (other than lateral)

1. These nuclei receive labyrinthine impulses (conveying information about the position and movements of the head) through the vestibular nerve. (The fibres of this nerve are constituted by central processes of bipolar neurons in the vestibular ganglion). The neurons of vestibular nuclei carry these impulses to the cortex of the vestibulo-cerebellum (flocculonodular lobe, and uvula). Many fibres of the vestibular nerve bypass the vestibular nuclei and project directly to the vestibulocerebellum. (Note that the vestibulo-cerebellum corresponds roughly to archicerebellum, but excludes the lingula, and includes part of the uvula).

2. The vestibulo-cerebellum projects to vestibular nuclei either directly, or after relay in the fastigial nucleus.

3. The vestibular nuclei are connected to cranial nerve nuclei supplying muscles that move the eyeballs through the medial longitudinal fasciculus. Some fibres of the medial longitudinal fasciculus ascend to the thalamus and others descend into the spinal cord.

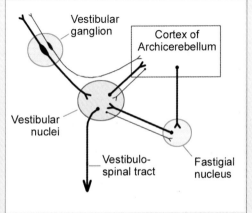

Fig. 12.10. Scheme to show vestibulo-cerebellar connections.

Through the connections described above the vestibulo-cerebellum (specially the flocculus) plays an important role in control of eye movements, particularly during movements of the head, and when the eyes are following a moving object (pursuit movements). [In this connection it is important to remember that visual information, and information about eye movements reach the flocculus through the reticular formation]. Also see page 181.

Connections of the lateral vestibular nucleus with the cerebellum

The lateral vestibular nucleus (of Dieter) does not receive fibres from the labyrinth, nor is it connected to the fastigial nucleus.

This nucleus receives a direct projection from the anterior part of the vermis (zone B). These impulses are relayed to the spinal cord through the lateral vestibulospinal tract (arising in the lateral vestibular nucleus).

The cerebellar cortex is able to influence muscles of the trunk and limbs through the lateral vestibular nucleus.

Olivocerebellar connections

The inferior olivary complex (made up of the main and accessory olivary nuclei) sends numerous fibres to the opposite half of the cerebellum (Fig. 12.11). Various parts of this complex exhibit a point to point relationship with the cerebellar hemisphere. The accessory olivary nuclei (lying most medially) project to the vermis and intermediate regions (zones A, B, C); while medial, intermediate and lateral parts of the (main) inferior olivary nucleus project to corresponding regions of the hemispheres (zone D).

Olivocerebellar fibres end within the cerebellar cortex as climbing fibres. Collaterals from these fibres terminate in cerebellar nuclei. There is a one to one relationship between cells of the inferior olive and Purkinje cells. Some details of olivocerebellar projections are given in Fig. 12.12.

The accessory olivary nuclei receive afferents from all levels of the spinal cord (spino-olivary tract, page 110) conveying both exteroceptive and proprioceptive impulses. These impulses reach the cerebellum through olivocerebellar fibres (which are completely crossed). We may, therefore, speak of a spino-olivo-cerebellar pathway. Exteroceptive and proprioceptive impulses also reach the olivary complex through the nucleus gracilis and cuneatus, and through the trigeminal nuclei. The inferior olivary nucleus also helps to connect the cerebral cortex (motor area), the thalamus, the corpus striatum, the red nucleus, and the reticular formation to the cerebellum.

Further details of olivocerebellar connections

1. The spinal sensory input to the inferior olivary nucleus is received mainly by the dorsal accessory olive. These inputs are relayed to the vermis and pars intermedia of the cerebellar cortex.

2. Visual related inputs reach the inferior olivary complex from the midbrain. Fibres from the superior colliculus reach the middle region of the medial accessory olive, and are relayed to the folium and tuber. These parts of the vermis are intimately involved in control of eye movements (saccades). Fibres also descend to the olivary complex from the vertical and horizontal gaze centres in the midbrain. These fibres reach outlying cell groups present in relation to the medial accessory olive; and are relayed to the flocculus.

3. Vestibular inputs reach outlying cell groups related to the medial accessory olive; and are relayed to the nodule.

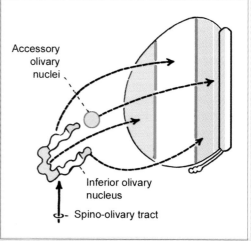

Fig. 12.11. Scheme to show the main features of olivocerebellar connections.

ADVANCED

Fig. 12.12. Details of olivoceebellar connections. Parts of the inferior Olivary complex and the parts of the cerebellum to which they project. The cerebellar nuclei give a GABA ergic feedback to the corresponding olivary nuclei.

Part of inferior olivary complex		Area of cerebellar cortex to which it projects	Cerebellar nuclei to which collaterals are given off
Principal inferior olivary nucleus		Hemisphere (Zone D)	Dentate
Medial acessory olive	Rostral part	Pars intermedia (Zone C2)	Globose
	Caudal part	Zone A of vermis	Fastigial
Dorsal accessory olive	Rostral part	Pars intermedia (Zones C1, C2)	Emboliform
	Caudal part	Zone B of vermis	Lat. vestibular nucleus

4. Fibres descending from the red nucleus project mainly to the main inferior olivary nucleus and the medial accessory olive. The inferior olivary complex is influenced by the cerebral cortex (motor, premotor) through the red nucleus. The cerebellum also influences the inferior olive through the red nucleus.

The fibres reaching the olivary complex from the red nucleus, and from the central grey matter of the midbrain, constitute the central tegmental tract (or fasciculus). On reaching the inferior olivary nucleus these fibres spread out as a thin layer around the inferior olivary nucleus, forming a layer called the ***olivary amiculum***.

Cerebello-olivary fibres

The cerebellar nuclei which receive collaterals from different parts of the inferior olivary complex (Fig. 12.12) give a GABAergic feed back to the corresponding part of the complex. The cerebellum also influences the olivo-cerebellar output directly through the red nucleus.

Connectons between cerebellum and reticular formation

Reticulo-cerebellar fibres

The cerebellum receives fibres from and sends fibres to the reticular formation (Fig. 12.13). Impulses passing from the cerebellum to the reticular formation are relayed to the spinal cord and to cranial nerve nuclei through reticulospinal and reticulonuclear pathways; and to the thalamus through reticulothalamic fibres. Details of these connections are as follows.

The cerebellum receives fibres mainly from three nuclei in the reticular formation. These are **(a)** the lateral reticular nucleus in the medulla, **(b)** the paramedian reticular nucleus (lying in the lower part of the medulla within the medial longitudinal fasciculus; not listed in Fig. 11.14), and **(c)** the reticular nucleus of the pontine tegmentum (Nucleus reticularis tegmenti pontis, NRTP).

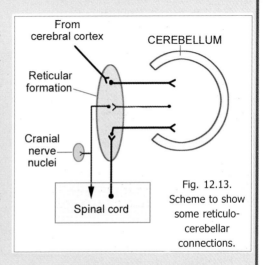

Fig. 12.13. Scheme to show some reticulo-cerebellar connections.

Fibres from the lateral reticular nucleus reach the anterior lobe and the biventral lobule (paramedian lobule of cats), bilaterally. Fibres from the NRTP reach almost all parts of the cerebellar cortex except the parts to which the lateral reticular nucleus projects.

The paramedian reticular nucleus sends fibres to the entire cerebellar cortex. The fibres from the lateral reticular nucleus and the NRTP give collaterals to cerebellar nuclei (mainly to the fastigial nucleus).

Cerebello-reticular connections

Cerebellar nuclei project to the lateral reticular nucleus and the NRTP. Fibres to the lateral reticular nucleus are mainly from the fastigial nucleus. Some of these fibres reach the reticular formation through the descending branch of the superior cerebellar peduncle. Fibres from the fastigial nucleus also reach the tegmentum of the midbrain (including the dorsal tegmental nucleus, the central grey, and the vertical gaze centre), the raphe nuclei and the locus coeruleus. Through some of these connections the cerebellum can influence visceromotor function.

Fibres from the dentate, emboliform and globose nuclei end in the medial reticular formation of the pons and medulla and in the NRTP (mainly from emboliform nucleus).

Cerebellorubral connections

Fibres arising in cerebellar nuclei (mainly emboliform and globose, with some from fastigial and dentate nuclei) pass through the superior cerebellar peduncle to reach the red nucleus (Fig.12.14). The significance of these connections is as follows.

(a) Neurons in the caudal magnocellular part of the red nucleus give origin to the rubrospinal tract (which is not prominent in man). Through this tract the cerebellum influences motor neurons in the spinal cord. In this cerebello-rubrospinal pathway there is a double decussation. The cerebellorubral fibres cross in the decussation of the superior cerebellar peduncle, while the rubrospinal fibres cross in the ventral tegmental decussation. As a result the cerebellum influences the same side of the spinal cord through this pathway.

(b) Fibres arising in the cranial parvicellular part of the red nucleus descend through the central tegmental tract to the inferior olivary complex. They can influence the activity of olivo-cerebellar fibres.

(c) Some fibres from the red nucleus project back to cerebellar nuclei. These nuclei are also influenced indirectly through collaterals reaching them from olivocerebellar fibres.

Cerebello-thalamic connections

Fibres arising in the dentate nucleus (and a few in the emboliform, globose and fastigial nuclei) pass through the superior cerebellar peduncle, to reach the thalamus of the opposite side, either directly, or after relay in the red nucleus.

Tecto-cerebellar connections

The superior and inferior colliculi send fibres to the cerebellum. The fibres terminate in vermal and paravermal regions. They are believed to carry auditory and visual impulses

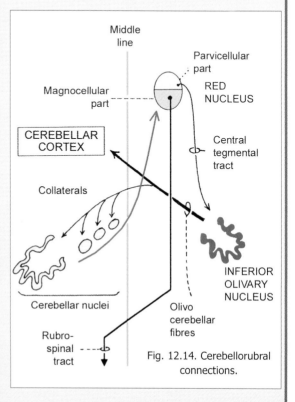

Fig. 12.14. Cerebellorubral connections.

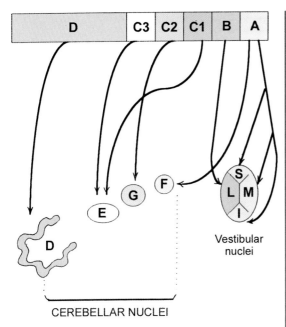

Fig. 12.15. Diagram showing projections from zones of cerebellar cortex to cerebellar and vestibular nuclei.

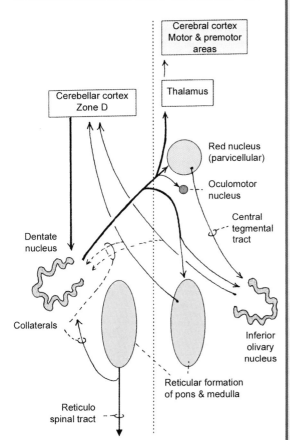

Fig. 12.16. Connections of the dentate nuclei.

to the cerebellum. Visual impulses may also reach the cerebellum through an occipito-ponto-cerebellar pathway, and through the inferior olivary complex.

Fibres ascending from the fastigial nucleus reach the tectum.

CONNECTIONS OF CEREBELLAR NUCLEI

In the preceding paragraphs mention has been made of many connections involving the cerebellar nuclei. We will now review the connections of each nucleus. The afferents to the nuclei follow a common pattern and will be considered together, but the efferents of each nucleus will be taken up separately.

Afferents to Cerebellar Nuclei

(a) Afferents from cerebellar cortex

The cerebellar nuclei receive the axons of Purkinje fibres. The zones of cortex from which each nucleus receives fibres are shown in Fig. 12.15. Note that in this figure projections to vestibular nuclei are also shown. These nuclei receive direct fibres from the cortex and are regarded as displaced cerebellar nuclei.

Zone A of the cerebellar cortex projects to the fastigial nucleus, and to vestibular nuclei (other than lateral). The projection to the vestibular nuclei is from the nodule, flocculus and part of the uvula. Fibres from the folium and tuber which are concerned with saccadic eye movements also reach vestibular nuclei.

Zone B projects to the lateral vestibular nucleus. Zones C_1 and C_3 project to the emboliform nucleus. Zone C_2 projects to the globose nucleus. The greater part of the cerebellar cortex (Zone D) projects to the dentate nucleus only.

(b) Collaterals of climbing fibres (olivocerebellar fibres)

The inferior olivary complex projects to all parts of the cerebellar cortex. Details of these connections have been summarised in Fig. 12.12. Note that climbing fibres meant for a given zone of cortex give collaterals to the cerebellar nucleus receiving cortical fibres from the same zone. For example:

1. The main inferior olivary nucleus projects to zone D.
2. These fibres give collaterals to the dentate nucleus.
3. Zone D projects to the dentate nucleus.

(c) Collaterals of mossy fibres

It may be recalled that all afferents to the cerebellum other than olivocerebellar end as mossy fibres. These fibres give collaterals to cerebellar nuclei.

1. Reticulocerebellar fibres and spino-cerebellar fibres give collaterals to the fastigial nucleus, the emboliform nucleus and the globose nucleus. Some reticulocerebellar fibres from the reticular nucleus of the pontine tegmentum give collaterals to the dentate nucleus.

2. Collaterals from pontocerebellar, cuneo-cerebellar and vestibulocerebellar fibres are traditionally described, but their presence is controversial. If present they are few in number.

Efferents of Cerebellar Nuclei

Efferents of dentate nucleus

Efferent fibres arising in the dentate nucleus constitute the greater part of the superior cerebellar peduncle (Fig. 12.16). On reaching the lower part of the midbrain most fibres cross the middle line (in the decussation of the peduncle) and divide into ascending and descending branches.

Most of the ascending fibres reach the thalamus, but some end in the red nucleus. Some ascending fibres end in the nucleus of the oculomotor nerve, and some in the tectum. The descending fibres end in the inferior olivary complex and in the reticular formation.

Some fibres of the superior cerebellar peduncle do not cross. Like the crossed fibres, the uncrossed fibres divide into ascending and descending branches all of which end in the reticular formation.

Efferents of the emboliform nucleus

To understand the connections of the emboliform nucleus think of it as a centre on pathways through which the cerebellar cortex controls motor neurons in the spinal cord. We have seen above that the emboliform nucleus receives afferents from the pars intermedia (paravermal area) of the cerebellar cortex (zones C_1, C_3). The efferents of the nucleus are as follows (Fig. 12.17).

Fibres arising in the emboliform nucleus pass through the superior cerebellar peduncle. They decussate and divide into ascending and descending branches.

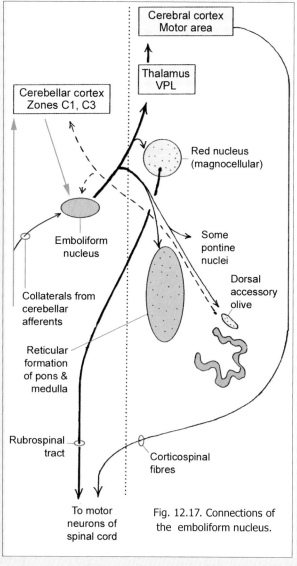

Fig. 12.17. Connections of the emboliform nucleus.

Some ascending fibres end in the red nucleus (magnocellular part). The emboliform nucleus can, therefore, influence motor neurons in the spinal cord through the rubrospinal tract. Other ascending fibres reach the ventral lateral nucleus of the thalamus (posterior part). From here they are relayed to the motor cortex. The cerebellum is, therefore, able to influence motor neurons through the corticospinal tracts also.

Some descending fibres end in the reticular formation (medial part, mainly the reticular nucleus of the pontine tegmentum). These fibres act on spinal neurons through reticulospinal fibres. Other descending fibres end in relation to pontine nuclei. They may influence activity of the ponto-cerebellar projection. Yet other descending fibres end in the (rostral half of the) dorsal accessory olivary nucleus (nucleo-olivary fibres).

Efferents of globose nucleus

Like those from the dentate and emboliform nuclei efferents from the globose nucleus pass through the superior cerebellar peduncle to reach the red nucleus and the thalamus (Fig. 12.18). Some fibres reach the superior colliculus, the central grey matter of the midbrain, raphe nuclei (in the reticular formation), and the nucleus of Darkschewitsch. The nucleus of Darkschewitsch projects to the upper part of the medial accessory olive through the medial tegmental tract.

Fibres passing into the descending division of the superior cerebellar peduncle connect the globose nucleus to the reticular nucleus of the pontine tegmentum. Spinal motor neurons can be influenced through this nucleus.

Connections of the fastigial nucleus

A general idea of the afferents to this nucleus has been given on page 177. We will now consider further details of both its afferents and efferents (Fig. 12.19). It is easier to understand the numerous connections of the fastigial nucleus if we consider them in relation to the functions they serve.

A. Control of muscle action (axial and proximal limb muscles) in response to labyrinthine stimuli.

1. Fibres of the vestibular nerve carrying labyrinthine impulses project to zone A of the cerebellar cortex. (The area includes the medial part of vermis, whole of posterior vermis and flocculus. The area corresponds roughly to the vestibulocerebellum of earlier descriptions).

These fibres may reach the cortex directly, or after relay in vestibular nuclei.

2. The vestibulocerebellum projects to the fastigial nucleus. Some vestibular fibres may reach the fastigial nucleus directly.

3. The fastigial nucleus projects to the (medial and spinal) vestibular nuclei. The medial vestibulospinal tract, arising in these nuclei descends to the spinal cord and ends in relation to motor neurons (bilaterally).

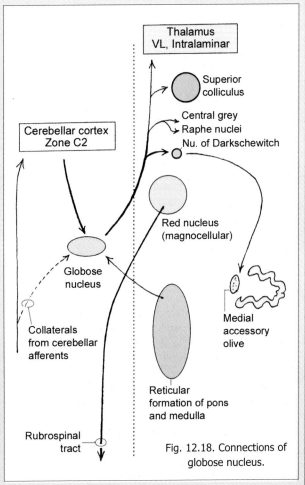

Fig. 12.18. Connections of globose nucleus.

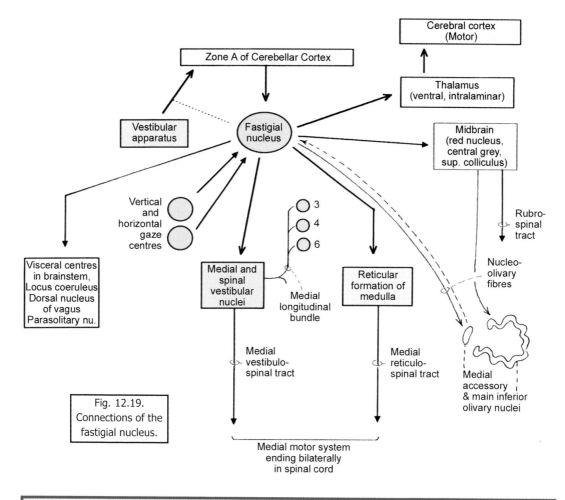

Fig. 12.19.
Connections of the
fastigial nucleus.

4. The fastigial nucleus also projects to the reticular formation of the medulla and influences motor neurons through the medial reticulospinal tract.

The two tracts (medial vestibulospinal and medial reticulospinal) through which the vestibulocerebellum influences spinal motor neurons is called the '*medial motor system*' (in distinction to the 'lateral' corticospinal system.

5. The fastigial nucleus sends efferents to the thalamus (ventral lateral and intralaminar nuclei). Fibres arising here reach the motor cortex and influence spinal motor neurons through corticospinal tracts.

B. Some fibres from the fastigial nucleus reach the midbrain. These fibres influence olivocerebellar output as follows.

(a) Some fibres end in the red nucleus. From here fibres passing through the central tegmental tract reach the medial accessory olive.

(b) Some fibres reach centres in the central grey matter (near the junction of the midbrain and the diencephalon). One of these is the nucleus of Darkschewitsch. Fibres arising in this region pass through the medial tegmental tract and reach the main inferior olivary nucleus. These inputs are excitatory for olivocerebellar impulses.

C. The fastigial nucleus plays a role in *visceromotor control* through connections with:

(a) the parasolitary nucleus (lying near the solitary nucleus);

(b) the locus coeruleus; and

(c) the dorsal nucleus of the vagus nerve.

D. *Control of eye movements*

This topic has been discussed on page 159. Here we will consider the role of the cerebellum in control of finer eye movements (saccades and pursuit movements. The pathways involved are as follows.

1. The folium and tuber (of the cerebellar vermis), and also the flocculus, receive impulses of vision and those related to eye movements (through the inferior olivary complex). From here fibres project to the fastigial nucleus.

2. The fastigial nucleus also receives fibres from the vertical gaze centre (midbrain) and the horizontal gaze centre (pons).

3. We have seen that the fastigial nucleus projects to the medial and spinal vestibular nuclei. Fibres arising here pass through the medial longitudinal fasciculus to reach the oculomotor, trochlear and abducent nuclei. Fibres of the medial longitudinal fasciculus also reach the cervical spinal cord and influence muscles that rotate the neck (sternocleidomastoid, trapezius).

4. The fastigial nucleus is connected to the superior colliculus and can influence eye movements through it.

E. *Control of olivocerebellar projection*

The fastigial nucleus plays a role in controlling flow of impulses from the inferior olivary complex to the cerebellum. Some fibres from the fastigial nucleus project to the medial accessory olivary nucleus. These fibres are inhibitory.

ADVANCED

Disorders of Equilibrium

We have seen that the maintenance of equilibrium, and of correct posture, is dependent on reflex arcs involving various centres including the spinal cord, the cerebellum, and the vestibular nuclei. Afferent impulses for these reflexes are carried by the posterior column tracts (fasciculus gracilis and fasciculus cuneatus), the spinocerebellar tracts, and others. Efferents reach neurons of the ventral grey column (anterior horn cells) through rubrospinal, vestibulospinal, and other 'extrapyramidal' tracts. Interruption of any of these pathways; or lesions in the cerebellum, the vestibular nuclei and other centres concerned; can result in various abnormalities involving maintenance of posture and coordination of movements.

Inability to maintain the equilibrium of the body, while standing, or while walking, is referred to as *ataxia.* This may occur as a result of the interruption of afferent proprioceptive pathways (*sensory ataxia*). Disease of the cerebellum itself, or of efferent pathways, results in more severe disability. Coordination of the activity of different groups of muscles is interfered with, leading to various defects. The person is unable to stand with his feet close together: the body sways from side to side and the person may fall. While walking, the patient staggers and is unable to maintain progression in the desired direction. Lack of proprioceptive information can be compensated to a considerable extent by information received through the eyes. The defects mentioned are, therefore, much more pronounced with the eyes closed (*Romberg's sign*). Lack of coordination of muscles also interferes with purposeful movements (*asynergia*). Movements are jerky and lack precision. For example, the patient finds it difficult to touch his nose with a finger, or to move a finger along a line. There is difficulty in performing movements involving rapid alternating action of opposing groups of muscles (e.g., tapping one hand with the other; repeated pronation and supination of the forearm). This phenomenon is called *dysdiadokokinesis.* Incoordination of the muscles responsible for the articulation of words leads to characteristic speech defects (*dysarthria*). For the same reason, the eyes are unable to fix the gaze on an object for any length of time. Attempts to bring the gaze back to the same point result in repeated jerky movements of the eyes. This is called *nystagmus.*

Apart from incoordination, cerebellar disease is characterised by diminished muscle tone (*hypotonia*). The muscles are soft, and tire easily (*asthenia*). Joints may lack stability (*flail joints*). Tendon reflexes may be diminished. Alternatively, tapping a tendon may result in oscillating movements of the part concerned, like a pendulum.

CLINICAL

Attempts have been made to correlate symptoms of cerbellar damage with different regions of the cerebellum, but without much success. Some correlations are as follows.

1. When the flocculus, nodule and uvula are damaged (*flocculonodular syndrome*) the main symptom is imbalance. Remember that the connections of the flocculonodular lobe are predominantly vestibular.

2. Small lesions in the cerebellar cortex may produce no effect. Extensive lesions are marked by hypotonia and incoordination (on the side of the lesion).

3. Intention tremor and staggering appear when the dentate nucleus or the superior cerebellar peduncle (which carries fibres from the nucleus) is damaged.

The role of the cerebellum in the control of eye movements has been discussed on page 181.

The Cerebellopontine angle

This is a small triangle interval bounded by the pons (anteromedialy), and the cerebellum (posteromedially). A tumour in this space produces characteristic symptoms.

(a) Pressure on the spinal nucleus of the trigeminal nerve leads to loss of sensations of pain and temperature over the face.

(b) Pressure on fibres and nucleus of the facial nerve results in facial paralysis.

(c) Pressure on the middle cerebellar peduncle leads to ataxia.

RELATED TOPICS IN OTHER CHAPTERS

The blood supply of the cerebellum is described in Chapter 21.

The cerebellum lies in close relation to the fourth ventricle. This is described in Chapter 20.

The development of the cerebellum is described on page 78.

Gross subdivisions of the cerebellum are given in Chapter 7.

13 : The Diencephalon

The diencephalon consists of the thalamus proper (or dorsal thalamus), the hypothalamus, the epithalamus, and the ventral thalamus (or subthalamus). The third ventricle may be regarded as the cavity of the diencephalon. The subdivisions of the diencephalon and the nuclei to be found in each division are summarised in Fig. 13.1.

The Thalamus (Dorsal Thalamus)

The thalamus (or dorsal thalamus) is a large mass of grey matter that lies immediately lateral to the third ventricle. It has two ends (or poles), anterior and posterior; and four surfaces, superior, inferior, medial and lateral.

The **anterior end (or pole)** lies just behind the interventricular foramen (Fig. 8.6). The **posterior end (or pole)** is called the pulvinar. It lies just above and lateral to the superior colliculus. The pulvinar is separated from the geniculate bodies by the superior brachium quadrigeminum.

The **medial surface** forms the greater part of the lateral wall of the third ventricle, and is lined by ependyma. The medial surfaces of the two thalami are usually interconnected by a mass of grey matter called the **interthalamic adhesion (connexus)**. Inferiorly, the medial surface is separated from the hypothalamus by the **hypothalamic sulcus**. This sulcus runs from the interventricular foramen to the aqueduct. The lateral surface of the thalamus is related to the internal capsule which separates it from the lentiform nucleus (Fig. 13.2). The **superior (or dorsal) surface** of the thalamus is related laterally to the caudate nucleus from which it is separated by a bundle of fibres called the **stria terminalis**, and by the thalamostriate vein. The thalamus and the caudate nucleus together form the floor of the central part of the lateral ventricle (Fig. 13.2). The medial part of the superior surface of the thalamus is, however, separated from the ventricle by the fornix, and by a fold of piamater called the **tela choroidea**.

At the junction of the medial and superior surfaces of the thalamus the ependyma of the third ventricle is reflected from the lateral wall to the roof. The line of reflection is marked by a line called the **taenia thalami.** Underlying it there is a narrow bundle of fibres called the **stria medullaris thalami** (not to be confused with the stria medullares present in the floor of the fourth ventricle). The **inferior surface** of the thalamus is related to the hypothalamus anteriorly (Fig. 8.5), and to the ventral thalamus posteriorly (Fig. 13.2). The ventral thalamus separates the thalamus from the tegmentum of the midbrain.

Note for teachers and students

On the basis of recent investigations the concepts regarding the nuclei to be included in each division of the diencephalon have undergone revision. The points to note are as follows.

1. The main part of the thalamus is described as the **dorsal thalamus**. The subthalamic region is now called the **ventral thalamus**.

2. The **reticular nucleus**, earlier included in the dorsal thalamus, is now regarded as a part of the ventral thalamus (on functional grounds).

3. The subthalamic nucleus is now included amongst the basal nuclei to which it is closely related functionally. It is not included in the ventral thalamus.

4. The medial and lateral geniculate bodies have traditionally been considered distinct from the other regions of the thalamus and have been grouped together as the metathalamus. However, they are now regarded as integral parts of the dorsal thalamus.

DIENCEPHALON : Subdivisions & Nuclei

A. DORSAL THALAMUS

LATERAL PART		OTHER PARTS
Ventral grup	*Lateral group*	Anterior nucleus (in anterior part)
Ventral anterior nucleus	Lateral dorsal nucleus	Intralaminar nuclei (main = centromedian nucleus)
Ventral lateral nucleus	Lateral posterior nucleus	Midiline nuclei
Ventral posterior nucleus (medial and lateral)	Pulvina	Metathalamus Medial geniculate body Lateral geniculate body

B. HYPOTHALAMUS		C. VENTRAL THALAMUS
Region	*Nuclei*	Reticular nucleus Ventral geniculate nucleus (or pregeniculate nucleus) Zona incerta
Preoptic region	Preoptic nucleus	
Supraoptic region	Paraventricular nucleus Suprachiasmatic nucleus Intermediate (anterior) nu. Supraoptic nucleus	Fields of Forel The upper ends of the red nucleus and the substantia nigra extend into this region
Tuberal region	Infundibular (arcuate) nu. Dorsimedial nucleus Ventrimedial nuceus Premamillary nuclei Lateral tuberal nucleus	**D. EPITHALAMUS** Paraventricular nuclei (anterior and posterior)
Mamillary region	Posterior nucleus Tuberomamillary nucleus	Habenular nuclei (medial and lateral)
Mamillary body		Stria medullaris thalami
Lateral region	Lateral nucleus	Pineal body

Fig. 13.1. Subdivisions and nuclei of the diencephalon

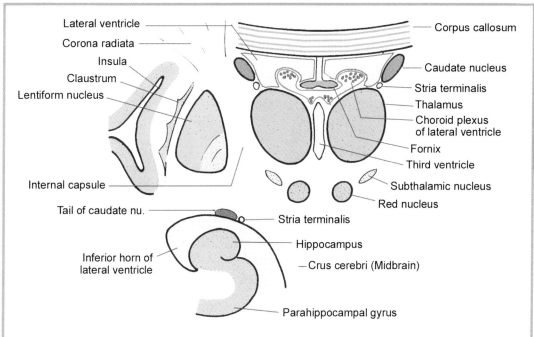

Fig. 13.2. Coronal section through the cerebrum to show structures related to the thalamus.

Internal Structure of the Thalamus

The thalamus consists mainly of grey matter. Its superior surface is covered by a thin layer of white matter called the ***stratum zonale;*** and its lateral surface by a similar layer called the ***external medullary lamina.***

The grey matter of the thalamus is subdivided into three main parts by a Y-shaped sheet of white matter which is called the ***internal medullary lamina*** (Fig. 13.3). This lamina is placed vertically. It divides the thalamus into a lateral part, a medial part, and an anterior part situated between the two limbs of the 'Y'.

A number of nuclei can be distinguished within each of these parts. Only the more important of these are listed below.

(a) Nuclei in the anterior part

A number of nuclei can be distinguished, but we shall refer to them collectively as the ***anterior nucleus.***

(b) Nuclei in the medial part

The largest of these is the ***medial dorsal nucleus.*** It is divisible into a magnocellular part (anteromedial) and a parvocellular part (posterolateral).

(c) Nuclei in the lateral part

The nuclei in the lateral part can be subdivided into a ***ventral group*** and a ***lateral group.***

The ***nuclei in the ventral group*** are as follows (in anteroposterior order).

1. ***Ventral anterior nucleus.***
2. ***Ventral lateral nucleus*** (also called the ***ventral intermediate nucleus***).

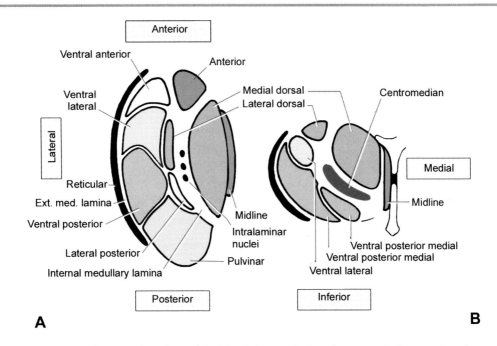

Fig. 13.3. Scheme to show the nuclei of the thalamus. A. Superior aspect. B. In coronal section.

3. *Ventral posterior nucleus*, which is further subdivided into a lateral part called the *ventral posterolateral nucleus*, and a medial part called the *ventral posteromedial nucleus* (Fig. 13.3B).

The *nuclei of the lateral group* are as follows (in anteroposterior order).

1. *Lateral dorsal nucleus* (or *dorsolateral nucleus*).

2. *Lateral posterior nucleus.*

3. *Pulvinar.*

(d) Other thalamic nuclei

In addition to the above the thalamus contains the following nuclei.

1. The *intralaminar nuclei* are embedded within the internal medullary lamina. There are several nuclei in this group. The most important of these is the *centromedian nucleus* (Fig. 13.3B).

2. The *midline nuclei* consist of scattered cells that lie between the medial part of the thalamus and the ependyma of the third ventricle. Several nuclei are recognised.

3. The *medial and lateral geniculate bodies* (traditionally described under metathalamus) are now included as part of the thalamus.

The reticular nucleus, earlier described as part of the dorsal thalamus, is now regarded as part of the ventral thalamus.

Connections of the Thalamus

Afferent impulses from a large number of subcortical centres converge on the thalamus (Fig. 13.4). Exteroceptive and proprioceptive impulses ascend to it through the medial lemniscus, the spinothalamic tracts, and the trigeminothalamic tract. Visual and auditory impulses reach the lateral and medial geniculate bodies respectively. Sensations of taste are conveyed to the thalamus through solitariothalamic fibres. Although the thalamus does not receive direct olfactory impulses they probably reach it through the amygdaloid complex. Visceral information is conveyed from the hypothalamus,

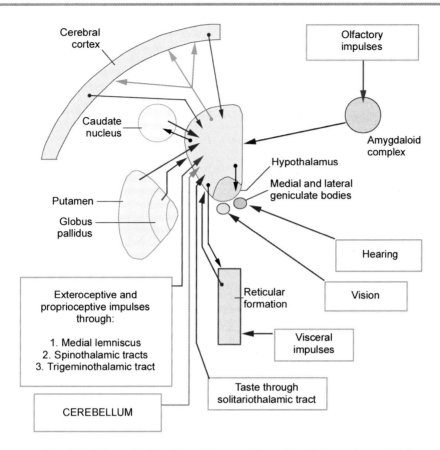

Fig. 13.4. Scheme to show the main connections of the thalamus (as a whole).

and probably through the reticular formation. In addition to these afferents, the thalamus receives profuse connections from all parts of the cerebral cortex, the cerebellum, and the corpus striatum. The thalamus is, therefore, regarded as a great integrating centre where information from all these sources is brought together. This information is projected to almost the whole of the cerebral cortex through profuse thalamocortical projections. The areas of cerebral cortex receiving fibres from individual thalamic nuclei are shown in Fig. 13.5a. Thalamocortical fibres form large bundles that are described as ***thalamic radiations*** or as ***thalamic peduncles***. These radiations are ***anterior*** (or ***frontal***), ***superior*** (or ***dorsal***), ***posterior*** (or ***caudal***), and ***ventral.*** Efferent projections from the thalamus also reach the corpus striatum, the hypothalamus, and the reticular formation. Besides its integrating function, the thalamus is believed to have some degree of ability to perceive exteroceptive sensations, specially pain.

Keeping these facts in mind we may now consider the connections of individual thalamic nuclei. These connections are numerous, and many are controversial. The description that follows is confined to better known connections.

Connections of Ventral Group of nuclei

1. From a clinical point of view the most important connections of the thalamus are those of the ***ventral posterior nucleus.*** We have seen that this nucleus is divisible into ventral posterolateral and ventral posteromedial parts (that are sometimes mentioned as separate nuclei). This nucleus

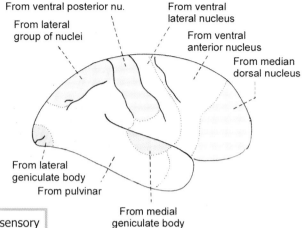

Fig. 13.5a. Diagram to show areas of cerebral cortex (superolateral surface) that are connected to individual thalamic nuclei. The connections are reciprocal. The anterior thalamic nuclei project mainly to the gyrus cinguli (not seen in this view).

BASIC

receives the terminations of the major sensory pathways ascending from the spinal cord and brainstem (Fig. 13.5b). These include the medial lemniscus, the spinothalamic tracts, the trigeminal lemniscus and the solitariothalamic fibres carrying sensations of taste. Within the nucleus fibres from different parts of the body terminate in a definite sequence. The fibres from the lowest parts of the body end in the most lateral part of the nucleus. The medial lemniscus and spinothalamic tracts carrying sensations from the limbs and trunk end in the ventral posterolateral part; while the trigeminal fibres (from the head) end in the ventral posteromedial part, which also receives the fibres for taste. Different layers of cells within the nucleus respond to different modalities of sensation.

All the sensations reaching the nucleus are carried primarily to the sensory area of the cerebral cortex (SI, areas 3,2,1) by fibres passing through the posterior limb of the internal capsule (superior thalamic radiation). They also reach the second somatosensory area (SII) located in the parietal operculum (of the insula).

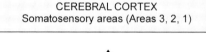
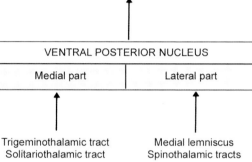

Fig. 13.5b. Connections of the ventral posterior nucleus of the thalamus.

ADVANCED

2. The ***ventral lateral nucleus*** is divisible into anterior, posterior and medial parts. Each part has distinct connections (Fig. 13.6).

The anterior part of the nucleus receives fibres from the globus pallidus and projects to the premotor and supplemental motor areas of the cerebral cortex.

The medial part receives afferents from the substantia nigra; and gives off a diffuse projection reaching many areas of the cerebral cortex.

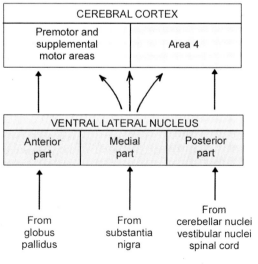

Fig.13.6. Connections of the ventral lateral nucleus of the thalamus.

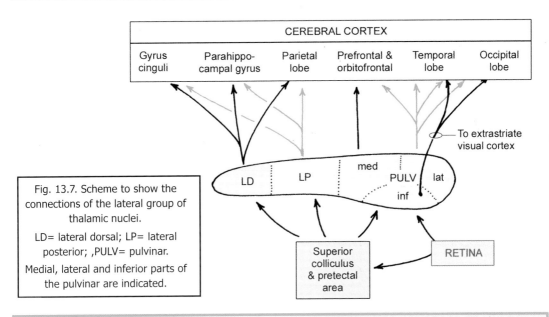

Fig. 13.7. Scheme to show the connections of the lateral group of thalamic nuclei.

LD= lateral dorsal; LP= lateral posterior; ,PULV= pulvinar.

Medial, lateral and inferior parts of the pulvinar are indicated.

The posterior part of the nucleus receives afferents from cerebellar nuclei and vestibular nuclei. It also receives some spinothalamic fibres. Efferents from this part of the ventral lateral nucleus project to area 4 of the cerebral cortex. Ablation of this part can reduce tremors in Parkinsonism.

3. The connections of the *ventral anterior nucleus* are largely unknown. It probably receives fibres from the globus pallidus and cerebellar nuclei, and sends efferents to the cerebral cortex (parietal lobe, anterior part). Its functions are unknown.

Connections of lateral group of nuclei

1. The *lateral dorsal nucleus* receives impulses from the superior colliculus (Fig. 13.7). Efferent projections reach the cingulate gyrus, the parahippocampal gyrus, and parts of the hippocampal formation. Some fibres reach the cortex of the parietal lobe.

2. The *lateral posterior nucleus* receives fibres from the superior colliculus. Efferents reach the cerebral cortex of the superior parietal lobule. They also reach the cingulate and parahippocampal gyri.

3. The *pulvinar* is divisible into medial, lateral, and inferior parts. (An anterior, or oral, part is also described). All parts receive fibres from the superior colliculus. The inferior part of the pulvinar also receives direct fibres from the retina. It is believed that the entire retina is represented in this part. Efferents from the pulvinar project to extrastriate visual areas in the occipital and parietal lobes; and to visual association areas in the posterior part of the temporal lobe. The inferior part of the pulvinar is thus a centre in an extrageniculate pathway from the retina to the cerebral cortex. However, the projections of the pulvinar to non-visual areas of the cerebral cortex suggest complex functions that may involve recognition and memory.

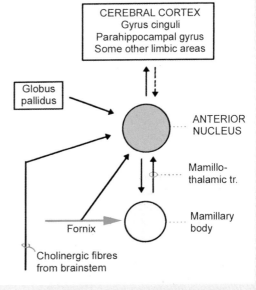

Fig.13.8.Connections of the anterior nucleus of the thalamus.

ADVANCED

Connections of other thalamic nuclei

1. The ***anterior nucleus*** receives fibres from the mamillary body through the mamillothalamic tract. Efferent fibres project to the gyrus cinguli (areas 23, 24, 32).

Integrity of this pathway is necessary for recent memory. Some other connections of the nucleus are shown in Fig. 13.8. Anterior thalamic nuclei are probably involved in functions involving attention and memory.

2. The ***medial dorsal nucleus*** is divisible into a smaller magnocellular part (placed anteromedially), and a larger parvocellular part (placed posterolaterally). The connections of the nucleus are shown in Fig. 13.9. The nucleus is involved in controlling emotional states. Damage to the nucleus leads to decrease in anxiety, tension and aggression. These functions are similar to those of the prefrontal cortex.

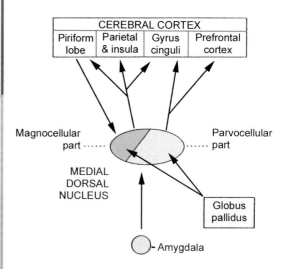

Fig. 13.9. Connections of the medial dorsal nucleus of the thalamus

3. ***Intralaminar nuclei:*** There are several nuclei in this group divided into subgroups, anterior and posterior. The posterior subgroup includes the large centromedian nucleus. The nuclei of this group receive inputs from the body through collaterals of spinothalamic tracts (Fig. 13.10). Fibres are also received from the reticular formation, the cerebellar nuclei, and the substantia nigra. The centromedian nucleus receives many fibres from the globus pallidus.

Efferents from intralaminar nuclei reach the cerebral cortex. Those from the anterior subgroup are diffuse reaching many parts of the cortex. Those from the posterior group project to the motor, premotor and supplemental motor areas. Efferents also reach the striatum. Functions of these nuclei are not known.

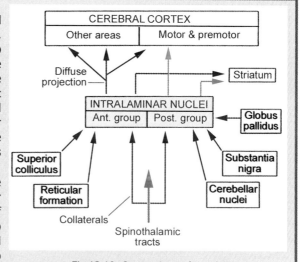

Fig.13.10. Connections of intralaminar thalamicnuclei

4. The ***midline nuclei*** consist of several small groups of neurons (but there is controversy regarding the groups to be included under this heading). The connections of the nuclei (shown in Fig. 13.11) are mainly with the limbic system. Afferents include noradrenergic, serotoninergic and cholinergic bundles ascending from the brainstem. The midline nuclei probably play a role in memory and arousal.

The intralaminar, midline and reticular nuclei, have in the past, been grouped together as ***nonspecific thalamic nuclei***. In the past they have been regarded as part of the ascending reticular activating system which is believed to be responsible for maintaining a state of alertness. They have been described as receiving afferents from the reticular formation (mainly gigantocellular nucleus and ventral reticular nucleus of the medulla; caudal reticular nucleus of pons) and projecting to all parts of the cerebral cortex. Recent investigations have shown, however, that there is no validity in dividing thalamic nuclei into specific and unspecific.

Sensory disorders (because of interruption of various ascending pathways) have been described on page 110. The thalamic syndrome is described on page 111.

Medial & Lateral Geniculate Bodies

The medial and lateral geniculate bodies are small oval collections of grey matter situated below the posterior part of the thalamus, lateral to the colliculi of the midbrain (Fig. 13.12). Each mass of grey matter is bent on itself, hence the term 'geniculate'. Traditionally, the geniculate bodies have been grouped together under the heading **meta-thalamus**; but because of functional relationships they are now included in the dorsal thalamus.

The Medial Geniculate Body

The medial geniculate body is a relay station on the auditory pathway. Medial, ventral and dorsal nuclei are described within it.

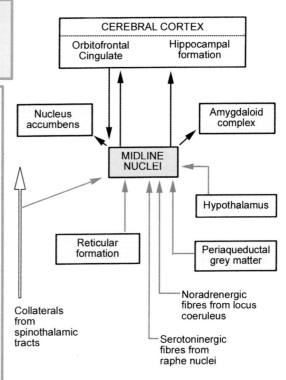

Fig. 13.11. Connections of the midline nuclei of the thalamus.

The medial geniculate body receives fibres of the lateral lemniscus either directly, or after relay in the inferior colliculus (Fig. 13.13). These fibres pass through the brachium of the inferior colliculus. Fibres arising in the medial geniculate body constitute the acoustic radiation. The acoustic radiation passes through the sublentiform part of the internal capsule to reach the acoustic areas of the cerebral cortex. Some other connections of the medial geniculate body are shown in Fig. 13.13.

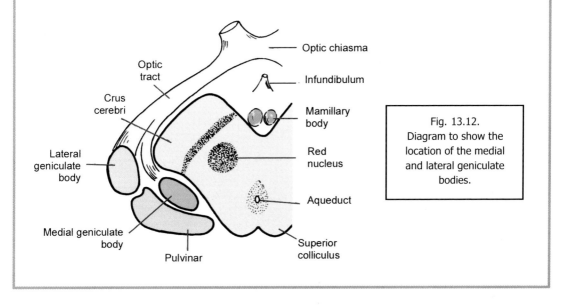

Fig. 13.12. Diagram to show the location of the medial and lateral geniculate bodies.

BASIC

Each medial geniculate body receives impulses from the cochleae of both sides. It also receives fibres from the auditory area of the cerebral cortex. These fibres form part of the ***descending acoustic pathway.***

Different neurons in the ventral nucleus of the medial geniculate body respond to different frequencies of sound (tonotopic organisation). The ventral nucleus projects to the primary auditory cortex. The neurons in the dorsal nucleus do not show tonotopic organisation. They project to auditory areas around the primary auditory area.

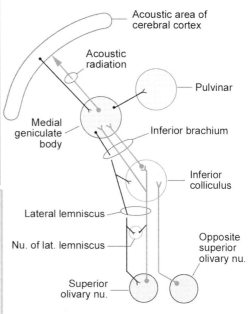

Fig. 13.13. Connections of the medial geniculate body. Also see Fig. 10.7.

The Lateral Geniculate Body

The lateral geniculate body is a relay station on the visual pathway. It receives fibres from the retinae of both eyes (Fig. 13.14). Efferents arising in this body constitute the optic radiation which passes through the retrolentiform part of the internal capsule to reach the visual areas of the cerebral cortex. Details of the visual pathway (including the representation of retinal quadrants in the lateral geniculate body) are described in Chapter 18.

Sections through the lateral geniculate body show that its grey matter is partially split to form six lamellae separated by nerve fibres (Fig. 13.15). These layers are numbered one to six from ventral to dorsal side. Laminae one, four and six receive fibres from the retina of the opposite side; while laminae two, three and five receive fibres from the retina of the same side. The fibres from different parts of the retinae project to specific parts of the lateral geniculate body, the whole of the retina being represented (visiotopic organisation). In turn these project to specific areas of the primary visual cortex (area 17).

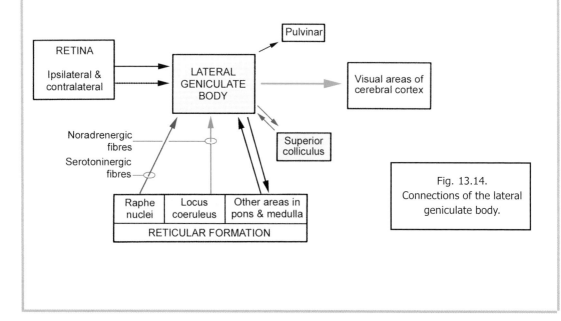

Fig. 13.14. Connections of the lateral geniculate body.

Apart from retinal fibres the lateral geniculate body receives fibres from the primary visual cortex, and from extrastriate visual areas. It also receives fibres from the superior colliculus, and from the reticular formation of the pons and medulla.

Noradrenergic fibres reach it from the locus coeruleus, and serotoninergic fibres from raphe nuclei (midbrain).

The various fibres reaching the lateral geniculate body form complicated synapses. The synaptic areas often form glomeruli somewhat similar to those in the cerebellum. In addition to neurons that relay retinal impulses to the visual cortex, the lateral geniculate body also contains some neurons that remain confined within it (Golgi type II neurons) and participate in the synapses.

The lateral geniculate body has traditionally been regarded as a simple relay station on the visual pathway. However, both anatomical and physiological evidence shows that considerable interaction of various impulses occurs in the geniculate body. However, the predominant view at present is that impulses from the right and left retinae are not integrated in the lateral geniculate body. Such integration takes place only in the cerebral cortex.

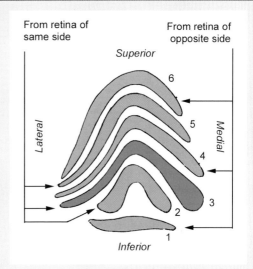

Fig. 13.15. Laminae of lateral geniculate body

The Hypothalamus

The hypothalamus is a part of the diencephalon. As its name implies it lies below the thalamus. On the medial side, it forms the wall of the third ventricle below the level of the hypothalamic sulcus. Laterally, it is in contact with the internal capsule, and (in the posterior part) with the ventral thalamus (subthalamus). Posteriorly, the hypothalamus merges with the ventral thalamus, and through it with the tegmentum of the midbrain. Anteriorly, it extends up to the lamina terminalis, and merges with certain olfactory structures in the region of the anterior perforated substance. Inferiorly, the hypothalamus is related to structures in the floor of the third ventricle. These are the tuber cinereum, the infundibulum, and the mamillary bodies, which are considered as parts of the hypothalamus.

Subdivisions of the Hypothalamus

For convenience of description the hypothalamus may be subdivided, roughly, into a number of regions (Figs. 13.16, 13.17). Some authorities divide it (from medial to lateral side) into three *zones* which are as follows.

(a) *Periventricular zone.*

(b) *Intermediate zone.*

(c) *Lateral zone.*

The periventricular and intermediate zones are often described collectively as the *medial zone* and we will follow this practice here. The column of the fornix lies between the medial and lateral zones. (The mamillothalamic tract and the fasciculus retroflexus also lie in this plane).

The hypothalamus is also subdivided anteroposteriorly into four *regions*. These are as follows.

(a) The *preoptic region* adjoins the lamina terminalis.

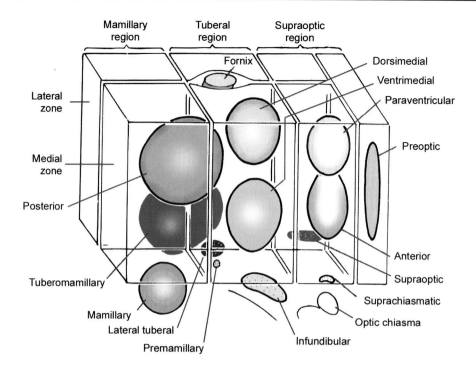

Fig. 13.16. Scheme to show the regions and zones of the hypothalamus and nuclei within them.

Fig. 13.17. Hypothalamic regions and nuclei in them.		
	Medial zone (Periventricular and intermediate)	Lateral zone
Preoptic region	Preoptic nucleus	
Supraoptic region	Paraventricular nu. Periventricular cell groups Suprachiasmatic nu. Intermediate cell groups (= anterior nucleus ?)	Supraoptic nucleus*
Tuberal region	Dorsimedial nucleus Ventrimedial nucleus Arcuate (infundibular) nucleus Premamillary nucleus	Lateral tuberal nucleus
Mamillary or posterior region	Posterior nucleus (lies partly in tuberal region)	Tuberomamillary nucleus*
Mamillary body	Mamillary nuclei	
*From a functional point of view the supraoptic and tuberomamillary nuclei are grouped with the nuclei of the intermediate zone.		

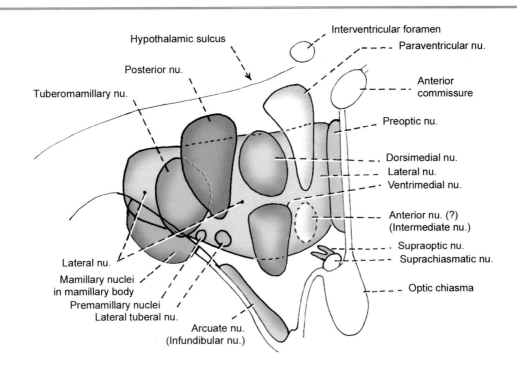

Fig. 13.18. Diagram to show the main hypothalamic nuclei as seen from the medial (ventricular) aspect.

(b) The ***supraoptic (or chiasmatic) region*** lies above the optic chiasma.

(c) The ***tuberal (or infundibulotuberal) region*** includes the infundibulum, the tuber cinereum and the region above it.

(d) The ***mamillary (or posterior) region*** consists of the mamillary body and the region above it.

The preoptic region differs from the rest of the hypothalamus in being a derivative of the telencephalon. (The lamina terminalis also belongs to the telencephalon).

Hypothalamic nuclei

The entire hypothalamus contains scattered neurons within which some aggregations can be recognized. These aggregations, termed the hypothalamic nuclei, are as follows (Figs. 13.16 to 13.18).

(1) The ***preoptic nucleus*** extends through the periventricular, intermediate, and lateral zones of the preoptic part.

(2) The ***mamillary nuclei*** lie within the mamillary body.

The remaining nuclei of the hypothalamus lie either in the periventricular, intermediate, or lateral zones. As the boundaries of nuclei are ill defined, different authors have allocated nuclei differently to these zones. To lessen confusion on this account we will consider the periventricular and intermediate zones collectively as the medial zone.

It has also been found that groupings of hypothalamic nuclei based on functional considerations do not necessary follow groupings according to the regions they lie in. The classification that follows is based on traditional teaching, and some comments on functional groupings are made below.

Nuclei in the medial zone

(3) The *paraventricular nucleus,* and

(4) the *suprachiasmatic nucleus,* lie in the supraoptic region.

(5) The *arcuate (or infundibular) nucleus* lies in the tuberal region.

(6) The *posterior nucleus* extends into both the tuberal and mamillary regions.

(7) The *anterior nucleus* occupies the supraoptic region.

(8) The *dorsimedial nucleus,* and

(9) the *ventrimedial nucleus* lie in the tuberal part, which also contains small aggregations of cells that constitute

(10) the *premamillary nuclei.*

Nuclei in the lateral zone

(11) The lateral zone contains a diffuse collection of cells that extend through the supraoptic, tuberal and mamillary regions. These cells constitute the *lateral nucleus.* The lateral zone also contains the following nuclei.

(12) The *supraoptic nucleus* lies in the supraoptic region (just above the optic tract).

(13) The *tuberomamillary nucleus* extends into the tuberal and mamillary regions.

(14) Small aggregations of neurons in the tuberal region constitute the *lateral tuberal nuclei.*

Some additional comments on grouping of hypothalamic nuclei

1. On the basis of functional considerations the supraoptic and tuberomamillary nuclei (of the lateral zone) are grouped along with nuclei in the medial zone.

2. The anterior nucleus is not mentioned in some recent texts. Instead a group of *intermediate nuclei* is described in this situation.

Neuromediators in the Hypothalamus

As many as 25 neuromediators have been located in the hypothalamus, and their distribution has been mapped out. The details are beyond the scope of this book.

Connections of the Hypothalamus

The hypothalamus is concerned with visceral function and is, therefore, connected to other areas having a similar function. These include the various parts of the limbic system, the reticular formation, and autonomic centres in the brainstem and spinal cord (Figs. 13.19, 13.20). Apart from its neural connections, the hypothalamus also acts by releasing secretions into the blood stream, and into CSF.

Afferent Connections

(1) The hypothalamus receives visceral afferents (including those of taste) through the spinal cord and brainstem. The exact pathways are not known. They probably pass through the reticular formation and consist of several relays.

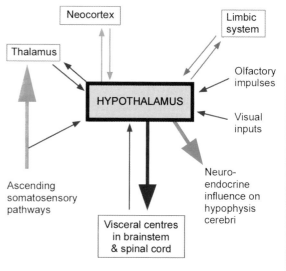

Fig. 13.19. Summary of main connections of the hypothalamus.

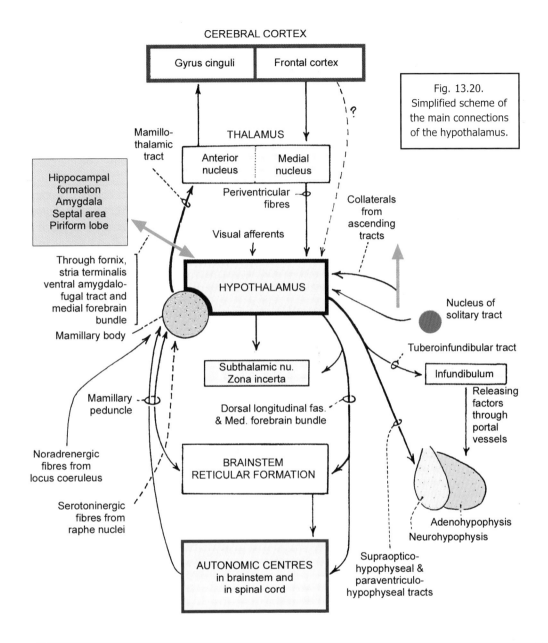

CEREBRAL CORTEX

Gyrus cinguli | Frontal cortex

?

Fig. 13.20.
Simplified scheme of
the main connections
of the hypothalamus.

Mamillo-
thalamic
tract

THALAMUS

Anterior
nucleus | Medial
nucleus

Hippocampal
formation
Amygdala
Septal area
Piriform lobe

Periventricular
fibres

Collaterals
from
ascending
tracts

Visual afferents

Through fornix,
stria terminalis
ventral amygdalo-
fugal tract and
medial forebrain
bundle

HYPOTHALAMUS

Nucleus of
solitary tract

Mamillary body

Tuberoinfundibular tract

Mamillary
peduncle

Subthalamic nu.
Zona incerta

Infundibulum

Releasing
factors
through
portal
vessels

Dorsal longitudinal fas.
& Med. forebrain bundle

Noradrenergic
fibres from
locus coeruleus

BRAINSTEM
RETICULAR FORMATION

Serotoninergic
fibres from
raphe nuclei

Adenohypophysis
Neurohypophysis

AUTONOMIC CENTRES
in brainstem and
in spinal cord

Supraoptico-
hypophyseal &
paraventriculo-
hypophyseal tracts

Many of these fibres pass through a bundle called the *mamillary peduncle*. Other fibres pass through a bundle called the *dorsal longitudinal fasciculus*. Fibres from the tegmentum of the midbrain also reach the hypothalamus through the *medial forebrain bundle.*

(2) Afferents from the nucleus of the solitary tract carry taste impulses (and other visceral sensations).

(3) Somatic afferents reach the hypothalamus through collaterals of major ascending tracts.

(4) The hypothalamus receives afferents from several centres connected to olfactory pathways, and to the limbic system.

These are the anterior perforated substance, the septal nuclei, the amygdaloid complex, the hippocampus and the piriform cortex. Many of these fibres reach the hypothalamus through the medial forebrain bundle. Fibres from the hippocampus travel through the fornix. Some fibres from the amygdaloid complex pass through the stria terminalis, and some through the ventral amygdofugal tract (Fig. 16.9).

Olfactory impulses are received after relay in the nucleus accumbens (in the ventral thalamus, near the anterior perforated substance); and through septal nuclei.

Visceral impulses reach the suprachiasmatic nucleus.

The locus coeruleus is connected to the hypothalamus through diffuse noradrenergic fibres. The raphe nuclei project to the hypothalamus through serotoninergic fibres. Some cholinergic and dopaminergic fibres also reach the hypothalamus.

(5) Cortico-hypothalamic fibres: In addition to fibres from the piriform cortex (mentioned above) the hypothalamus is believed to receive fibres from the cortex of the frontal lobe. Some of these are direct. Others relay in the thalamus (medial dorsal and midline nuclei) and reach the hypothalamus through periventricular fibres (so called because they travel just subjacent to the ependyma). The gyrus cinguli may influence the hypothalamus indirectly through the hippocampal formation. Some fibres from the orbital cortex may reach the hypothalamus through the medial forebrain bundle.

(6) The hypothalamus also receives fibres from the subthalamic nucleus, and the zona incerta.

Efferent Connections

(1) The hypothalamus sends fibres to autonomic centres in the brainstem and spinal cord. Centres in the brainstem receiving such fibres include the nucleus of the solitary tract, the dorsal nucleus of the vagus, the nucleus ambiguus, and the parabrachial nucleus. Fibres descending to the spinal cord end in neurons in the intermediolateral grey column. It also sends fibres to the hippocampal formation, the septal nuclei, the amygdaloid complex, and the tegmentum of the midbrain, and autonomic centres in the brainstem and spinal cord. These fibres pass through the same bundles that convey afferent fibres from these centres.

(2) Fibres from the mamillary body pass through the mamillothalamic tract to reach the anterior nucleus of the thalamus. New fibres arising here project to the gyrus cinguli. Fibres from the mamillary nuclei also reach the subthalamic region and the tegmentum. (through the mamillo-tegmental tract).

(3) Fibres from the hypothalamus project widely to the neocortex. They play a role in maintaining cortical arousal.

Control of hypophysis cerebri by the hypothalamus.

Neurons in some hypothalamic nuclei produce bioactive peptides that are discharged in the neighbourhood of capillaries; or in some cases into CSF. The process of the production of such bioactive

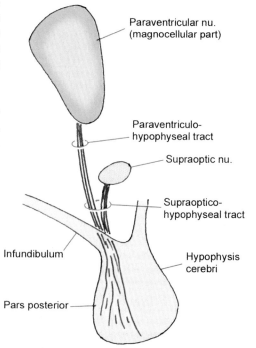

Fig. 13.21. Paraventriculo-hypophyseal and supraoptico-hypophyseal tracts.

	Hypothalamic nuclei producing them			
Fig. 13.22. Releasing factors produced by hypothalamic nuclei	Arcuate nucleus	Periventricular cell groups	Paraventricular nucleus	Ventrimedial nu. Dorsimedial nu.
GHRH (Growth hormone releasing hormone)	+			
Somatostatin (inhibits GH and TSH)		+		
GnRH (gonadotropin releasing hormone)	+	+		
CRH (corticotropin releasing hormone)			+	
TRH (thyrotropin releasing hormone)		+		+
Dopamine (inhibits prolactin and TSH)	+			

substances by neurons (as distinct from release of neurotransmitters at synapses or efferent nerve endings) is referred to as **neurosecretion**.

The peptides (hormones) are synthesised by the neuron and are seen as membrane bound granules. Each peptide is associated with a **neurophysin** which binds the peptide. The granules move along axons to their terminations. Neurosecretory material in cell somata and in axons can be demonstrated by suitable staining. Release of peptide is triggered by activity of the neuron (and is associated with influx of Ca_{++} ions at the terminals). The released peptides are absorbed into blood. The release of peptides depends on inputs to the neurons concerned. Neurosecretory cells are influenced by temperature and osmolarity of blood, and by concentrations in it of hormones and of nutrients.

Control of Neurohypophysis

It is now known that **vasopressin** (antidiuretic hormone) and **oxytocin**, associated with the neurohypophysis, are really neurosecretory products synthesised in the paraventricular and supraoptic nuclei of the hypothalamus. The cells concerned are large (magnocellular secretion). Axons of the paraventricular nucleus descend towards the supraoptic nucleus as the **paraventriculohypophyseal tract** (Fig. 13.21). They join axons arising from the supraoptic nucleus to form the **supraoptico-hypophyseal tract**. The axons of the tract pass down into the infundibulum and from there into the neurohypophysis. Here the axons branch

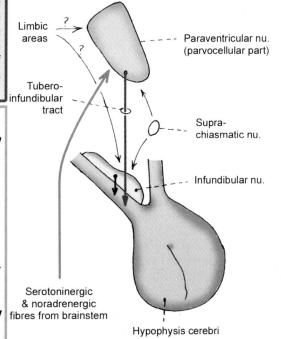

Fig. 13.23. Some areas concerned in production of releasing factors.

profusely and end in relation to capillaries around which they release their secretion.

The neurons producing vasopressin and oxytocin are distinct. Although both types of neurons are found in each nucleus, the supraoptic nucleus is believed to mainly produce vasopressin, and the paraventricular nucleus is believed to mainly produce oxytocin.

Control of the adenohypophysis by the hypothalamus

The hypothalamus controls secretion of hormones by the adenohypophysis by producing a number of *releasing factors*. Axons of cells in the infundibular (arcuate) nucleus end in the median eminence and infundibulum. They travel through the *tuberohypophyseal tract* which also receives fibres from several other hypothalamic nuclei. The axon terminals of the fibres in these tracts are closely related to capillaries in the region. The cells of the arcuate (infundibular) nucleus produce releasing factors that travel along their axons and are released into the capillaries. These capillaries carry these factors into the pars anterior of the hypophysis cerebri through the *hypothalamo-hypophyseal portal system*. In the pars anterior these factors are responsible for release of appropriate hormones. It may be noted, however, that in the case of some hormones their secretion is inhibited by such factors.

In addition to the arcuate nucleus some other hypothalamic nuclei are also involved in production of releasing factors. The nuclei and the releasing factors produced by them are shown in Fig. 13.22. Fig. 13.23 shows some pathways through which the production of releasing factors may be controlled.

Fibre bundles associated with the hypothalamus

In considering the connections of the hypothalamus reference has been made to a number of fibre bundles not described earlier. These are briefly considered below.

Medial forebrain bundle

The medial forebrain bundle begins in the anterior olfactory areas. It runs caudally through the lateral zone of the hypothalamus, to reach the tegmentum of the midbrain. It contains both ascending and descending fibres. Cholinergic, noradrenergic and dopaminergic fasciculi pass through this bundle. Various other neuromediators have also been demonstrated in relation to this bundle.

Mamillary peduncle

The mamillary peduncle is a bundle of fibres that connects the tegmentum of the midbrain to the mamillary body. The fibres in it carry visceral impulses to the hypothalamus (Fig. 13.20).

Dorsal longitudinal fasciculus

The dorsal longitudinal fasciculus (of Schultz) runs vertically within the brainstem, in close relation to the central grey matter. It is made of unmyelinated fibres and is, therefore, also called the *unmyelinated longitudinal fasciculus*. It connects centres in the midbrain, pons, and the upper part of the medulla with the hypothalamus and thalamus. The fibres in it are both ascending and descending.

Central tegmental tract

This tract descends through the midbrain. It lies lateral to the medial longitudinal fasciculus, dorsolateral to the red nucleus. When traced upwards it ascends through the ventral thalamic (subthalamic) region to reach the lentiform nucleus. Some fibres even reach the motor cortex. Traced downwards the tract extends to the medulla where it reaches the inferior olivary complex, and the reticular formation.

In the brainstem, most the fibres in the tract are those arising in the parvocellular part of the red nucleus. These fibres descend to the inferior olivary complex. The central tegmental tract connects the motor cortex and red nucleus to the reticular formation and the inferior olivary complex.

Some fibres in the tract are serotoninergic, noradrenergic or cholinergic. The noradrenergic fibres arise from the nucleus coeruleus.

Functions of the Hypothalamus

The hypothalamus plays an important role in the control of many functions that are vital for the survival of an animal. In exercising such control the hypothalamus acts in close coordination with higher centres including the limbic system and the prefrontal cortex, and with autonomic centres in the brainstem and spinal cord. The main functions attributed to the hypothalamus are as follows.

Regulation of eating and drinking behaviour

The hypothalamus is responsible for feelings of hunger and of satiety, and this determines whether the animal will accept or refuse food. It has been observed that stimulation of the lateral zone of the hypothalamus stimulates hunger while stimulation of the medial zone produces satiety. The lateral zone is also responsible for thirst and drinking. Based on such studies a **feeding centre** has been described in the lateral hypothalamic nucleus, and a **satiety centre** in the ventromedial nucleus.

Correlate this with the fact that some neurons in the hypothalamus are sensitive to osmolarity (preoptic nucleus), glucose content and fatty acid content of blood.

Regulation of sexual activity and reproduction

The hypothalamus controls sexual activity, both in the male and female. It also exerts an effect on gametogenesis, on ovarian and uterine cycles, and on the development of secondary sexual characters. These effects are produced by influencing the secretion of gonadotropic hormones by the hypophysis cerebri.

Control of autonomic activity

The hypothalamus exerts an important influence on the activity of the autonomic nervous system, and thus has considerable effect on cardiovascular, respiratory and alimentary functions. Sympathetic activity is said to be controlled, predominantly, by caudal parts of the hypothalamus; and parasympathetic activity by cranial parts, but there is considerable overlap between the regions concerned.

Emotional behaviour

The hypothalamus has an important influence on emotions like fear, anger and pleasure. Stimulation of some areas of the hypothalamus produces sensations of pleasure, while stimulation of other regions produces pain or other unpleasant effects.

Control of endocrine activity

The influence of the hypothalamus in the production of hormones by the pars anterior of the hypophysis cerebri, and the elaboration of oxytocin and the antidiuretic hormone by the hypothalamus itself, have been described above. Through control of the adenohypophysis, the hypothalamus indirectly influences the thyroid gland, the adrenal cortex, and the gonads.

Response to stress.

Through control over the autonomic nervous system, and hormones, the hypothalamus plays a complex role in the way a person responds to stress.

Temperature regulation

Some neurons in the preoptic nucleus of the hypothalamus act as a thermostat to control body temperature. When body temperature rises or falls, appropriate mechanisms are brought into play to bring the temperature back to normal.

Biological clock

Several functions of the body show a cyclic variation in activity, over the twenty four hours of a day. The most conspicuous of these is the cycle of sleep and waking. Such cycles (called *circadian rhythms*) are believed to be controlled by the hypothalamus, which is said to function as a biological clock. The suprachiasmatic nucleus is believed to play an important role in this regard. Lesions of the hypothalamus disturb the sleep-waking cycle.

Pressure on the hypothalamus can give rise to the *hypothalamic syndrome* that is marked by diabetes insipidus.

The Epithalamus

The epithalamus lies in relation to the posterior part of the roof of the third ventricle, and in the adjoining part of its lateral wall. The structures included in the epithalamus are as follows.

1. Pineal body.   **2.** Paraventricular nuclei, anterior and posterior. (Do not confuse these with the paraventricular nucleus in the hypothalamus).   **3.** Habenular nuclei, medial and lateral.   **4.** Stria medullaris thalami. **5.** Posterior commissure.

The Pineal body

The pineal body (or pineal gland) is a small piriform structure present in relation to the posterior wall of the third ventricle of the brain. It has for long been regarded as a vestigeal structure of no functional importance. However, it is now known to be an endocrine gland of considerable significance. The pineal body is made up of cells called *pinealocytes.* Pinealocytes are separated from one another by neuroglial cells that resemble astrocytes in structure (For details see the author's HUMAN HISTOLOGY). The pineal body produces a number of hormones (chemically indolamines or polypeptides). These hormones have an important regulatory influence on many endocrine organs including the hypophysis cerebri, the thyroid, the parathyroids, the adrenals, and the gonads. The hormones of the pineal body reach the hypophysis cerebri both through blood and through the cerebrospinal fluid.

The attachment of the pineal body to the posterior wall of the third ventricle is through a stalk that has two laminae, superior and inferior. The superior lamina is traversed by fibres of the *habenular commissure*; and the inferior lamina by fibres of the *posterior commissure.*

The pineal body is innervated by postganglionic sympathetic neurons located in the superior cervical sympathetic ganglia. The fibres travel through the *nervus conarii*. The fibres of this nerve end in the habenular nuclei. Fibres arising in these nuclei form the *habenulopineal tract.* A ganglion (*ganglion conarii)* has been described at the apex of the pineal body.

Some activities of the pineal body (e.g., the secretion of the hormone *melatonin*) show a marked circadian rythm, which appears to be strongly influenced by exposure of the animal to light. Activity of the pineal body is greater in darkness. It has been suggested that the suprachiasmatic nucleus of the hypothalamus plays an important role in the cyclic activity of the pineal body. This nucleus receives fibres from the retina. In turn it projects to the tegmental reticular nuclei. Reticulospinal fibres arising in these nuclei influence the sympathetic preganglionic neurons in the first thoracic segment of the the spinal cord. Axons of these neurons reach the superior cervical sympathetic ganglia from which the nervus conarii arises and supplies the pineal body.

A tumour of the pineal body can produce *precocious puberty*. Melatonin is believed to regulate the onset of puberty.

Paraventricular nuclei of epithalamus

These are groups of neurons lying deep to ependyma of the dorsal part of the third ventricle (close to the midline thalamic nuclei). Some connections of these nuclei are shown in Fig. 13.24.

The Habenular Nuclei

The habenular nuclei (medial and lateral) are situated in relation to a triangular depression in the wall of the third ventricle called the **habenular trigone.** The trigone lies in relation to the dorsomedial part of the thalamus. It is medial to the pulvinar, separated from it by the sulcus habenulae. The superior colliculus lies just behind the trigone. The habenular nuclei of the two sides are connected by fibres that form the habenular commissure (see below).

These nuclei have been regarded as cell stations in olfactory and visceral pathways but their function is not understood. The habenular nuclei receive afferents from several areas included in the limbic system (Fig. 13. 25). Most of these fibres travel through the stria medullaris thalami (see below). Ascending fibres from the tegmentum of the midbrain reach the habenular nuclei through ascending

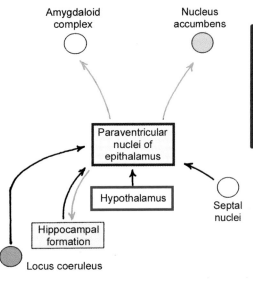

Fig. 13.24. Connections of paraventricular nuclei of the epithalamus.

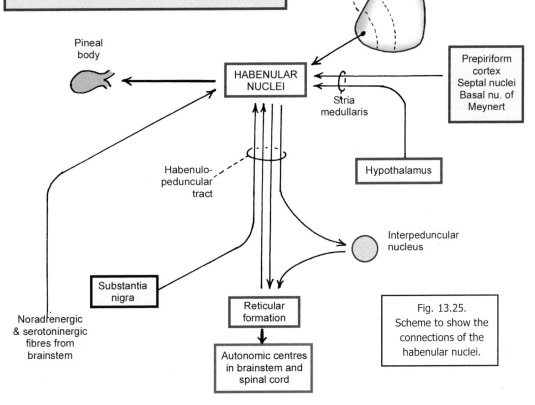

Fig. 13.25. Scheme to show the connections of the habenular nuclei.

noradrenergic and serotonergic bundles that travel through the habenulopeduncular tract (see below).

Efferents from the habenular nuclei reach the pineal body through the ***habenulopineal tract***. The main outflow from these nuclei reaches the interpeduncular nucleus through the ***habenulopeduncular tract*** which is also called the ***fasciculus retroflexus.*** Other efferents are shown in Fig. 13.25. The habenular nuclei influence neurons concerned with various visceral and endocrine functions. They may be involved in control of sleep, and in temperature regulation.

Stria Medullaris Thalami & Habenular commissure

The ***stria medullaris thalami*** is a bundle of fibres lying deep to the taenia thalami (along the junction of the medial and superior surfaces of the thalamus). It begins near the anterior pole of the thalamus and runs backwards to reach the habenular region. Many afferents to the habenular nuclei pass through the stria medullaris thalami.

Some fibres of the stria medullaris thalami cross in the superior (or anterior) lamina of the pineal stalk to reach the habenular nuclei of the opposite side. These fibres constitute the ***habenular commissure.***

Some of the fibres passing through this commissure are true commissural fibres that connect the amygdaloid complex and the hippocampal cortex of the right and left cerebral hemispheres. Some tectohabenular fibres also pass through the commissure.

Several neuromediators have been demonstrated in the fibres of the stria medullaris. These include acetylcholine, noradrenalin, serotonin and GABA.

Posterior Commissure

The posterior commissure lies in the inferior lamina of the stalk of the pineal body. A number of small nuclei are present in relation to the commissure. These include the interstitial and dorsal nuclei of the posterior commissure, the nucleus of Darkschewitsch, and the interstitial nucleus of Cajal. Some fibres arising from these nuclei pass through the posterior commissure. Other fibres continue into it from the medial longitudinal bundle. Some fibres arising in the thalamus, the tectum, and the pretectal nuclei also pass through the posterior commissure.

Teachers and students who have read some earlier editions of this book should note that the subthalamic region is now called the ventral thalamus. They will find the list of structures included in this region unusual. The following clarifications are necessary.

1. The subthalamic nucleus is closely related topographically, to this region. However, on functional considerations it is now considered to be one of the basal nuclei.

2. The reticular nucleus was previously included as one of the nuclei of the dorsal thalamus. However, on the basis of its connections it is now considered as part of the ventral thalamus.

3. From the above it will be seen that the term ventral thalamus is applied to a functionally related group of nuclei and not just to structures lying ventral to the dorsal thalamus.

The Ventral Thalamus

The part of the diencephalon that is called the ventral thalamus lies below the posterior part of the thalamus, behind and lateral to the hypothalamus. In the past it has been referred to as the subthalamic region.

Inferiorly, the ventral thalamus is continuous with the tegmentum of the midbrain (the upper ends of the red nucleus and the substantia nigra reaching it). Laterally, it is related to the lowest part of the internal capsule.

The main masses of grey matter that are included in the ventral thalamus are the reticular nucleus (previously described as part of the dorsal thalamus), the zona incerta and the perigeniculate nuclei.

The Reticular Nucleus

The reticular nucleus is made up of a thin layer of neurons covering the lateral aspect of the (dorsal) thalamus, separated from the latter by the external medullary velum. Laterally, the nucleus is related to the internal capsule. Inferiorly, it becomes partially continuous with the zona incerta.

Most fibres emerging from the dorsal thalamus have to traverse the reticular nucleus. (The fibres crossing through it give the nucleus a reticulated appearance, and hence the name). As they pass through it the fibres give collaterals to the reticular nucleus.

In this way the nucleus receives somatic, visceral and auditory impulses. The main efferents of the reticular nucleus pass back into the dorsal thalamus. These fibres are GABAergic. They may influence conduction through the dorsal thalamus (Fig. 13.26). The reticular nucleus also receives fibres from the nucleus cuneiformis (in the reticular formation of the midbrain).

The Pregeniculate Nucleus

This nucleus has connections similar to those of the lateral geniculate nucleus. Its visual connections include fibres from the retina, pretectal region and superior colliculus. It has numerous other connections. The nucleus appears to have some role in vision and in eye movements.

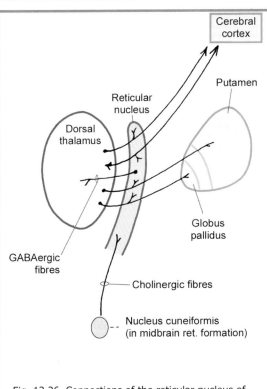

Fig. 13.26. Connections of the reticular nucleus of the thalamus.

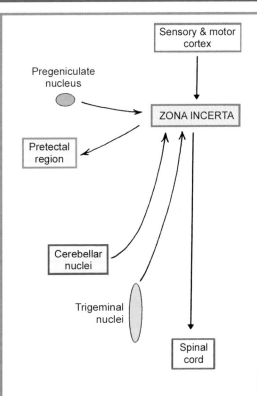

Fig. 13.27. Connections of the zona incerta.

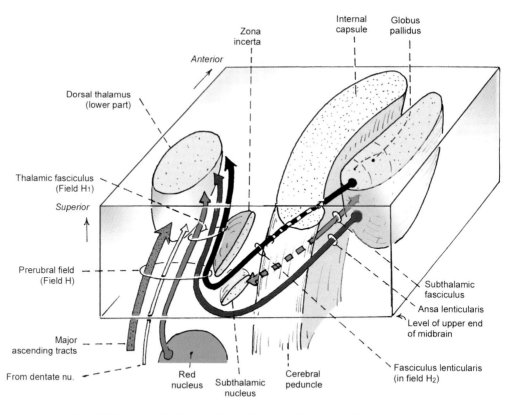

Fig. 13.28. Schematic 3-dimensional diagram of the ventral thalamic region
to show some of its features.

The Zona Incerta

The zona incerta is a thin lamina of grey matter continuous with the reticular nucleus of the thalamus. It intervenes between the subthalamic nucleus and the thalamus. Its functions are not known. Some of its connections are shown in Fig. 13.27.

ADVANCED

Lying near the zona inserta there are two groups of neurons that need mention.

(a) Some neurons lie along the lower edge of the zona inserta (near the upper end of the red nucleus). These are termed the nuclei of the prerubral field.

(b) Some neurons lying within the fibres of the ansa lenticularis (see below) constitute the entopeduncular nucleus.

Both these nuclei receive fibres from the globus pallidus and relay them to the reticular formation of the midbrain. Some fibres descend to the inferior olivary complex and to other brainstem nuclei.

BASIC

Fibre Bundles passing through the Subthalamic Region

In addition to its grey matter the subthalamic region contains a number of fibre bundles (Fig. 13.28,). Ascending tracts (medial lemniscus, spinal lemniscus, trigeminal lemniscus) pass through it on their way from the midbrain to the thalamus. They are accompanied by dentato-thalamic and rubrothalamic fibres.

The subthalamic region also contains two bundles of fibres that connect the globus pallidus to the thalamus. These are the ***ansa lenticularis*** and the ***fasciculus lenticularis***. Associated with these bundles there are certain regions called the fields of Forel (H, H_1, and H_2) shown in Fig. 13.28.

Starting from the globus pallidus, the ***ansa lenticularis*** winds round the ventral and posterior border of the internal capsule to reach the subthalamic region, where it lies ventral and medial to the subthalamic nucleus. Fibres of the ***fasciculus lenticularis*** intersect those of the internal capsule to reach the subthalamic region. Here they pass medially above the subthalamic nucleus and below the zona incerta. This region is field H_2 of Forel.

The ***subthalamic fasciculus*** (connecting the globus pallidus to the subthalamic nucleus) occupies a position intermediate between the ansa lenticularis and the fasciculus lenticularis. The fibres of the ansa lenticularis and of the fasciculus lenticularis join together medial to the subthalamic nucleus (in field H of Forel) to form the ***thalamic fasciculus*** (which is also joined by dentatothalamic and rubrothalamic fibres). The thalamic fasciculus passes above the zona incerta (field H_1 of Forel) to reach the thalamus.

THE SUBTHALAMIC NUCLEUS

As explained above the subthalamic nucleus which has traditionally been described as a part of the subthalamic region is now grouped functionally with the basal nuclei which are considered in Chapter 14.

The subthalamic nucleus is shaped like a biconvex lens. It lies between the thalamus above, and the substantia nigra below (Figs. 13.2, 13.28). The upper end of the red nucleus is close to it. The nucleus is closely related to the zona incerta, the fascicularis lenticularis intervening between the two.

The fibres connecting the subthalamic nucleus to the globus pallidus form a bundle called the ***subthalamic fasciculus*** which passes through the internal capsule. For connections of the subthalamic nucleus see Chapter 14.

DEVELOPMENT OF THE DIENCEPHALON

The establishment of the diencephalon has been described on page 71. On page 87 we have seen that with the great enlargement of the telencephalon, the diencephalon comes to lie on the medial side of the cerebral hemisphere. The lateral wall of the diencephalon is subdivided by the appearance of the epithalamic and hypothalamic sulci. The central part lying between the two sulci enlarges to form the thalamus. The part above the epithalamic sulcus remains small and forms the epithalamus which is represented by the habenular nuclei and the pineal body. The part below the hypothalamic sulcus forms the hypothalamus.

RELATED TOPICS

The third ventricle which is the cavity of the diencephalon is described in Chapter 20.
The bood supply of the region is given in Chapter 21.

14 : The Basal Nuclei

The basal nuclei (or basal ganglia) are large masses of grey matter situated in the cerebral hemispheres. Classically, the following have been included under the definition of basal nuclei (Fig. 13.2). All these are telencephalic in origin.

(a) *Caudate nucleus.*

(b) *Lentiform nucleus*, which consists of two functionally distinct parts, the *putamen* and the *globus pallidus*.

(c) *Amygdaloid nuclear complex*.

(d) The *claustrum* is often included among the basal ganglia.

Various other terms commonly used for some of the above nuclei are as follows. The caudate nucleus and the lentiform nucleus together constitute the *corpus striatum.* This consists of two functionally distinct parts. The caudate nucleus and the putamen form one unit called the *striatum,* while the globus pallidus forms the other unit, the *pallidum.*

Recent researches have shown that a number of masses of grey matter, other than those listed above, are very closely related functionally to the basal nuclei. These are as follows.

1. The *subthalamic nucleus* (which is of diencephalic origin) is so closely linked to the basal nuclei that it is now regarded as belonging to this group.

2. The *substantia nigra* (midbrain) is also closely linked, functionally, to the basal nuclei.

3. Some masses of grey matter found just below the corpus striatum (near the anterior perforated substance) are described as the *ventral striatum*. The part of the globus pallidus which lies below the level of the anterior commissure is designated as the *ventral pallidum*.

The Caudate Nucleus

The caudate nucleus is a C-shaped mass of grey matter (Fig.14.1). It consists of a large head, a body and a thin tail. The nucleus is intimately related to the lateral ventricle. The head of the nucleus bulges into the anterior horn of the ventricle and forms the greater part of its floor (Fig.20.3). The body of the nucleus lies in the floor of the central part (Fig. 20.2); and the tail in the roof of the inferior horn of the ventricle (Fig. 20.5). The anterior part of the head of the caudate nucleus is fused, inferiorly, with the lentiform nucleus. This region of fusion is referred to as the *fundus striati*. The fundus striati is continuous, inferiorly, with the anterior perforated substance. The anterior end of the tail of the caudate nucleus ends by becoming continuous with the lentiform nucleus. It lies in close relation to the amygdaloid complex.

The body of the caudate nucleus is related medially to the thalamus, and laterally to the internal capsule which separates it from the lentiform nucleus (Fig. 14.2). Some other relationships of the caudate nucleus are shown in Fig. 13.2.

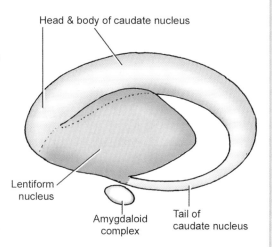

Fig. 14.1. The corpus striatum viewed from the lateral aspect.

The Lentiform Nucleus

The lentiform nucleus lies lateral to the internal capsule. Laterally, it is separated from the claustrum by fibres of the external capsule. (Note that these capsules are so called because they appear, by naked eye, to form a covering for the lentiform nucleus). Superiorly, the lentiform nucleus is related to the corona radiata, and inferiorly to the sublentiform part of the internal capsule. Some other relationships are evident in Fig. 13.2. The lentiform nucleus appears triangular (or wedge shaped) in coronal section. It is divided, by a thin lamina of white matter, into a lateral part, the **putamen;** and a medial part, the **globus pallidus.** The globus pallidus is further subdivided into medial and lateral (or internal and external) segments.

The Claustrum

This is a thin lamina of grey matter that lies lateral to the lentiform nucleus. It is separated from the latter by fibres of the external capsule. Laterally, it is separated by a thin layer of white matter from the cortex of the insula. Its connections and functions are unknown.

The Amygdaloid Complex

This complex (also called the amygdaloid body, amygdala) lies in the temporal lobe of the cerebral hemisphere, close to the temporal pole. It lies deep to the uncus, and is related to the anterior end of the inferior horn of the lateral ventricle.

Connections of the Basal Nuclei

The various basal nuclei have numerous connections, but no useful purpose is served by enumerating the afferents and efferents of each nucleus. An integrated view of the corpus striatum, along with the substantia nigra and the subthalamic nucleus, is necessary. A scheme showing the main connections is given in Fig. 14.3.

The striatum (caudate nucleus and putamen) receive afferents from the following.

(**1**) The entire cerebral cortex. These fibres are glutamatergic.

(**2**) The intralaminar nuclei of the thalamus.

(**3**) The pars compacta of the substantia nigra. These fibres are dopaminergic. (Some dopaminergic fibres arise from the retrorubral nuclei lying behind the red nucleus).

(**4**) Noradrenergic fibres are received from the raphe nuclei (in the reticular formation of the midbrain).

(**5**) Serotoninergic fibres are received from the locus coeruleus.

The afferents from the cerebral cortex and from the thalamus provide the striatum with various modalities of sensory information (other than olfactory). The main output of the striatum is concentrated upon the pallidum, and on the

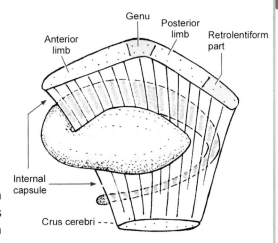

Fig. 14.2. Relationship of the corpus striatum to the internal capsule.

substantia nigra (pars reticularis). Fibres also reach the substantia nigra from the pallidum directly, or after relay in the subthalamic nucleus or in the pedunculo-pontine nucleus.

The efferents of the pallidum are as follows.

1. Like the striatum, the pallidum projects to the substantia nigra. These fibres take three main routes. Some reach the substantia nigra directly. Others are relayed in the subthalamic nucleus; while still others are relayed in the pedunculopontine nucleus.

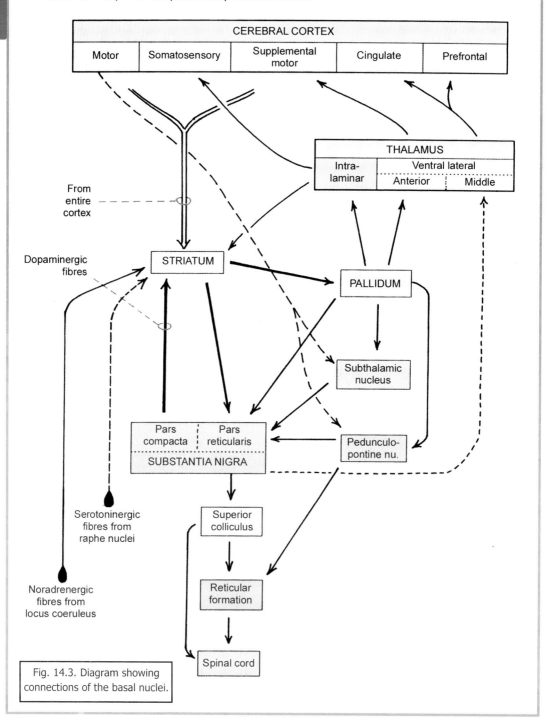

Fig. 14.3. Diagram showing connections of the basal nuclei.

2. The pallidum projects to the intralaminar nuclei of the thalamus, from where impulses are relayed to the somatosensory area of the cerebral cortex.

3. The pallidum also projects to the anterior part of the ventral lateral nucleus of the thalamus. These inputs are relayed to the supplemental motor area.

Connections of substantia nigra

As shown in Fig. 14.3 the pars compacta of the substantia nigra sends a dopaminergic projection to the striatum. A projection from the striatum ends in the pars reticularis of the substantia nigra. This part also receives fibres from the pallidum directly, or after relay in the subthalamic nucleus or in the pedunculo-pontine nucleus.

The pars reticularis projects to the (middle part of the) ventral lateral nucleus of the thalamus. These impulses are relayed to cingulate and prefrontal areas of the cerebral cortex. Other efferents of the pars reticularis reach the superior colliculus. They are relayed from there to the reticular formation of the medulla, and to the spinal cord. These regions also receive fibres descending from the pedunculopontine nucleus.

In summary note the following.

(**a**) The various basal nuclei are interconnected. The substantia nigra, the subthalamic nucleus, and the pedunculo-pontine nucleus form an integral part of this interconnected system.

(**b**) Cranially, the system receives fibres from the cerebral cortex; and send back impulses to it through the thalamus.

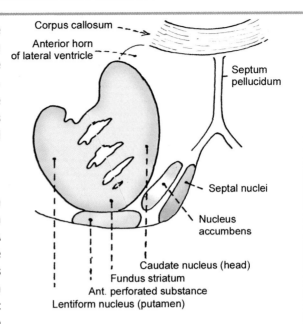

Fig. 14.4. Coronal section passing through the anterior part of the corpus striatum.

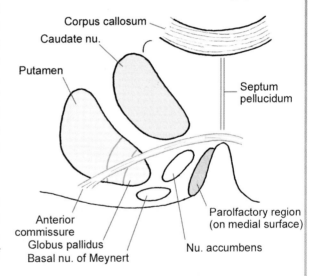

Fig. 14.5. Composite diagram showing the region of the ventral thalamus. Actually, all structures shown cannot be seen in any one vertical plane.

(**c**) Descending fibres from the system influence the superior colliculus, the reticular formation of the medulla, and the spinal cord.

Ventral striatum and pallidum

On the basis of recent investigations some masses of grey matter lying in the region of the anterior perforated substance are now described as the ventral striatum. In Fig. 14.4 we see the anterior part

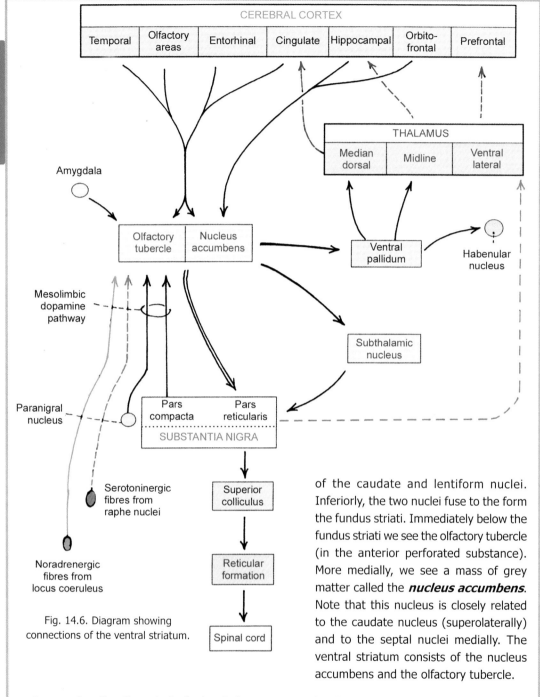

Fig. 14.6. Diagram showing connections of the ventral striatum.

of the caudate and lentiform nuclei. Inferiorly, the two nuclei fuse to the form the fundus striati. Immediately below the fundus striati we see the olfactory tubercle (in the anterior perforated substance). More medially, we see a mass of grey matter called the ***nucleus accumbens***. Note that this nucleus is closely related to the caudate nucleus (superolaterally) and to the septal nuclei medially. The ventral striatum consists of the nucleus accumbens and the olfactory tubercle.

A coronal section through the brain a little posterior to the plane of Fig. 14.4 is shown in Fig. 14.5. Note the anterior commissure running laterally just below the head of the caudate nucleus. It cuts through the globus pallidus. The part of the globus pallidus lying inferior to the anterior commissure is called the ventral pallidum. Identify the olfactory tubercle in Fig. 14.5. Medial to it there is a collection of neurons that form the ***basal nucleus of Meynert***. In this figure the position of the nucleus accumbens is shown diagrammatically: it actually lies more anteriorly.

The reason for considering the nucleus accumbens and the olfactory tubercle as parts of the striatum is that their connections are very similar to those of the main part of the striatum (or dorsal striatum). These are shown in Fig. 14.6 which should be compared with Fig. 14.3.

Abnormal Movements

CLINICAL

Various kinds of abnormal movements are seen in neurological disorders involving the basal nuclei (basal ganglia), the subthalamic nucleus and the cerebellum. These may take the form of involuntary shaking (*tremor*) of the hands, head or other parts of the body, because of rapid alternating contraction of opposing groups of muscles. In some instances the tremor comes on when the patient tries to perform voluntary movement (*intention tremor*). Another type of abnormal movement consists of a slow twisting of a limb, or of the face or neck (*athetosis*). Sudden, jerky, shock-like movements involving any part of the body (*myoclonus*) may also occur. These can cause objects held in the hand to be thrown away (*hemiballism*). Sometimes different, complex, involuntary movements occur in succession, particularly in the distal parts of the limbs (*chorea*).

It has not been possible to precisely correlate specific abnormal movements with disease in specific regions of the basal nuclei and neighbouring structures. The movements are not a result of inactivity of the diseased centres but are, on the contrary, to be regarded as release phenomena, due to abolition of inhibitory influences. Hemiballism is known to be produced by lesions in the subthalamic nucleus. Intention tremor is seen in disorders of the cerebellum.

In many cases, abnormal movements are accompanied by rigidity of muscles, because of increased muscle tone. The increased tone is also a release phenomenon. One common syndrome characterised by rigidity and abnormal movements is called *Parkinsonism* or *paralysis agitans* (shaking palsy). It is characterised by marked rigidity which leads to a stooped posture, a slow shuffling gait, difficulty in speech, and a mask-like face. Characteristic involuntary 'pill-rolling' movements of the hands are seen. The condition is believed to be due to degenerative changes in the striatum and the substantia nigra.

In patients of Parkinsonism positron emission tomography reveals deficit of dopamine in the striatum. Grafting of embryonic ventral mesencephalic tissue, which is rich in dopamine producing neurons, has been tried as a treatment of Parkinsonism with limited success. Further refinements of the technique may make this a clinically valuable treatment. It has also been found that in some disorders of the striatum (e.g., progressive supranuclear gaze palsy) adequate amounts of dopamine reach the striatum from the substantia nigra, but receptors for dopamine are deficient in striatal neurons.

DEVELOPMENT OF THE CORPUS STRIATUM

DEVELOPMENT

The corpus striatum is a derivative of the thickened basal part of the telecephalon. Nerve fibres of the developing internal capsule cut through the developing corpus striatum and divide it into medial and lateral parts. The medial part becomes the caudate nucleus. The lateral part forms the lentiform nucleus.

RELATED TOPICS

The blood supply of the diencephalon is described in Chapter 21.

15 : Further Consideration of the Cerebral Cortex

The division of the cerebral cortex in terms of sulci and gyri has been considered in Chapter 8. The classical concepts regarding the functional areas of the cortex have also been described therein. These should be reviewed before reading the account that follows.

Structure of the Cerebral Cortex

Because of the presence of a large number of sulci, only about one third of the total area of cerebral cortex is seen on the surface of the brain. The total area of the cerebral cortex has been estimated to be about 2000 cm².

Like other masses of grey matter the cerebral cortex contains the cell bodies of an innumerable number of neurons along with their processes, neuroglia and blood vessels. The neurons are of various sizes and shapes. They establish extremely intricate connections with each other and with axons reaching the cortex from other masses of grey matter. In spite of a very large volume of work done on the subject, it is not yet possible to explain the neuronal patterns within the cerebral cortex in terms of function. In any case such considerations are beyond the scope of this book.

Neurons in the Cerebral Cortex

Cortical neurons vary in size, in the shape of their cell bodies, and in the lengths, branching patterns and orientation of their processes. Some of these are described below (Fig. 15.1).

(**1**) The most abundant type of cortical neurons are the *pyramidal cells*. (In contrast all other neurons in the cortex are referred to as non-pyramidal neurons). About two thirds of all cortical neurons are pyramidal. Their cell bodies are triangular, with the apex generally directed towards the surface of the cortex. A large dendrite arises from the apex. Other dendrites arise from basal angles. The axon arises from the base of the pyramid. The processes of pyramidal cells extend vertically through the entire thickness of cortex and establish numerous synapses. The axon of a pyramidal cell may terminate in one of the following ways.

(**a**) It may travel to other regions like the basal ganglia, the brainstem or the spinal cord. Fibres that leave the cortex commonly give off collaterals that terminate within the cortex.

(**b**) It may cross to the opposite side (through a commissure) and reach the corresponding region of the opposite hemisphere. Sometimes it may reach a different region of the opposite hemisphere.

(**c**) It may enter the white matter to travel to another part of the cortex.

(**d**) It may be short and may terminate within the same area of cortex.

(**2**) The *stellate neurons* are relatively small and multipolar. They form about one third of the total neuronal population of the cortex. Under low magnifications (and in preparations in which their processes are not demonstrated) these neurons look like granules. They have, therefore, been termed *granular neurons* by earlier workers. Stellate cells are of various types depending on their location, and on the pattern of ramification of their processes. Their axons are short and end within the cortex. Their processes extend chiefly in a vertical direction within the cortex, but in some cases they may be orientated horizontally. Some cells included under the term stellate may be fusiform rather than stellate, with one large process arising at either end. Some varieties of stellate cells are illustrated in Fig. 15.1. Depending on the density of synaptic spines on their dendrites, stellate neurons are classified as *spiny* and *nonspiny*.

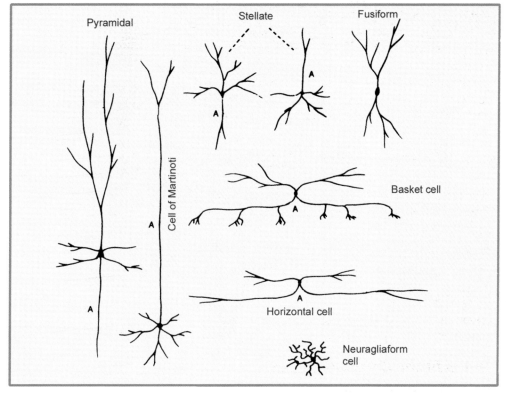

Fig. 15.1. Some of the cell types to be seen in the cerebral cortex. A=axon. Other varieties not shown include bipolar cells, chandelier cells and double bouquet cells.

In addition to the stellate and pyramidal neurons the cortex contains numerous other cell types some of which are illustrated in Fig. 15.1.

The neurotransmitter used by pyramidal cells is either glutamate or aspartate. In spiny stellate cells it is glutamate, while in most nonspiny stellate cells it is GABA.

Laminae of Cerebral Cortex

On the basis of light microscopic preparations stained by methods in which the cell bodies are displayed (e.g., Nissl method) and those where myelinated fibres are stained (e.g., Weigert method) the cerebral cortex is described as having six layers or laminae (Fig. 15.2). From the superficial surface downwards these laminae are as follows.

1. Plexiform or molecular layer. **2**. External granular layer. **3**. Pyramidal cell layer. **4**. Internal granular layer. **5**. Ganglionic layer **6**. Multiform layer.

The plexiform layer is made up predominantly of fibres although a few cells are present. All the remaining layers contain both stellate and pyramidal neurons as well as other types of neurons. The external and internal granular layers are made up predominantly of stellate (granular) cells. The predominant neurons in the pyramidal layer and in the ganglionic layer are pyramidal. The largest pyramidal cells (giant pyramidal cells of Betz) are found in the ganglionic layer. The multiform layer contains cells of various sizes and shapes.

In addition to the cell bodies of neurons the cortex contains abundant nerve fibres. Many of these are vertically orientated. Some of these fibres represent afferents entering the cortex. In addition to the vertical fibres the cortex contains transversely running fibres that form prominent aggregations in certain situations. One such aggregation, present in the internal granular layer is called the **external band of Baillarger**. Another, present in the ganglionic layer is called the **internal band of Baillarger**. The space between the cell bodies of neurons is permeated by a dense plexus formed by their processes. This plexus is referred to as the **neuropil**. (Some workers use the term neuropil for the entire mass of nervous tissue including grey matter as well as white matter).

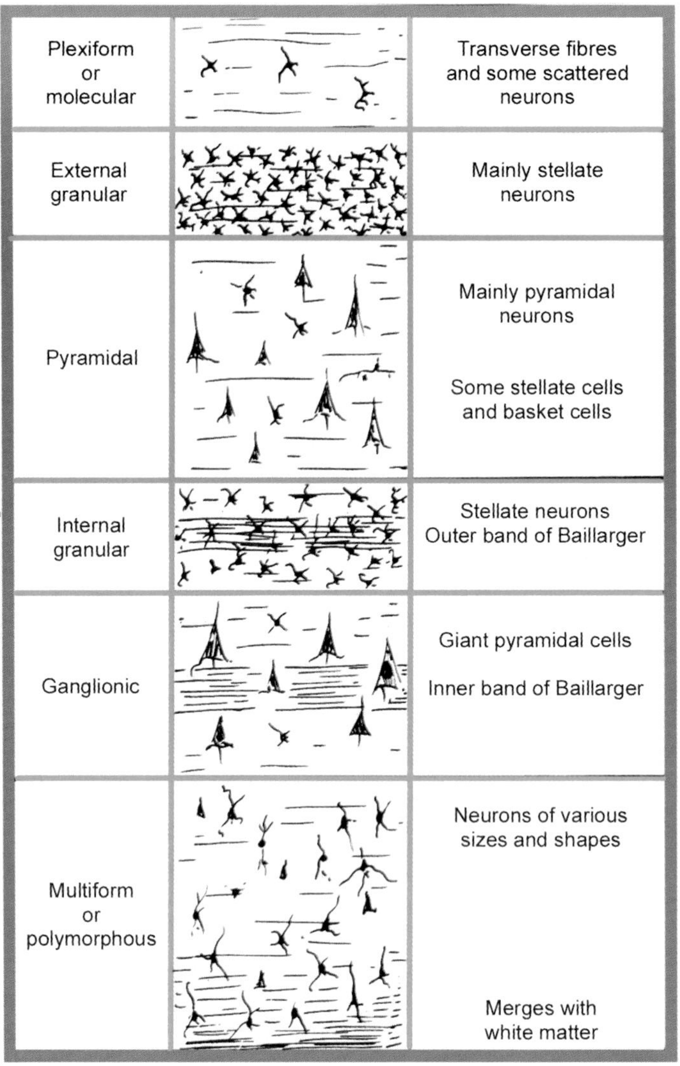

Layer		Description
Plexiform or molecular		Transverse fibres and some scattered neurons
External granular		Mainly stellate neurons
Pyramidal		Mainly pyramidal neurons Some stellate cells and basket cells
Internal granular		Stellate neurons Outer band of Baillarger
Ganglionic		Giant pyramidal cells Inner band of Baillarger
Multiform or polymorphous		Neurons of various sizes and shapes Merges with white matter

Fig. 15.2. Laminae of cerebral cortex.

Variations in Cortical Structure

The structure of the cerebral cortex shows considerable variation from region to region, both in terms of thickness and in the prominence of the various laminae described above. As already mentioned finer variations form the basis of the subdivisions into Brodmann's areas. Other workers divide the cortex into five broad varieties. These are as follows.

(**1**) In the **agranular cortex** the external and internal granular laminae are inconspicuous. This type of cortex is seen most typically in the precentral gyrus (area 4) and is, therefore, believed to be typical of 'motor' areas. It is also seen in areas 6, 8, 44 and in parts of the limbic system.

(**2**) In the **granular cortex** the granular layers are highly developed while the pyramidal and ganglionic layers are poorly developed or absent. This type of cortex is seen most typically in 'sensory' areas including the postcentral gyrus, the visual cortex, and the acoustic areas (see below). In the visual area the external band of Baillarger is prominent and forms a white line that can be seen with the naked eye when the region is freshly cut across. This **stria of Gennari** gives the name **striate cortex** to the visual cortex.

Between the two extremes represented by the agranular and granular varieties of cortex, three intermediate types are described as follows.

(**3**) **Frontal cortex** (**4**) **Parietal cortex** and (**5**) **Polar cortex**

The frontal type is nearest to the agranular cortex, the pyramidal cells being prominent; while the polar type is nearest to the granular cortex. The terms frontal and parietal are unfortunate as these types are not confined to the regions suggested by their names. The approximate distribution of the five types of cortex described above, on the superolateral surface of the cerebral hemisphere, is shown in Fig. 15.3.

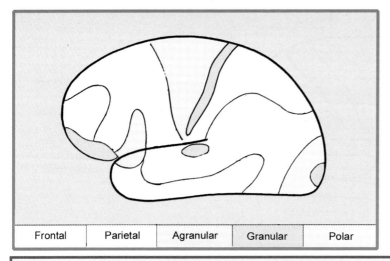

Fig. 15.3.
Superolateral
surface of the
cerebral hemisphere
showing the
distribution of areas
of cortex having
different types of
histological
structure.

| Frontal | Parietal | Agranular | Granular | Polar |

Before terminating this section on the structure of the cerebral cortex it is necessary to emphasise the following facts, revealed by both anatomical and physiological studies.

(**a**) From the point of view of function one has to think in terms of 'vertical columns' of cortex rather than in terms of laminar structure.

(**b**) The *similarities* between different regions of the cortex, in terms of the total neuronal population per unit volume of cortex, and in terms of the ratios of pyramidal and stellate (granular) neurons, are more striking than differences in laminar structure. Counts of neurons in delimited zones of cortex have shown that the total number of neurons is remarkably constant over different areas. However, the striate area (area 17) is an important exception, the neurons being much more numerous (about two and a half times) here as compared to other parts of cortex. In a given area of cortex about two thirds of neurons are pyramidal, and one third non-pyramidal.

Further Consideration of Functional Areas of the Cerebral Cortex

The classical concept of the functional areas of the cerebral cortex has been presented on page 88. Recent work has shown that these concepts need modification in some areas and elaboration in others.

According to classical teaching the cerebral cortex has been divided into the following:

(a) Motor areas

When these areas are stimulated electrically movements occur in various parts of the body. Anatomically, these areas give origin to projection fibres that form the corticospinal and corticonuclear tracts.

(b) Sensory areas

Electrical activity can be recorded in these areas of cortex when a suitable sensory stimulus is applied to a part of the body. Stimulation of these areas of cortex can produce certain sensations in corresponding parts of the body. These sensory areas of the cortex receive fibres from thalamic nuclei in which major sensory pathways terminate.

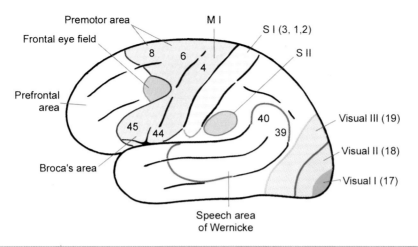

Fig. 15.4. Recent concept of functional areas on the superolateral aspect of the cerebral hemisphere.

(c) Association areas

Areas in which a direct motor or sensory function cannot be demonstrated have been considered to be association areas where information from various sources is presumably integrated, and used to direct appropriate responses.

More recent investigations have shown that the division of the cortex into motor, sensory and association areas is an over-simplification. Many areas previously described as association areas are now known to have 'motor' or 'sensory' functions. Further it has been shown that motor and sensory functions overlap in the same areas of the cortex.

Motor and Premotor Areas

As described on page 89 the motor area lies in the precentral gyrus (area 4). This is the ***primary motor area*** (MI). This area has the lowest threshold of stimulation for producing contralateral body movements.

A supplemental motor area (MII) is present on the medial aspect of the cerebral hemisphere, in the medial frontal gyrus, anterior to the paracentral lobule (areas 6, 8). In this area the body is represented with the area for the lower limb posteriorly, that for the face anteriorly, the area for the upper limb lying between these two. Additional motor areas have been described in the adjoining part of the cingulate gyrus.

On the superolateral surface, the premotor area lies anterior to the motor area occupying areas 6 and 8. (We have seen that on the medial aspect of the hemisphere areas 6 and 8 are occupied by the supplemental motor area.)

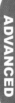

The distinction between motor and premotor areas is vague, and the entire area is sometimes described as the primary motor area. Studies on areas of the cortex giving origin to corticospinal fibres show that they arise from a wide area covering the main and supplemental motor areas, the premotor area, and many areas in the parietal lobe (SI including areas 3, 2, 1; area 5; and SII in the parietal operculum). It is obvious that this area is not coextensive with the definition of motor areas. Some studies claim that only 20 - 30% of corticospinal fibres arise from area 4; and that as many as 50% may have their origin in the parietal lobe. In relation to motor function the site of termination of corticospinal fibres in spinal grey matter becomes significant. Most fibres that descend from the parietal lobe end in the dorsal grey column; while those ending in the ventral grey column are predominantly from the frontal lobe. The latter appear to be the ones most important for motor control.

The premotor area appears to be responsible for programming intended movements, and control of movements in progress. It is divisible into a dorsal and a ventral area. The dorsal area appears to

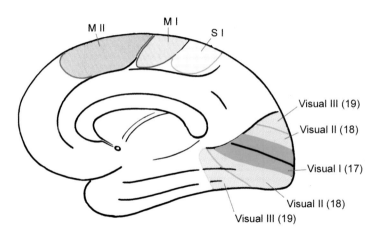

Fig. 15.5.
Functional areas
on the medial
aspect of the
cerebral
hemisphere
(recent
concept)

be concerned with movements initiated by the individual, while the ventral area appears to be concerned with control of movements that take place in response to external stimulation.

The cortex of the motor area is characterised by the presence of large pyramidal cells (giant pyramidal cells of Betz). At one time these cells were considered to be the source of all corticospinal fibres but, as discussed above, this if now known to be incorrect.

It has been estimated that the size of the soma of a neuron is proportional to the total volume of its processes. It follows that neurons having very long axons will have large somata. Purkinje cells that give origin to corticospinal fibres descending to sacral segments of the spinal cord can, therefore, be expected to be among the largest pyramidal cells.

Apart from its corticospinal output, the motor area is connected (in a point to point manner) with the main sensory cortex (SI). This explains why neurons in area 4 are responsive to peripheral stimulation. Area 4 receives afferents from the posterior part of the ventral lateral nucleus of the thalamus. This nucleus receives fibres from cerebellar nuclei. In this way the cerebellum projects to area 4. Area 4 also receives fibres from some other parts of the thalamus, the hypothalamus, and some other parts of the cerebral cortex (including the primary sensory area SI).

The frontal eye field and the motor speech area (of Broca) are parts of the premotor area. These are described on page 89.

Apart from the motor speech area of Broca there are two other areas concerned with motor control of speech. One of these is located in the temporal and parietal lobes (motor speech area of Wernicke) while the other is located in the supplemental motor area (MII) (Figs. 15.4, 15.5).

In summary note the following:

(a) A localised lesion of the primary motor area normally produces contralateral monoplegia. An extensive lesion can cause hemiplegia.

(b) Lesions of the premotor area have an adverse effect on skilled movements.

(c) Lesions of the frontal eye field result in deviation of both eyes to the side of lesion.

(d) Lesions of the motor speech area destroy the ability to speak.

(e) Lesions of the prefrontal areas lead to personality changes.

Sensory Areas

The sensory area of classical description is also called the first somatosensory area (SI). It has been described on page 90. It receives projections from the ventral posteromedial and ventral posterolateral nuclei of the thalamus, conveying impulses received through the medial, spinal and trigeminal lemnisci. We have seen that different parts of the body have a definite representation within this area.

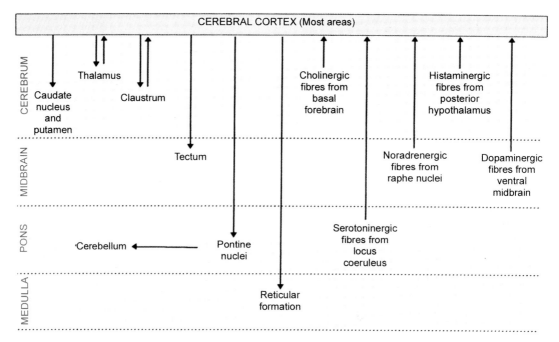

Fig. 15.6. Regions to which most parts of the cerebral cortex are connected.

It has also been shown that different sensations may be represented in different parts within the area. Unit recordings show that area 2 is concerned mainly with proprioceptive impulses, while area 3 responds only to cutaneous stimuli.

A second area predominantly somatosensory in function (second somatosensory area or SII) has been described in relation to the superior lip of the posterior ramus of the lateral sulcus (Fig. 15.4).

The sensory speech area of Wernicke lies in the posterior part of the superior and middle temporal gyri. It extends into areas 39 and 40 of the parietal lobe. This area is responsible for interpretation of speech.

Parts of the superior parietal lobule (areas 5, 7) help us to recognise shape, size and texture of objects

Like area SI, SII receives fibres from the ventral posterior nucleus of the thalamus. It also receives fibres from SI. Descending fibres from SII reach the spinal cord, the nucleus gracilis and cuneatus and the main trigeminal nucleus. Neurons in SII respond best to intermittent stimulation e.g., vibration. SII may be responsible for perception of pain and temperature.

A small part of the primary sensory area, probably within area 2, is believed to serve as a *cortical vestibular area*.

The effects of damage to sensory areas are as follows.

(a) Damage to the first somatosensory area causes loss of sensation (both exteroceptive and prioprioceptive) from the opposite side of the body.

(b) Damage to the second sensory area may lead to inability to appreciate pain and temperature.

(c) Damage to some areas behind the main sensory area (areas 5, 7) interferes with ability to identify objects by feeling them.

(d) Damage to the area of Wernicke leads to failure to understand speech.

Visual Areas

The classical visual area has been described on page 90. This area receives fibres of the optic radiation. It is also called the *striate cortex*. In addition to the striate cortex additional areas of cortex responding to visual inputs are described. Area 18 (*peristriate area*) is the second visual area; and area 19 (*parastriate area*) is the third visual area.

A modified nomenclature recognising five visual areas has been described as follows.

1. First visual area (V1) in area 17.

2. Second visual area (V2) occupying the greater part of area 18, but not the whole of it.

3. Third visual area (V3) occupying a narrow strip over the anterior part of area 18.

4. Fourth visual area (V4) within area 19.

5. Fifth visual area (V5) at the posterior end of the superior temporal gyrus.

The visual areas give off efferent fibres also. These reach various parts of the cerebral cortex in both hemispheres. In particular, they reach the frontal eye field which is concerned with eye movements. Like other 'sensory' areas the visual areas are, therefore, to be regarded as partly motor in function. This view is substantiated by the fact that movements of the eyeballs and head can be produced by stimulation of areas 17 and 18 which constitute an *occipital eye field.* Efferents from the visual areas also reach the superior colliculus, the pretectal region, and the nuclei of cranial nerves supplying muscles that move the eyeballs. There is physiological evidence of a corticogeniculate projection. Fibres also reach the thalamus (pulvinar).

The total number of neurons to be seen in delimited vertical areas of cortex is remarkably constant in different regions. The cortex of the visual area is an exception and has a much greater density of neurons than other parts of the cortex.

For effects of damage to the visual pathway see Chapter 18.

Auditory (acoustic) Areas

The classical area for hearing (primary auditory area, A1) has been described on page 90. As in the case of the visual areas it has been shown that fibres of the acoustic radiation end not only in the classical or first auditory area, but extend into some neighbouring areas as well. These include a second acoustic area lying in the superior temporal gyrus anterior to A1. A number of other auditory areas have been described.

Efferent fibres arising in the acoustic areas project to the medial geniculate body, and to the inferior colliculus, and may possibly reach motor nuclei of cranial nerves. Some of these efferents may influence the state of contraction of the stapedius and tensor tympani muscles. The acoustic areas are also connected with other parts of the cerebral cortex.

It may be remembered that the fibres of each lateral lemniscus are bilateral. Hence, the acoustic areas in each cerebral cortex receive fibres from both the right and left cochleae. The close relationship of the acoustic areas to Wernicke's speech area may be noted. The association is significant in view of the obvious relationship between hearing and speech.

As the auditory areas receive impulses from both sides, a lesion on one side produces only partial loss of hearing. Lesions in the secondary auditory area (area 22) interferes with interpretation of speech (*word deafness*).

Prefrontal Areas

The part of the frontal lobe excluding the motor and premotor areas is referred to as the prefrontal area. It includes the parts of the frontal gyri anterior to the premotor area, the orbital gyri, most of the medial frontal gyrus, and the anterior part of the gyrus cinguli.

The prefrontal area has numerous connections with the thalamus, the corpus striatum, the limbic system, the hypothalamus, the reticular formation, the cranial nerve nuclei, and the pontine nuclei. These connections suggest that this area is concerned with both somatic and visceral activity. Injury to some parts of this region makes the person more docile, but also negligent and lacking in concentration. The prefrontal area appears to be concerned with normal expression of emotions, and the ability to predict consequences of actions. The medial part of the prefrontal area is associated with auditory and visual functions.

Disorders of Memory and Behaviour

Some neurological disorders are associated with impairment of memory. It is now known that discrete areas of the brain are involved in memory, and that different areas influence different modalities of memory. The observations given below should be regarded as tentative and may well need modification.

1. The best known 'system' damage of which leads to defects of memory consists of the hippocampus (including the subiculum), the fimbria and fornix, the mamillary bodies, the mamillothalamic tract, the anterior nuclei of the thalamus, and the gyrus cinguli (and the fibres of the cingulum). It has been shown that damage anywhere along this pathway results in loss of memory of events, leaving general knowledge of the person intact.

2. In contrast, ablation (in monkeys) of the perirhinal cortex (a strip of cortex lying lateral to the rhinal sulcus) leads to loss of knowledge about objects (as distinct to knowledge of events).

3. Other regions of the brain important in memory probably include the amygdala and the prefrontal cortex. The amygdala are probably responsible for evaluating the significance of environtal events, for example in recognising what objects are edible, or in recognising attributes of the opposite sex. Damage to the amygdala leads to the **Kluver Bucy syndrome** in which such ability is disorganised. This results in marked changes in ingestive behaviour, the animal ingesting material (like foeces) not normally eaten. Abnormalities in sexual behaviour are also seen probably because of the failure to distinguish between male and female animals.

The **nucleus accumbens**, located in the ventral striatum is a part of the mesolimbic dopamine system. It has acquired importance following the recognition that this nucleus is concerned with the stimulating and pleasure giving effects of addictive drugs (including nicotine and alcohol).

SOME FEATURES OF CORTICAL CONNECTIONS

Recent investigations have brought to light some interesting features of cortical connections that are briefly summarised below.

A. Relationship of cortical laminae to incoming and outgoing fibres

The main fibres entering or leaving a given area of cortex can be described as follows.

1. Fibres projecting from one area of cortex to another are referred to as **feed forward** fibres. They arise mainly in lamina 3, with some from lamina 2. They terminate mainly in lamina 4 (but also in 1, 6 and others) of the receiving area of cortex (Fig. 15.7).

2. The receiving area sends a **feedback** to the area of cortex from it receives a feed forward projection. These feedback fibres arise in lamina 5 (of receiving cortex) and end in lamina 1 of the cortex from which the feed forward projection was received.

3. The projections to the striatum (corticostriate fibres), to the spinal cord (corticospinal fibres), to pontine nuclei (corticopontine fibres), and to the medulla

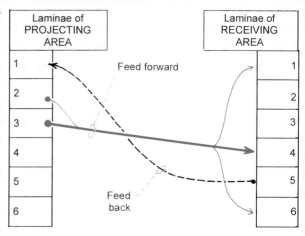

Fig. 15.7. Concept of feed forward and feedback cortical connections.

(corticobulbar fibres) all arise mainly from lamina 5 of the cortex.

4. Corticothalamic projections arise from lamina 6.

5. Major afferent fibres entering the cortex (e.g., from the thalamus; or feed forward fibres from other cortical areas) end mainly in lamina 4. Some reach laminae 1 and 6, while a few reach the remaining laminae.

B. Pattern of cortico-cortical connections

It has been recognised for long that cortical areas have numerous connections with other parts of the cerebral cortex. Recent investigations show that there is a pattern in these connections, and that the pattern has important physiological implications.

(a) The first feature of this concept is that major sensory areas of cortex send feed forward projections to adjoining areas of cortex; and the latter in turn project to other contiguous areas. Through a series of such connections the sensory areas get connected to the limbic cortex.

(b) The second feature of the concept is that main sensory areas (in the parietal, occipital and temporal lobes) are reciprocally connected to areas in the frontal lobe.

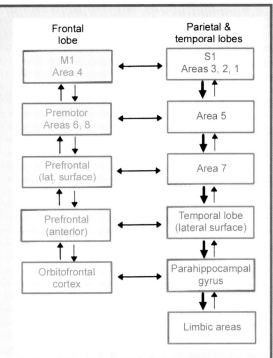

Fig. 15.8. Scheme to show the pattern of interconnections between areas of cerebral cortex

These features can be clarified by considering the connections of the primary sensory area (SI) as follows.

1. The primary sensory area (SI) sends a feed forward projection to area 5 (lying in the superior parietal lobule). Area 5 projects to area 7 (lying further back in the parietal lobe). Area 7 projects to the temporal lobe in the region of the superior temporal sulcus. This region projects to the parahippocampal gyrus which in turn projects to the limbic cortex. Note the series of steps in this scheme. Although the main connection is in the 'forward' direction, all connections are reciprocal (Fig. 15.8).

2. Each 'step' of progression (from the main sensory area) is connected to an area in the frontal lobe. SI is connected to MI. Note that these areas are contiguous to one another. Step 2, represented by area 5, is connected to the premotor area. In a similar manner each 'step' (in the parietal and temporal lobes) is connected to an area in the frontal lobe progressively farther removed from the motor area. This would appear to indicate a close functional linking of sensory and motor regions at various levels. All connections are reciprocal.

3. As with the somatosensory area, the visual and auditory areas are also connected to the limbic cortex through a series of 'steps'. These are also connected reciprocally to the frontal lobe.

It is, therefore, not surprising that neurons responding to somatic, visual, and auditory impulses are widely scattered in the cerebral cortex; and that these are closely linked with motor responses.

RELATED TOPICS

The blood supply of the cerebrum, and associated clinical conditions, are considered in Chapter 21.

The lateral ventricle is described in Chapter 20.

The Olfactory Region

A major difficulty in considering the olfactory pathways is that these involve numerous, rather obscure and small, structures and areas. For a proper understanding it is necessary that the names and positions of these areas be introduced at the outset.

The peripheral end organ for smell is the **olfactory mucosa** that lines the upper and posterior parts of the nasal cavity. Nerve fibres arising in this mucosa collect to form about twenty bundles that together constitute an **olfactory nerve.** The bundles pass through foramina in the cribriform plate of the ethmoid bone to enter the cranial cavity where they terminate in the **olfactory bulb** (Figs. 16.1, 16.3).

The olfactory bulb is an elongated oval structure that lies just above the cribriform plate. It is continuous posteriorly with the **olfactory tract** through which it is connected to the base of the cerebral hemisphere. When traced posteriorly the olfactory tract divides into **medial and lateral olfactory striae** (Figs. 16.1, 16.2). The point of bifurcation is expanded and forms the **olfactory trigone.** An **intermediate stria** is sometimes present. The olfactory striae are intimately related to a mass of grey matter called the **anterior perforated substance**. The medial and lateral striae form the anteromedial and anterolateral boundaries of this substance. The intermediate stria extends into the anterior perforated substance and ends in a slight elevation (in the anterior part of the substance) called the **olfactory tubercle**. Posterolaterally, the anterior perforated substance is related to the uncus (Fig. 16.1), while posteromedially it is bounded by a bundle of fibres called the **diagonal band** (of Broca)(Fig. 16.2).

The uncus is a part of the cerebral hemisphere that lies on the tentorial surface a little behind and medial to the temporal pole. It represents the anterior end of the **parahippocampal gyrus** and is separated from the temporal pole by the rhinal sulcus.

The anterior part of the parahippocampal gyrus, including the uncus, is referred to as the **entorhinal area** (area 28). Some other areas present in the region are shown in Fig. 16.2.

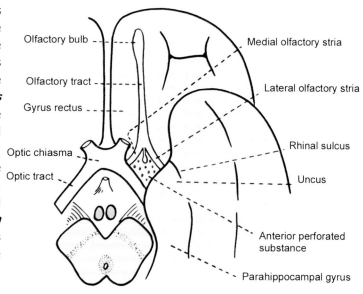

Fig. 16.1. Some structures related to the anterior part of the base of the brain.

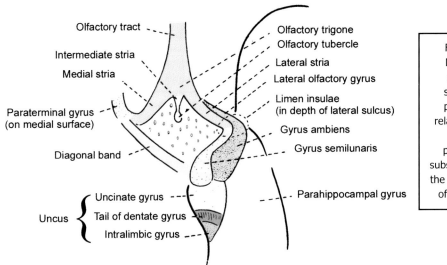

Olfactory tract

Intermediate stria

Medial stria

Paraterminal gyrus
(on medial surface)

Diagonal band

Olfactory trigone
Olfactory tubercle
Lateral stria
Lateral olfactory gyrus
Limen insulae
(in depth of lateral sulcus)
Gyrus ambiens
Gyrus semilunaris

Parahippocampal gyrus

Uncus { Uncinate gyrus
Tail of dentate gyrus
Intralimbic gyrus

Fig. 16.2.
Details of
olfactory
structures
present in
relation to the
anterior
perforated
substance. Note
the subdivisions
of the uncus

The uncus is subdivided into three parts. From anterior to posterior side these are (Fig. 16.2) the *uncinate gyrus,* the *tail of the dentate gyrus* (band of Giacomini) and the *intralimbic gyrus.*

When traced backwards the lateral olfactory stria reaches the *limen insulae* (in the depth of the stem of the lateral sulcus). Here it bends sharply to the medial side and becomes continuous with a small area of grey matter lying anterior to the uncus and called the *gyrus semilunaris* (or periamygdaloid area). The gyrus semilunaris is closely related to the *amygdaloid complex* which lies deep (i.e., superior) to it. The lateral olfactory stria is covered by a thin layer of grey matter called the *lateral olfactory gyrus.* When traced backwards this gyrus becomes continuous with a part of the cortex called the *gyrus ambiens.* The gyrus ambiens lies lateral to the gyrus semilunaris. Posteriorly, it becomes continuous with the entorhinal area. The lateral olfactory gyrus and the gyrus ambiens collectively form the *prepiriform region* (or area).

The term *piriform lobe* is applied collectively to the following parts that have been identified above.

(**1**) Prepiriform region (lateral olfactory gyrus and gyrus ambiens).

(**2**) Gyrus semilunaris (or periamygdaloid region).

(**3**) Lateral olfactory stria (?).

(**4**) Anterior part of parahippocampal gyrus, including the uncus (entorhinal area, Brodmann's area 28: See Fig. 8.10).

When traced medially, the medial olfactory stria, and the diagonal band, both reach the medial surface of the hemisphere, where they end near the paraterminal gyrus (which lies just in front of the lamina terminalis: Fig. 16.10).

The Olfactory Pathway

The fibres of the olfactory nerves are processes of *olfactory receptor cells* lying in the epithelium lining the olfactory mucosa (Fig. 16.3). These receptor cells are homologous to sensory neurons located in sensory ganglia. In other words, the first order sensory neurons of the olfactory pathway are located within the olfactory epithelium itself. (In the course of evolution *all* neurons have arisen by modification of epithelial cells and their migration, in most cases, into deeper tissues. The olfactory receptor cells retain their position in the epithelium and are, therefore, regarded as primitive).

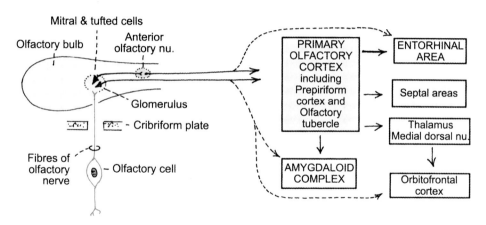

Fig. 16.3. Scheme to show the main features of the olfactory pathway

Each receptor cell consists of a cell body and of two processes i.e., it is a bipolar cell. The peripheral process (dendrite) reaches the surface of the olfactory epithelium and ends in a small swelling. A number of cilia are attached to this swelling. The central process (axon) enters the submucosa, and forms one fibre of the olfactory nerve. The olfactory nerve fibres terminate in the olfactory bulb.

Olfactory Bulb

The olfactory bulb receives fibres of the olfactory nerves, arising from olfactory cells (or olfactory sensory neurons). These incoming fibres synapse with neurons within the bulb. Fibres arising from the latter form the olfactory tract.

Several types of cells are present in the olfactory bulb. The most important of these are:

(**a**) The *mitral cells* and *tufted cells* that give origin to fibres of the olfactory tract.

Other cells present are as follows:

(b) *Periglomerular cells* and *granule cells* have processes that remain confined to the bulb.

The olfactory bulb is made up of a number of concentric layers which are shown in Fig. 16.4.

(**1**) Incoming fibres of olfactory nerves occupy the most superficial layer.

(**2**) The second, or glomerular, layer contains synaptic glomeruli in which terminals of olfactory nerve fibres synapse with dendrites of mitral cells, tufted cells and periglomerular cells.

(**3**) The third layer is in the form of a plexus formed by dendrites of mitral and tufted cells. Somata of tufted cells also lie in this layer.

(**4**) The fourth layer contains somata of mitral cells.

(**5**) The fifth layer is made up mainly of axons of mitral and tufted cells.

(**6**) The sixth layer contains clusters of granule cells.

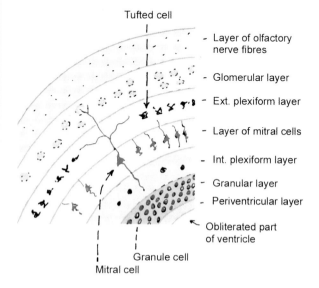

Fig. 16. 4. Layers of the olfactory bulb.

Apart from olfactory nerve fibres, the olfactory bulb receives centrifugal fibres from a number of sources as shown in Fig. 16.5. It is believed that perception of smell can be considerably modulated through these inputs.

Many neuropeptides are present in the olfactory bulb. These include GABA, dopamine, glutamate, aspartate, enkephalin, luteinising hormone releasing hormone (LHRH) and substance P.

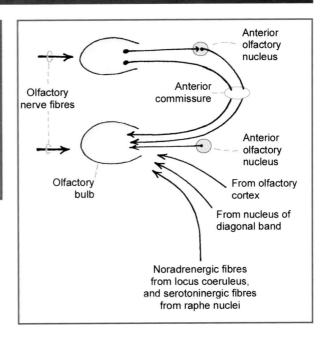

Fig. 16.5. Diagram to show the afferents of the olfactory bulb.

Olfactory tract

The olfactory tract is made up predominantly of axons of mitral and tufted cells of the olfactory bulb. Some scattered neurons are also present within the tract. They collectively constitute **the anterior olfactory nucleus**. Some axons of mitral and tufted cells relay in this nucleus.

The olfactory tract also contains centrifugal fibres travelling to the olfactory bulb from various centres in the brain. These are shown in Fig. 16.5.

Olfactory cortex

The term olfactory cortex is applied to all areas of the cerebral cortex that receive direct fibres from the olfactory bulb.

In the past it has been held that olfactory pathways differ from those for other sensations in that there is no relay in the thalamus. This concept needs modification in that while most olfactory fibres reach their cortical destinations without relay (ignoring relay of some in the anterior olfactory nucleus), some others are now believed to reach the thalamus.

Primary Olfactory Projection

The main regions receiving direct fibres from the olfactory bulb are:

(**1**) The prepiriform cortex (including the lateral olfactory gyrus and the gyrus ambiens).

(**2**) The gyrus semilunaris (periamygdaloid area).

Some direct fibres also reach the following:

(**3**) Anterior olfactory nucleus which relays them to other regions.

(**4**) Olfactory tubercle (in the anterior perforated substance).

(**5**) Entorhinal area.

BASIC

The term ***piriform cortex or primary olfactory cortex*** is rather loosely applied to these regions, the areas included varying in different accounts. Apart from the above, some direct olfactory axons also reach some parts of the cortex of the insula; and the main (central) nuclei of the amygdaloid complex.

Secondary olfactory projection

1. Apart from primary olfactory fibres the entorhinal area receives numerous olfactory fibres after relay in other parts of the piriform cortex.

2. It has been recently recognised that the piriform cortex sends a major projection to the medial dorsal nucleus of the thalamus. From here olfactory impulses are relayed to the cortex on the orbital aspect of the frontal lobe (orbito-frontal cortex, centro-posterior part).
3. Another region of the orbitofrontal cortex (latero-posterior) receives direct projections from the piriform cortex. This projection by-passes the thalamus. Studies on alterations in brain blood flow in response to olfactory stimuli suggest that appreciation of such stimuli takes place bilaterally in the piriform cortex, but only in the right frontal lobe.

The primary olfactory cortex is connected to various other areas. In the past, many of these areas have been included under the term ***rhinencephalon*** or smell brain. It is now recognised, however, that although these areas might receive olfactory impulses their primary functions are not olfactory. Some of these areas and their connections are considered below as part of the limbic system.

The Limbic Region

The term ***limbic system*** has been applied, in the past, to certain regions of the brain that are believed to play an important role in the control of visceral activity. Many of these areas have been considered as having a predominantly olfactory function; but it is now realised that this is not so. The areas of cerebral cortex included in the region are often referred to as the ***limbic lobe***.

Some of the functions attributed to the so called limbic system are as follows.
(**a**) Integration of olfactory, visceral, and somatic impulses reaching the brain.
(**b**) Control of activities necessary for survival of the animal, including the procuring of food and eating behaviour.
(**c**) Control of activities necessary for survival of the species including sex behaviour.
(**d**) Emotional behaviour.
(**e**) Retention of recent memory.
These can be interfered with in lesions of the region.

However, at present concepts regarding the unity of the so called limbic system are being seriously questioned, and the concept of these structures forming a "system" may well be discarded in future. It is for this reason that the heading for this section has been changed from the limbic system (in the previous edition) to the limbic region.

The areas to be included under the heading limbic system are not completely agreed upon. The following are generally included.

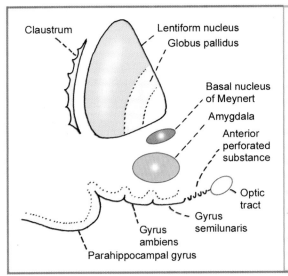

Fig. 16.6. Some relations of the amygdala as seen in a coronal section.

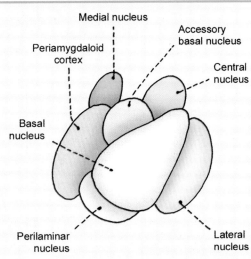

Fig. 16.7. Subdivisions of the amygdaloid complex as seen in a coronal section.

BASIC

Areas forming the limbic cortex

One of the problems in identifying the areas to be included under this heading arises from the fact that much information has been derived from experiments on animals. The areas included, in the brains of higher primates, include the following.

(**a**) Hippocampus (Ammon's horn), and dentate gyrus.

(**b**) Entorhinal cortex.

(**c**) Gyrus cinguli (some parts of which are excluded), and paraterminal gyrus.

(**d**) Part of the parahippocampal gyrus.

(**e**) The indusium griseum may be regarded as a vestigial part of the limbic cortex.

(**f**) The amygdaloid nuclei are included under the limbic cortex. (This may appear strange as these nuclei are not part of the cerebral cortex. However, it has been found that the connections of these nuclei are similar to those of the cortex).

2. Bordering the limbic cortex there are ***perilimbic areas***. These include those parts of the gyrus cinguli and the parahippocampal gyrus that are not included in the limbic cortex. The retrosplenial gyrus (or gyrus fasciolaris) is also included.

3. Some authors include some of the olfactory areas in the region of the anterior perforated substance, and the septal region.

Fibre bundles related to the limbic region

These include the following.

1. Olfactory nerves, tract and striae.

2. Fornix, stria terminalis, stria medullaris thalami, diagonal band, and anterior commissure.

Some of these regions are considered in detail below. It is relevant to know that some regions not included in the limbic region, are nevertheless closely related to it functionally. These include the hypothalamus, and the reticular formation of the midbrain. The medial part of the thalamus, and the frontal cortex are also closely related functionally to the limbic system. Several of the areas included in the limbic region have been considered along with the olfactory pathway. The hypothalamus has been considered on page 193. We shall now consider some other areas.

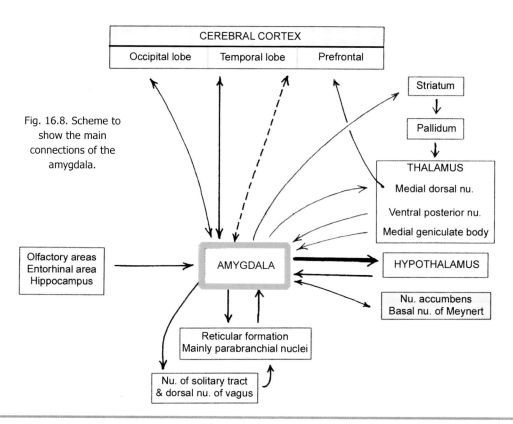

Fig. 16.8. Scheme to show the main connections of the amygdala.

Amygdaloid Nuclear Complex

This region is also called the amygdaloid body or amygdala. Some features of this region have been considered on page 209. It is situated near the temporal pole of the cerebral hemisphere in close relation to the anterior end of the inferior horn of the lateral ventricle. Superiorly, the complex is related to the anterior part of the lentiform nucleus. Inferiorly, the complex is related to the gyrus semilunaris, the gyrus ambiens and the uncinate gyrus. It lies just below the anterior end of the tail of the caudate nucleus. The lower end of the stria terminalis lies in relation to the amygdaloid complex (Figs. 14.1 and 16.9).

In the region between the amygdaloid complex and the lentiform nucleus there is a region of substriatal grey matter within which there is a collection of cholinergic neurons. These neurons form the **basal nucleus of Meynert**. Some relationships of the amygdaloid complex are shown in Fig. 16.6.

The amygdaloid complex is divided into a number of nuclei that have a complex terminology. A simplified version is shown in Fig. 16.7. Identify the **lateral, medial, basal** and **central** nuclei, and the **periamygdaloid cortex**. The basal and lateral nuclei are collectively referred to as the **basolateral nucleus**. Cells of the central and medial nuclei spread backwards along the stria terminalis and, along with this extension, they are referred to as the **extended amygdala**.

CONNECTIONS OF THE AMYGDALOID NUCLEI

(a) Connections with the brainstem

1. The amygdala receive fibres from, and send fibres to, the reticular formation, particularly the parabrachial nucleus (Fig. 16.8).

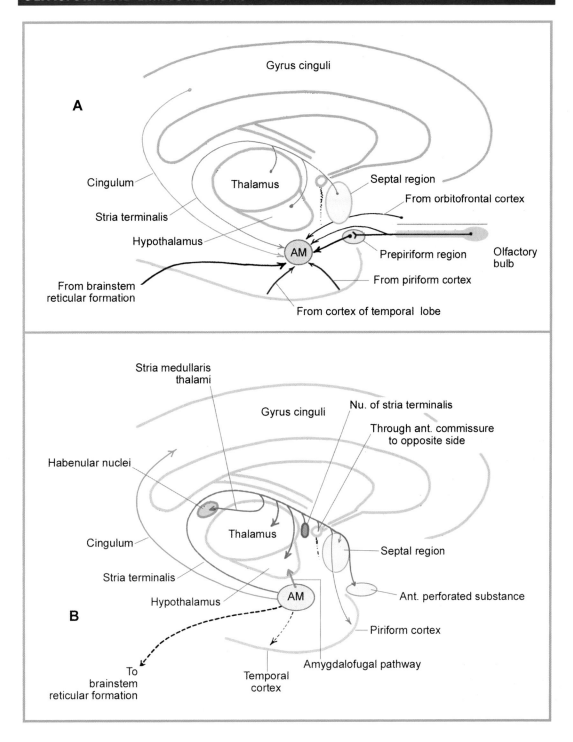

Fig. 16.9. Scheme to show the routes taken by fibres to and from the amygdaloid complex.
A. Afferents. B. Efferents.

ADVANCED

2. Noradrenergic fibres from the locus coeruleus, and serotoninergic fibres from the raphe nuclei reach the amygdala through the medial forebrain bundle. Dopaminergic fibres ascend from the ventral tegmental area of the midbrain.

3. Some fibres from the amygdala reach the nucleus of the solitary tract, and the dorsal nucleus of the vagus. The nucleus of the solitary tract projects back to the amygdala through the parabrachial nuclei. Through these connections the amygdala receive gustatory and visceral information can influence cardiovascular and respiratory functions.

(b) Connections with the diencephalon
1. The amygdala send a major projection to various nuclei in the hypothalamus. Some fibres are also received from the hypothalamus.

2. Fibres projecting to the thalamus end mainly in the medial dorsal nucleus. The impulses are relayed to the prefrontal cortex. Afferents are received from the ventral posterior nucleus (gustatory sensations), and from the medial geniculate body.

(c) Connections with the corpus striatum
A prominent projection is sent to the striatum (caudate nucleus and putamen). Many fibres also reach the nucleus accumbens (which is a nucleus in the ventral striatum). Through the striatum the amygdaloid complex indirectly influences the pallidum, which in turn projects to the medial dorsal nucleus of the thalamus. The amygdaloid complex sends many fibres to the basal nucleus of Meynert (lying in the region ventral to the corpus striatum), This projection is cholinergic. The nucleus projects back to the amygdala.

(d) Cortical connections of amygdala
It is now known that in addition to its connections to olfactory areas, entorhinal area and hippocampus, the amygdaloid complex has numerous connections with widespread areas of neocortex. The areas include the cingulate gyrus, and parts of the frontal, temporal and occipital lobes, including the visual and auditory areas.

CLINICAL

On the basis of all the connections described above, and on the basis of experimental studies it appears probable that the amygdala play an important role in the control of emotional behaviour. Lesions of the amygdaloid complex lead to the ***Kluver-Bucy syndrome***. The experimental animals appear to be unable to correctly evaluate its environment leading to gross and bizarre alterations in eating behaviour, and in sex behaviour.

BASIC

Septal Region
This term is used to designate certain masses of grey matter that lie immediately anterior to the lamina terminalis and the anterior commissure (Fig. 16.10). The cerebral cortex of this region shows two small vertical sulci called the anterior and posterior ***parolfactory sulci.***

The region between the lamina terminalis and the posterior sulcus is the ***paraterminal gyrus.*** The anterior part of this region which adjoins the posterior parolfactory sulcus is called the ***prehippocampal rudiment.*** The region between the anterior and posterior parolfactory sulci is the ***subcallosal area*** (or ***parolfactory gyrus***). Most workers agree that the paraterminal gyrus (along with the prehippocampal rudiment) forms part of the septal region. Some include the subcallosal area as well. The cortex of this region is referred to as the ***septal area*** in distinction to the ***septal nuclei*** which lie deep to the cortex.

Phylogenetically, the septal region is divided into a ***precommissural septum*** and a ***supra-commissural septum***. The septal area is the precommissural septum. The supracommissural septum is represented by the septum pellucidum. The septal nuclei are divided into dorsal, ventral, medial and caudal groups.

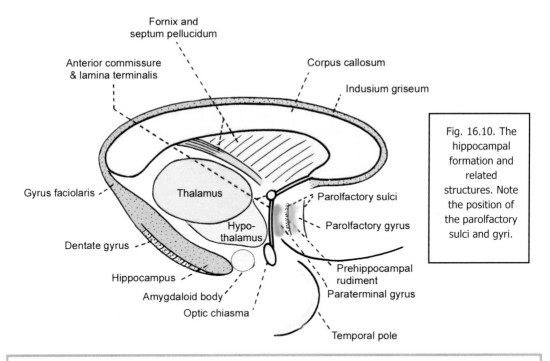

Fig. 16.10. The hippocampal formation and related structures. Note the position of the parolfactory sulci and gyri.

The septal area is continuous inferiorly with the diagonal band and with the medial olfactory stria (Fig. 16.2). Superiorly, it is continuous with the indusium griseum (Fig. 16.10). The septal nuclei are related inferiorly to the anterior perforated substance.

The **connections of the septal region** are shown in Fig. 16.11. From these connections it is seen that the septal region is linked mainly to the hippocampus and to the hypothalamus, and is functionally associated with both these regions. It is also linked to the brainstem reticular formation through noradrenergic, serotoninergic, and dopaminergic fibres. Cholinergic and GABAergic efferents are given off to the cingulate cortex.

Hippocampal Formation

In the human embryo, the hippocampal formation develops in relation to the medial surface of each cerebral hemisphere close to the choroid fissure of the lateral ventricle. It is at first approximately C-shaped in accordance with the outline of the body and inferior horn of the ventricle. The upper part of the formation is, however, separated from the ventricle because of the development of the corpus callosum between the two. For the same reason, this part of the formation remains underdeveloped and is represented by a thin layer of grey matter lining the upper surface of the corpus callosum. This layer is the **indusium griseum.**

Within the indusium griseum are embedded two bundles of longitudinally running fibres called the **medial and lateral longitudinal striae** (on each side of the midline). Posteriorly, the indusium griseum is continuous with a thin layer of grey matter related to the inferior aspect of the splenium of the corpus callosum. This grey matter is the **splenial gyrus** or **gyrus faciolaris.** The splenial gyrus runs forwards to become continuous with the **dentate gyrus** present in relation to the inferior horn of the lateral ventricle.

In the region of the inferior horn of the lateral ventricle, the developing hippocampus is pushed into the cavity of the ventricle because of the great development of the neighbouring neocortex. The hippocampal formation is best developed in this region and forms the **hippocampus.** This term includes the dentate gyrus.

BASIC

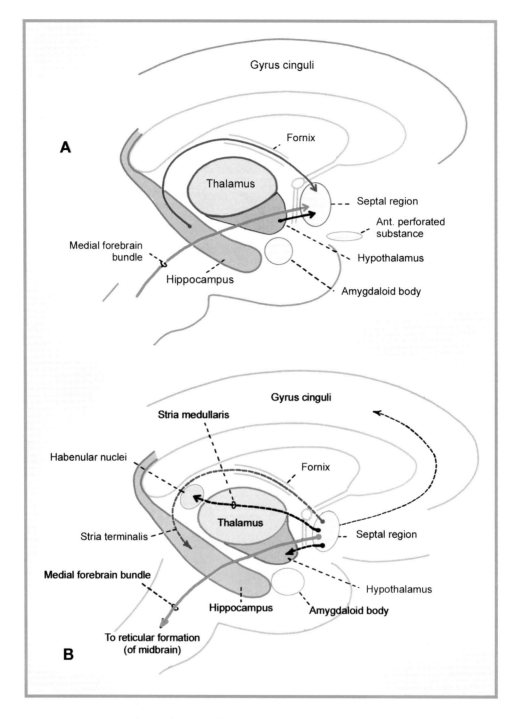

Fig. 16.11. Schemes to show the connections of the septal region.
A. Afferents. B. Efferents.

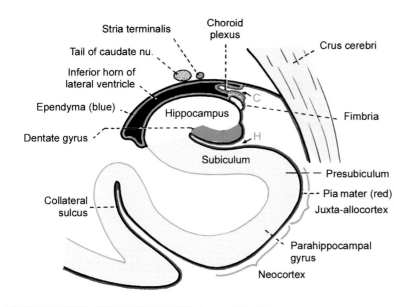

Stria terminalis

Tail of caudate nu.

Inferior horn of lateral ventricle

Ependyma (blue)

Dentate gyrus

Choroid plexus

Hippocampus

Subiculum

Crus cerebri

C

Fimbria

H

Collateral sulcus

Presubiculum

Pia mater (red)

Juxta-allocortex

Parahippocampal gyrus

Neocortex

Fig. 16.12. Coronal section through the cerebral hemisphere in the region of the inferior horn of the lateral ventricle to show the hippocampus and related structures. C=choroid fissure. H=hippocampal fissure.

Several subdivisions of the region are described. These are illustrated in Fig. 16.12 which represents a coronal section through the inferior horn of the lateral ventricle. In this figure note that the cavity of the inferior horn is closed, on the medial side, only by apposed layers of pia mater and ependyma. A fold of pia mater (tela choroidea) projects into the ventricle and encloses a bunch of capillaries that constitute the choroid plexus. This fissure through which the tela choroidea projects into the ventricle is the ***choroid fissure.*** The cerebral cortex that lies below the choroid fissure is S-shaped in cross section. The upper and middle limbs of the 'S' are separated by the ***hippocampal fissure.*** The superior limb of the 'S' forms the hippocampus. The hippocampus consists of two parts. The part that forms the superior convex surface is called ***Ammon's horn*** or ***cornu ammonis.*** (This is the hippocampus proper). The deeper part which lies below and medial to Ammon's horn, and forms the upper wall of the hippocampal fissure, is the ***dentate gyrus.*** The middle limb of the 'S' connects the cornu ammonis to the parahippocampal gyrus which forms the lower limb of the 'S'. The middle limb is an area of transition between the parahippocampal gyrus and the cornu ammonis. It is called the ***subiculum.***

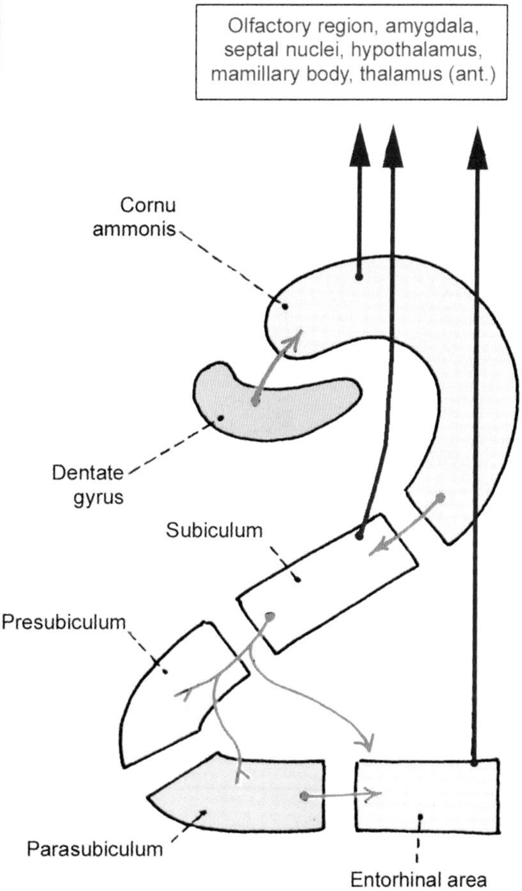

Olfactory region, amygdala, septal nuclei, hypothalamus, mamillary body, thalamus (ant.)

Cornu ammonis

Dentate gyrus

Subiculum

Presubiculum

Parasubiculum

Entorhinal area

Fig. 16.13. Intrinsic connections of the hippocampus. Also see Fig. 16.14.

Some further subdivisions of the region are as follows. Ammon's horn is divided into zones CA1, CA2 and CA3, CA3 being nearest the dentate gyrus, and CA1 being towards the subiculum. The subicular region is subdivided into subiculum (proper), the presubiculum, and the parasubiculum. The parasubiculum is continuous with the anterior part of the parahippocampal gyrus (entorhinal area).

The hippocampus forms a longitudinal projection that occupies the greater part of the floor of the inferior horn of the lateral ventricle. Its anterior end is expanded and notched and resembles a foot. It is therefore called the ***pes hippocampi.***

The ventricular surface of the hippocampus is covered by a layer of nerve fibres that constitute the ***alveus.*** The fibres of the alveus pass medially and collect to form a bundle of fibres, the ***fimbria,*** that projects above the medial part of the hippocampus (Fig. 16.12).

The fimbria runs backwards along the medial side of the hippocampus to become continuous with the fornix (see below).

The ***dentate gyrus*** is a longitudinal strip of grey matter. Laterally, it is fused with the cornu ammonis. Its medial margin is free, and bears a series of notches that give it a dentate appearance

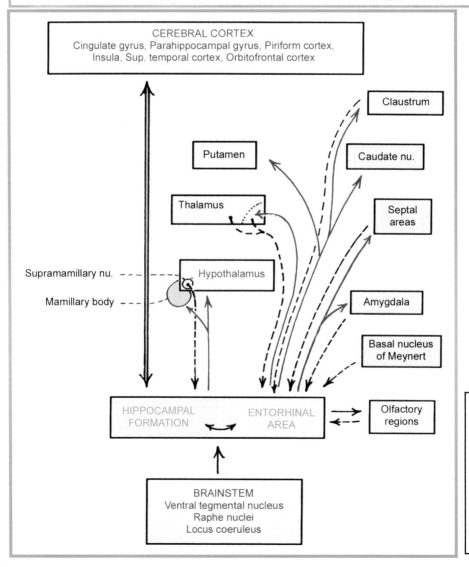

Fig. 16.14. Scheme to show the connections of the hippocampal formation and entorhinal area.

(Fig. 16.12): hence the name dentate gyrus. When traced anteriorly the dentate gyrus runs medially across the inferior surface of the uncus. This part is called the ***tail of the dentate gyrus*** (Fig. 16.2). As stated above, the posterior end of the dentate gyrus is continuous with the splenial gyrus (gyrus faciolaris) (Fig.16.10). Because of its close relationship to the dentate gyrus the uncus is sometimes regarded as part of the hippocampal formation.

The structure of the hippocampus is different from that of the rest of the cerebral cortex. While most of the cerebral cortex is six layered the hippocampal cortex is made up of three layers only. The subiculum is a transitional zone in which a gradual reduction in the number of layers takes place. Further details of the structure of the hippocampus are beyond the scope of this book.

ADVANCED

Connections of the hippocampus

In previous editions of this book the connections of the hippocampus described were those shown in Fig. 16.15. In recent years the hippocampus has been studied in great detail and concepts regarding its connections have undergone considerable revision the main features of which are as follows.

1. Apart from its olfactory connections, the entorhinal area (area 28) is closely linked functionally to the hippocampus, the two having numerous interconnections, and sharing their inputs and outputs (see below).

2. ***Intrinsic connections***: The various parts of the hippocampal region are closely linked to each other (Fig. 16.13). The dentate gyrus sends fibres to the cornu ammonis, which in turn sends fibres to the subiculum. The subiculum projects to the entorhinal area, directly or through relays in the presubiculum and parasubiculum.

3. ***Extrinsic connections with subcortical centres***:

(**a**) The hippocampus and entorhinal area send fibres to the amygdaloid complex and septal areas, the hypothalamus including the mamillary body, and the anterior (and some other) nuclei of the thalamus. Some fibres reach the striatum (caudate nucleus and putamen), the claustrum, and the basal nucleus of Meynert (Fig. 16.14).

(**b**) The hippocampus and entorhinal area receive fibres from some of the subcortical centres to which they send fibres. These include the amygdaloid complex and septal areas, the thalamus (anterior region), and the claustrum. They also receive fibres from some other regions of the thalamus and from the supramamillary nucleus (in the hypothalamus).

(**c**) The entorhinal area receives and gives fibres to olfactory areas.

(**d**) Fibres ascend to the hippocampus and entorhinal area from the brainstem (ventral tegmental nucleus, raphe nuclei, locus coeruleus).

4. ***Cortical Connections:*** The hippocampus and entorhinal area send fibres to and receive fibres from various parts of the cortex including the cingulate gyrus, the parahippocampal gyrus, the piriform cortex, the cortex of the insula, the superior temporal gyrus and the orbitofrontal cortex. In addition the region is brought into communication with many other areas of the brain through the parahippocampal gyrus.

Fibre bundles of limbic region

Stria Terminalis

BASIC

This bundle of fibres is closely related to the inferior horn and central part of the lateral ventricle. It begins in the amygdaloid complex and runs backwards in the roof of the inferior horn. It then winds upwards and forwards to lie in the floor of the central part of the ventricle. Finally, it terminates near the interventricular foramen and anterior commissure by dividing into various smaller bundles. Throughout its course, it is closely related to the medial side of the caudate nucleus (Fig. 13.1). In the inferior horn it is related to the tail of this nucleus. In the central part of the ventricle it lies medial to the body of the caudate nucleus. Here the thalamus is medial to it. A group of neurons located just

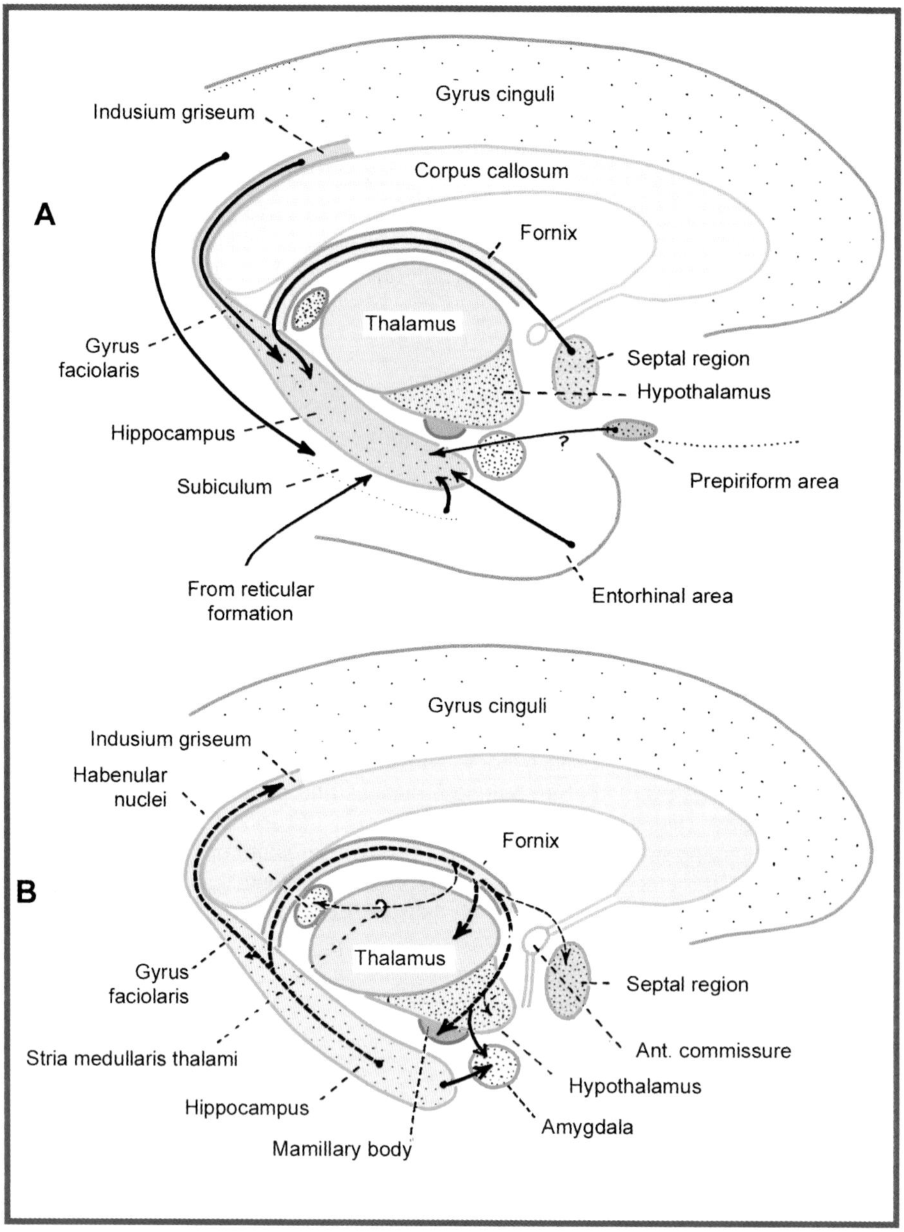

Fig. 16.15. Diagrams to show some fibres passing through the fornix.

behind the anterior commissure is sometimes described as the nucleus of the stria terminalis (Fig. 16.9B).

The stria terminalis contains the following fibres (as traditionally described, Figs. 16.9 and 16.11).
   1. Fibres from the amygdaloid complex to the septal region, the hypothalamus, the anterior perforated substance, the piriform lobe and the nucleus of the stria terminalis.
   2. Fibres from the amygdaloid nucleus to the habenular nuclei. These fibres leave the stria at its anterior end and reach the habenular nuclei through the stria medullaris thalami.

3. Some fibres from the amygdaloid complex run forwards in the stria, cross to the opposite side in the anterior commissure, and then run backwards in the stria of the opposite side to reach the opposite amygdaloid complex.

4. Fibres from the septal areas and adjoining regions possibly run backwards in the stria to reach the amygdaloid complex.

Anterior Commissure

The anterior commissure is situated in the anterior wall of the third ventricle at the upper end of the lamina terminalis (Fig. 16.10).

When traced laterally, it divides into anterior and posterior bundles. The posterior bundle passes below the lentiform nucleus. Fibres passing through the commissure interconnect the regions of the two cerebral hemispheres concerned with the olfactory pathway. These include the olfactory bulb, the anterior olfactory nucleus, the prepiriform cortex, the entorhinal area, the anterior perforated substance, the amygdaloid complex and related structures. Other fibres interconnect the parahippocampal gyri and other parts of the two temporal lobes. Some fibres interconnect the frontal lobes of the two sides.

ADVANCED

The Fornix

The fornix is a prominent bundle of fibres seen on the medial aspect of the cerebral hemisphere. It is made up, predominantly, of fibres arising in the hippocampus. The **body** of the fornix is suspended from the corpus callosum by the septum pellucidum (Figs. 13.1, 8.6) and comes into close relationship with the tela choroidea in the roof of the third ventricle. When traced posteriorly, the body of the fornix divides into two parts called **crura.** Each crus of the fornix becomes continuous with the fimbria of the corresponding side. The two crura are interconnected by fibres passing from one to the other. These crossing fibres constitute the **hippocampal commissure** or **commissure of the fornix.** The anterior end of the body of the fornix also divides into right and left halves called the **columns** of the fornix. Each column turns downwards just in front of the interventricular foramen and passes through the hypothalamus to reach the mamillary body (Fig. 16.15B).

BASIC

Most of the fibres of the fornix lie behind the anterior commissure and are, therefore, referred to as the **postcommissural fornix.** In contrast some fibres of the fornix that descend in front of the anterior commissure constitute the **precommissural fornix.** Some of the fibres of the fornix pass above the splenium of the corpus callosum to reach structures above the latter. These fibres constitute the **dorsal fornix.**

The fibres contained in the fornix are as follows (Fig. 16.8):

1. Fibres interconnecting the hippocampi of the two sides through the hippocampal commissure.

2. Fibres from the hippocampus that pass through the postcommissural fornix to reach the mamillary body. These are then relayed to the anterior nucleus of the thalamus. Some fibres of the fornix end directly in this nucleus and some in the hypothalamus.

3. Fibres from the hippocampus that pass through the precommissural fornix reach the septal region. Some of these fibres turn backwards to enter the stria medullaris thalami and reach the habenular nuclei.

4. Fibres entering the dorsal fornix reach the splenial gyrus and the gyrus cinguli.

ADVANCED

17 : Internal Capsule and Commissures of the Brain

The Internal Capsule

A preliminary description of the internal capsule is given on page 91. This should be read before studying the details of the fibres passing through the capsule.

The fibres passing through the capsule may be ascending (to the cerebral cortex) or descending (from the cortex). The arrangement of fibres is easily remembered if it is realized that any group of fibres within the capsule **takes the most direct path** to its destination. Thus fibres to and from the anterior part of the frontal lobe pass through the anterior limb of the internal capsule. Those to and from the posterior part of the frontal lobe, and from the greater part of the parietal lobe, occupy the genu and posterior limb of the capsule. Fibres to and from the temporal lobe occupy the sublentiform part (Fig. 17.3), while those to and from the occipital lobe pass through the retrolentiform part. Some fibres from the lowest parts of the parietal lobe accompany the temporal fibres through the sublentiform part.

Ascending Fibres

These are **predominantly thalamocortical fibres** which go from the thalamus to all parts of the cerebral cortex (Figs. 17.1, 17.2B).

Fibres to the frontal lobe constitute the **anterior thalamic radiation** (or **frontal thalamic peduncle**). They pass through the anterior limb of the internal capsule. The fibres arise mainly from the medial and anterior nuclei of the thalamus. The anterior thalamic radiation also carries fibres from the hypothalamus and limbic structures to the frontal cortex.

Fibres travelling from the ventral posterior nuclei of the thalamus to the somatosensory area (in the postcentral gyrus) constitute the **superior thalamic radiation** (or the **superior, or dorsal, thalamic peduncle**). These fibres occupy the genu and posterior limb of the capsule. It should be noted that these fibres are third order sensory neurons responsible for conveying somesthetic sensations to the cerebral cortex. The superior thalamic radiation also contains some fibres that go from the thalamus to parts of the frontal and parietal lobes adjoining the postcentral gyrus.

Fibres from the thalamus to the occipital lobe constitute the **posterior thalamic radiation** (or the **posterior, or caudal, thalamic peduncle**). This includes the **optic radiation** from the lateral geniculate body to the visual cortex. These radiations lie in the retrolentiform part of the internal capsule. The retrolentiform part also contains some fibres passing from the thalamus to the posterior part of the parietal lobe.

Fibres from the thalamus to the temporal lobe constitute the **inferior thalamic radiation** (or **ventral thalamic peduncle**). It includes the **acoustic radiation** from the medial geniculate body to the acoustic area of the cerebral cortex. These fibres pass through the sublentiform part of the internal capsule.

BASIC

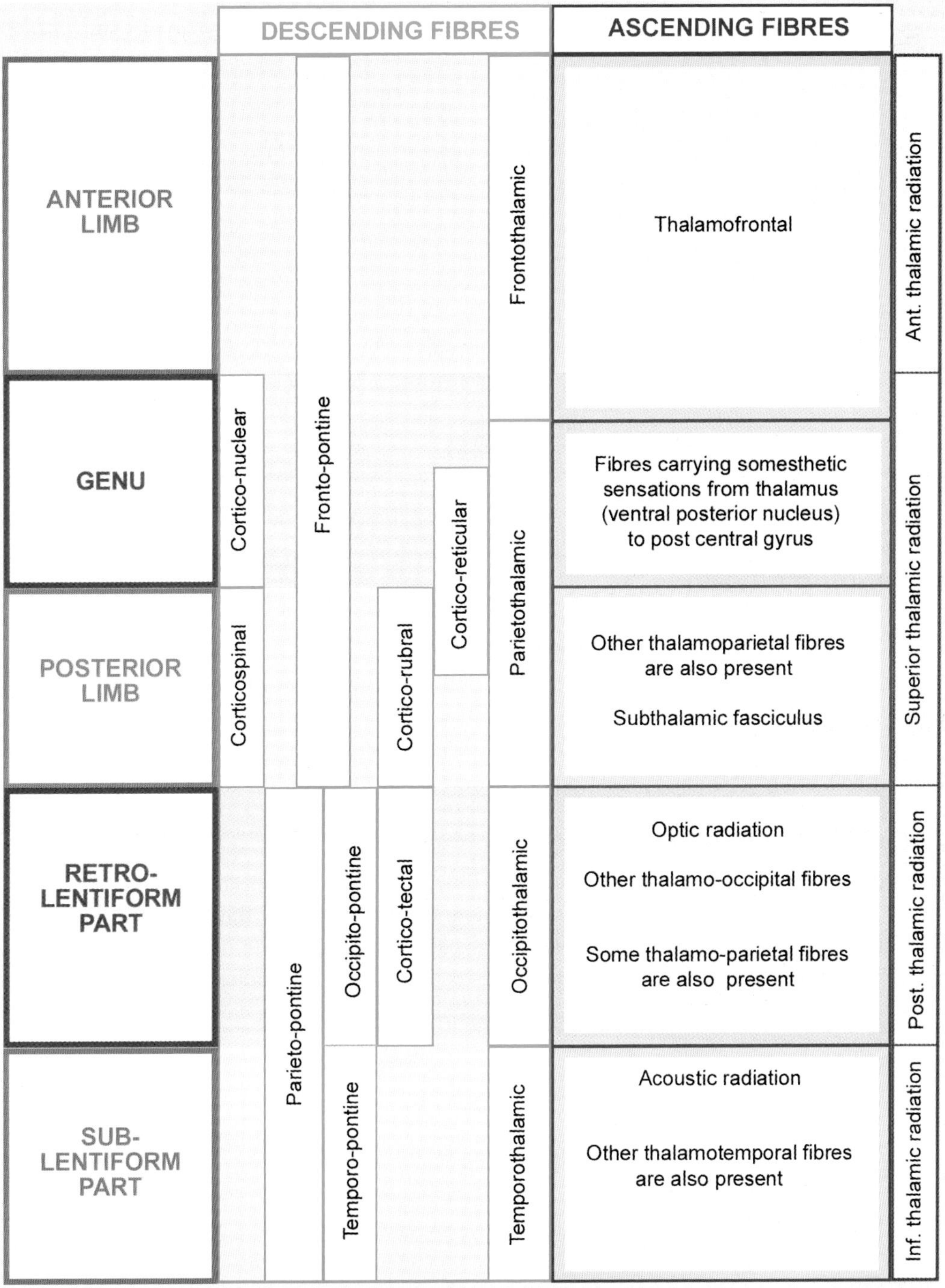

	DESCENDING FIBRES					ASCENDING FIBRES	
ANTERIOR LIMB			Fronto-pontine		Frontothalamic	Thalamofrontal	Ant. thalamic radiation
GENU	Cortico-nuclear			Cortico-reticular	Parietothalamic	Fibres carrying somesthetic sensations from thalamus (ventral posterior nucleus) to post central gyrus	Superior thalamic radiation
POSTERIOR LIMB	Corticospinal			Cortico-rubral		Other thalamoparietal fibres are also present Subthalamic fasciculus	
RETRO-LENTIFORM PART		Parieto-pontine	Occipito-pontine	Cortico-tectal	Occipitothalamic	Optic radiation Other thalamo-occipital fibres Some thalamo-parietal fibres are also present	Post. thalamic radiation
SUB-LENTIFORM PART			Temporo-pontine		Temporothalamic	Acoustic radiation Other thalamotemporal fibres are also present	Inf. thalamic radiation

Fig. 17.1. Scheme to show the fibres passing through the internal capsule.

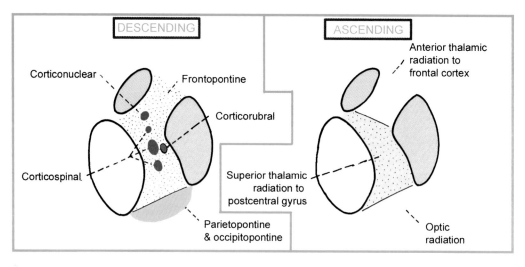

Fig. 17.2. Fibres passing through the internal capsule. A. Descending fibres. B. Ascending fibres.

Descending Fibres

(1) Corticospinal and corticonuclear fibres

Corticonuclear fibres (for motor cranial nerve nuclei) pass through the genu of the internal capsule (Figs. 17.1, 17.2A).

Corticospinal fibres form several discrete bundles in the posterior limb of the capsule. The fibres for the upper limb are most anterior, followed (in that order) by fibres for the trunk and lower limb.

(2) Corticopontine fibres

Frontopontine fibres are the most numerous. They pass through the anterior limb, genu, and posterior limb of the internal capsule. Parietopontine fibres pass mainly through the retrolentiform part. Some fibres pass through the sublentiform part. Temporopontine fibres pass through the sublentiform part (Fig.17.3). Occipitopontine fibres pass through the retrolentiform part.

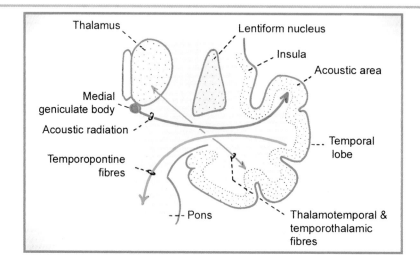

Fig. 17.3. Fibres passing through the sublentiform part of the internal capsule

(3) Corticothalamic fibres

These pass from various parts of the cerebral cortex to the thalamus. They form part of the thalamic radiations described above.

(4) Fibres from Cerebral Cortex to Brainstem nuclei

(a) **Corticonuclear fibres** to cranial nerve nuclei have been mentioned above.

(b) **Corticorubral fibres** pass through the posterior limb.

(c) **Corticoreticular fibres** pass through the genu and posterior limb.

(d) **Occipitotectal** and **occipitocollicular** fibres pass through the retrolentiform part.

(5) Fibres of the **subthalamic fasciculus** pass transversely through the posterior limb (intersecting the vertically running fibres). The fibres connect the subthalamic nucleus to the globus pallidus.

The blood supply of the internal capsule is described in Chapter 21. Thrombosis in an artery supplying the internal capsule (cerebral thrombosis) leads to a stroke that results in hemiplegia. The opposite side of the body is affected (See page 104). As the tracts passing through the internal capsule are closely packed even a small lesion can cause extensive paralysis. Sensations can also be lost. Reflexes are exaggerated as in a typical upper motor neuron paralysis. Rupture of one of the arteries leads to cerebral haemorrhage that is often fatal. (See page 104).

Commissures of the Brain

The two halves of the brain and spinal cord are interconnected by numerous fibres that cross the middle line. In some situations such fibres form recognisable bundles that are called commissures. Strictly speaking commissural fibres are those that connect corresponding regions of the two sides. Many of the fibres passing through the socalled commissures do not fulfill this criterion as they connect different regions of the two sides. Such fibres are really association fibres. We have seen that several tracts passing through the spinal cord and brainstem cross from one side to the other. These crossings are **decussations**, but collections of such fibres are sometimes loosely referred to as commissures e.g., the ventral white commissure of the spinal cord.

The Corpus Callosum

The corpus callosum is the largest commissure connecting the right and left cerebral hemispheres. Its subdivisions have been described on page 92.

The fibres passing through the corpus callosum are generally believed to interconnect corresponding regions of the entire neocortex of the right and left sides. However, some important exceptions are now known.

(i) The greater parts of the visual areas are not interconnected. Only those parts of visual areas that receive impulses from a narrow strip along the vertical meridian of the retina are interconnected. The band of cortex concerned lies at the junction of areas 17 and 18. Similar bands are also present in relation to other visual areas.

(ii) The parts of the sensorimotor areas (SI and SII) concerned with the hands and feet are not interconnected.

The corpus callosum can be congenitally absent. As the two cerebral hemispheres are not connected there is a *split brain effect*. If one hand is trained to perform an act the other hand may not be able to do so.

Other Commissures

Other commissures connecting the two cerebral hemispheres are the *anterior commissure* (page 239), the *posterior commissure* (page 202), the *hippocampal commissure* or *commissure of the fornix* (page 239) and the *habenular commissure* (page 202).

In close relationship to the optic chiasma a number of commissures carrying fibres not concerned with vision are described. These include the *ventral supraoptic commissure* (of Gudden), the *dorsal supraoptic commissure* (of Meynert) and the *anterior hypothalamic commissure* (of Ganser). The constitution of these commissures is controversial and will not be considered.

Commissural fibres also interconnect the two halves of the cerebellum, and the colliculi of the midbrain.

BASIC

FOR CHAPTER 18

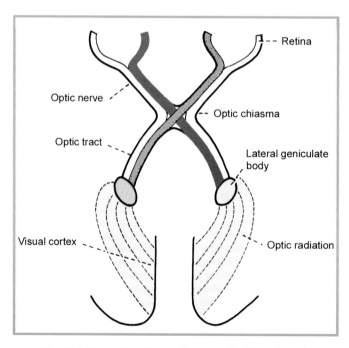

Fig. 18.1. The optic pathway. Note that the fibres from the medial (or nasal) half of each retina cross over to the optic tract of the opposite side.

18 : The Visual Pathway

The peripheral receptors for light are situated in the **retina**. Nerve fibres arising in the retina constitute the **optic nerve**. The right and left optic nerves join to form the **optic chiasma** in which many of their fibres cross to the opposite side. The uncrossed fibres of the optic nerve, along with the fibres that have crossed over from the opposite side form the **optic tract**.

The optic tract terminates predominantly in the **lateral geniculate body**. Fresh fibres arising in this body form the **geniculo-calcarine tract** or **optic radiation** which ends in the visual areas of the cerebral cortex (Fig. 18.1, on page 244)).

The Retina

The retina has a complex structure. It contains photoreceptors that convert the stimulus of light into nervous impulses. These receptors are of two kinds, **rods** and **cones** (Fig. 18.2). There are about seven million cones in each retina. The rods are far more numerous, and number more than 100 million.

The cones respond best to bright light. They are responsible for sharp vision and for discrimination of colour. They are most numerous in the central region of the retina which is responsible for sharp vision. This area is about 6mm in diameter. Within this region there is a yellowish area called the **macula lutea**. The centre of the macula shows a small depression called the **fovea centralis**.

Medial to the central area, there is a circular area called the **optic disc**. This area is devoid of photoreceptors and is, therefore, called the **blind spot**. The fibres of the optic nerve leave the eyeball through the region of the optic disc.

The macula lies exactly in the optical axis of the eyeball. When any object is viewed critically its image is formed on the macula. The fovea centralis is believed to contain cones only. Rods, on the other hand, predominate in peripheral parts of the retina. They can respond to poor light and specially to movement across the field of vision.

Each rod or cone may be regarded as a modified neuron. It consists of a cell body, a peripheral process and a central process. The cell body contains a nucleus. The peripheral process is rod shaped in the case of rods, and cone shaped in the case of cones (hence the names rods and cones). The ends of these peripheral processes are separated from one another by processes of pigment cells. The central processes of rods and

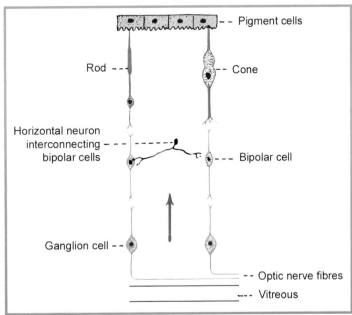

Fig. 18.2. Simplified scheme of the neurons within the retina. The red arrow indicates the direction of light falling on the retina.

cones are like those of neurons. They end by synapsing with other neurons within the retina. For details of the structure of rods and cones, see the author's HUMAN HISTOLOGY.

The basic neuronal arrangement within the retina is shown in Fig. 18.2. The central processes of rods and cones synapse with the peripheral processes of ***bipolar cells***. The central processes of bipolar cells synapse with dendrites of ***ganglion cells***. Axons arising from ganglion cells form the ***fibres of the optic nerve***.

The various elements mentioned above form a series of layers within the retina. The outermost layer (towards the choroid) is formed by the pigments cells, followed in sequence by the rods and cones, the bipolar cells, the ganglion cells, and a layer of optic nerve fibres. The layer of optic nerve fibres is apposed to the vitreous. It will be obvious that light has to pass through several of the layers of the retina to reach the rods and cones. This 'inverted' arrangement of the retina is necessary as passage of light in the reverse direction would be obstructed by the layer of pigment cells.

The pigment cells are important in spacing the rods and cones and in providing them with mechanical support. They absorb light and prevent back reflection. A nutritive and phagocytic role has also been attributed to them.

At this stage it must be emphasised that the structure of the retina is very much more complex than the highly simplified description above would suggest. Some points worthy of note are as follows.

(1) Rods and cones are of various types. Intermediate forms between them are also present. The rods and cones have a complicated ultrastructure. Their outer segments contain photopigments which appear to be concerned in converting the stimulus of light into a nervous impulse.

(2) Bipolar cells and ganglion cells are of various types. They vary in size and in their connections. Some bipolar cells are connected with cones, some with rods, and others with both rods and cones.

(3) The vertically orientated elements of the retina (i.e., rods and cones, bipolar cells, ganglion cells) are interconnected by horizontally disposed neurons. Some of these appear to be devoid of axons and are called ***amacrine cells***.

(4) The number of rods and cones (over 100 million) greatly exceeds the number of ganglion cells (about one million). It is, therefore, obvious that the impulses from several rods and cones must be concentrated on a single ganglion cell; and must, therefore, travel along a single optic nerve fibre. The one to one relationship between rods and cones, bipolar cells and ganglion cells shown in Fig. 18.2 is only for sake of simplicity.

(5) According to some authorities, the retina receives some fibres through the optic nerve although their source is uncertain. Other authorities however, deny the presence of such fibres.

(6) Besides the nervous elements, the retina contains supporting cells which are believed to represent a specialised type of neuroglia.

The Visual Field and Retinal Quadrants

When the head and eyes are maintained in a fixed position, and one eye is closed, the area seen by that eye constitutes the ***visual field*** for that eye. Now if the other eye is also opened the area seen is more or less the same as was seen with one eye. In other words the visual fields of the two eyes overlap to a very great extent. On either side, however, there is a small area seen only by the eye of that side. Although the two eyes view the same area, the relative position of objects within the area appears somewhat dissimilar to the two eyes as they view the object from slightly different angles. The difference though slight, is of considerable importance as it forms the basis for the perception of depth (***stereoscopic vision***).

For convenience of description, the visual field is divided into right and left halves. It may also be divided into upper and lower halves so that the visual field can be said to consist of four quadrants (Fig. 18.3). In a similar manner each retina can also be divided into quadrants. Images of objects in

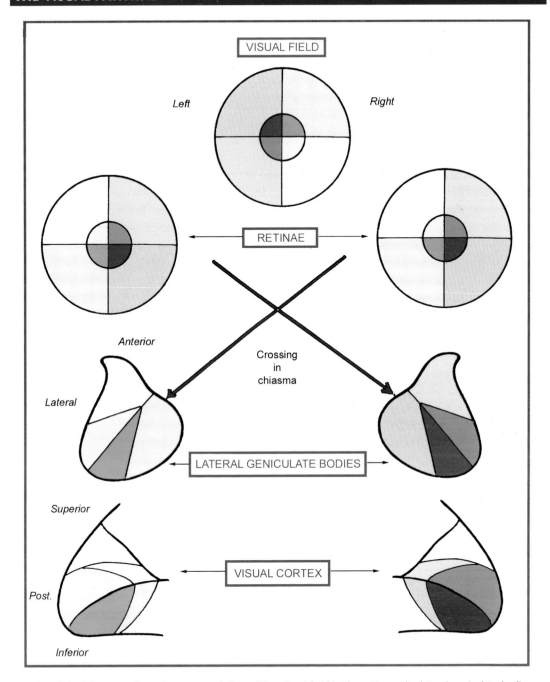

Fig. 18.3. Scheme to show the representation of the visual field in the retinae, the lateral geniculate bodies and the visual cortex of the two sides. The peripheral parts of the visual field are represented by light colours while the corresponding macular areas are represented by dark colours.

the field of vision are formed on the retina by the lens of the eyeball. As with any convex lens the image is inverted. If an object is placed in the **right** half of the field of vision its image is formed on the **left** half of the retina and **vice versa**. Unfortunately, instead of using the words right and left, the two halves of the retina are usually referred to as **nasal** (= medial) and **temporal** (= lateral) halves. This introduces a complication as the left half of the left eye is the temporal half, while in the

BASIC

case of the right eye it is the nasal half. Thus the image of an object placed in the right half of the field of vision falls on the temporal half of the left retina, and on the nasal half of the right retina.

Optic Nerve, Optic Chiasma & Optic Tract

The optic nerve is made up of axons of the ganglion cells of the retina. These axons are at first unmyelinated. The fibres from all parts of the retina converge on the optic disc. In this region the sclera has numerous small apertures and is, therefore, called the *lamina cribrosa* (crib = sieve). Bundles of optic nerve fibres pass through these apertures. Each fibre acquires a myelin sheath as soon as it pierces the sclera. The fibres of the nerve arising from the four quadrants of the retina maintain the same relative position within the nerve. The fibres arising from the macula are numerous and form the *papillomacular bundle*. Close to the eyeball, the macular fibres occupy the lateral part of the nerve, but by the time they reach the chiasma they lie in the central part of the nerve.

The fibres of the optic nerve arising in the nasal half of each retina enter the optic tract of the opposite side after crossing in the chiasma. Fibres from the temporal half of each retina enter the optic tract of the same side (Fig. 18.1). Thus the right optic tract comes to contain fibres from the right halves of both retinae, and the left tract from the left halves. In other words, all optic nerve fibres carrying impulses relating to the left half of the field of vision are brought together in the right optic tract and vice versa. We have already noted that each optic tract carries these fibres to the lateral geniculate body of the corresponding side.

The Lateral Geniculate Body

Some aspects of the structure of the lateral geniculate body have been considered on page 192. It has been seen that the grey matter of this body is split into six laminae (Fig. 13.17). Fibres from the eye of the same side end in laminae 2, 3, and 5; while those from the opposite eye end in laminae 1, 4, and 6. The macular fibres end in the central and posterior part of the lateral geniculate body, and this area is relatively large (Fig. 18.3). Fibres from the peripheral parts of the retina end in the anterior part of the lateral geniculate body. The upper half of the retina is represented laterally, and the lower half of the retina is represented medially. Specific points on the retina project to specific points in the lateral geniculate body. In turn, specific points of this body project to specific points in the visual cortex. In this way a point to point relationship is maintained between the retinae and the visual cortex.

Recent studies of synaptic patterns within the lateral geniculate body indicate that this nucleus is not to be regarded as a simple relay station and that various influences may modify the conduction of impulses through it. In this connection it may be noted that the lateral geniculate body receives afferents from the visual cortex.

Geniculocalcarine Tract and Visual Cortex

Fibres arising from cells of the lateral geniculate body constitute the geniculocalcarine tract or optic radiation. These fibres pass through the retrolentiform part of the internal capsule. The optic radiation ends in the visual areas of the cerebral cortex (areas 17, 18, 19).

Some fibres of the radiation loop forwards and downwards into the temporal lobe before turning backwards into the occipital lobe. The highest fibres may loop into the parietal lobe.

The cortex of each hemisphere receives impulses from the retinal halves of the same side (i.e., from the opposite half of the field of vision). The upper quadrants of the retina are represented above the calcarine sulcus, and the lower quadrants below it. The cortical area for the macula is larger than that for peripheral areas. It occupies the posterior part of the visual area. The cortical area for the peripheral part of the retina is situated anterior to the area for the macula.

Injuries to different parts of the visual pathway can produce various kinds of defects. Loss of vision in one half (right or left) of the visual field is called *hemianopia*. If the same half of the visual field is lost in both eyes the defect is said to be *homonymous* and if different halves are lost the defect is said to be *heteronymous*. Note that the hemianopia is named in relation to the *visual field* and not to the retina.

Injury to the optic nerve will obviously produce total blindness in the eye concerned. Damage to the central part of the optic chiasma (e.g., by pressure from an enlarged hypophysis) interrupts the crossing fibres derived from the nasal halves of the two retinae resulting in *bitemporal heteronymous hemianopia*. It has been claimed that macular fibres are more susceptible to damage by pressure than peripheral fibres and are affected first. When the lateral part of the chiasma is affected a *nasal hemianopia* results. This may be unilateral or bilateral. Complete destruction of the optic tract, the lateral geniculate body, the optic radiation or the visual cortex of one side, results in loss of the opposite half of the field of vision. A lesion on the right side leads to *left homonymous hemianopia*.

Partial injury may affect only one quadrant. The resulting condition is called *quadrantic anopia*. Injury to looping fibres of the geniculocalcarine tract may lead to blindness in the upper quadrant when the lesion is in the temporal lobe; and in the lower quadrant when the lesion is in the parietal lobe.

It may be noted that in lesions of the visual pathway macular vision is often spared. This is so because of the large size of the macular area, and because some areas have a double blood supply (from posterior and middle cerebral arteries).

Lesions confined to areas 18 and 19 (peristriate and parastriate areas) may not result in loss of vision, but the patient may be unable to interpret images seen. This is *visual agnosia*.

Lesions anterior to the lateral geniculate body also interrupt fibres responsible for the *pupillary light reflex* (see below).

CLINICAL

Reflexes related to the Eyeball

Pupillary reflexes

Light thrown on an eye causes the pupil of that eye to contract. This is called the *direct pupillary light reflex.* At the same time the pupil of the other eye also contracts. This is called the *consensual light reflex.* The pathway for the light reflex is shown in Fig. 18.4. Impulses from the retina (of the eye on which light is thrown) travel through the optic nerve, chiasma and optic tracts. Near the lateral geniculate body the fibres concerned pass into the midbrain and end in the pretectal nucleus. Axons arising from this nucleus reach the Edinger Westphal nuclei of both sides. Fibres arising in these nuclei supply the sphincter pupillae after relay in the ciliary ganglion. The consensual reflex may be explained by the following.

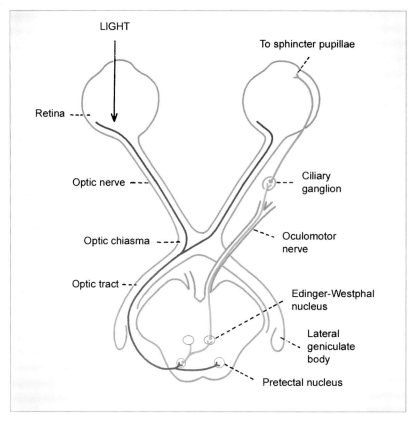

Fig. 18.4. Pathway for the light reflex. Note that all structures shown are bilateral. Some of them are shown only on one side for sake of clarity.

(**a**) Fibres of each optic nerve enter both optic tracts as a result of partial crossing in the chiasma.

(**b**) Fibres from each optic tract end in both pretectal nuclei.

(**c**) Fibres from each pretectal nucleus reach the Edinger Westphal nuclei of both sides.

Constriction of the pupil also takes place when we look at a near object i.e., during accommodation. The pathway for this *accommodation reflex* is different from that for the light reflex, and is believed to involve the visual cortex. In certain diseases (notably syphlitic infection) of the nervous system the pupillary light reflex may be abolished, but pupillary constriction in response to accommodation remains. This condition is called *Argyll-Robertson-pupil.* In such cases the lesion is believed to be in the pretectal area.

Corneal Reflex

If the cornea is touched with a small wisp of cotton this results in closing of both eyes. This is called the *corneal reflex*. Impulses from the cornea travel along branches of the ophthalmic division of the trigeminal nerve to the sensory nuclei of this nerve. Secondary fibres establish connections with the motor nuclei of the facial nerve of both sides. Fibres arising in the facial nuclei, and reaching the muscles closing the palpebral aperture, complete the reflex arc. In the case of injury to the ophthalmic division of the trigeminal nerve, the corneal reflex cannot be elicited from that side, but a bilateral response is obtained by stimulating the cornea of the normal side. In facial paralysis the response is seen only on the normal side.

Introduction

The autonomic nervous system is made up of nerves supplying the viscera (and blood vessels) along with the parts of the brain and spinal cord related to them. It is subdivided into two divisions, *sympathetic* and *parasympathetic*. Both these divisions contain efferent as well as afferent fibres. The efferent fibres supply smooth muscle throughout the body. The influence may be either to cause contraction or relaxation. In a given situation, the sympathetic and parasympathetic nerves generally produce opposite effects. For example, sympathetic stimulation causes dilatation of the pupil, whereas parasympathetic stimulation causes constriction. In hollow viscera like the stomach or urinary bladder, parasympathetic stimulation produces movement and inhibits the sphincters. An opposite sympathetic effect is usually described. In the case of blood vessels, the influence on smooth muscle may result in vasoconstriction or in vasodilatation.

In addition to supplying smooth muscle autonomic nerves innervate glands. Such nerves are described as *secretomotor*. The secretomotor nerves to almost all glands are parasympathetic. The only exception are the sweat glands which have a sympathetic supply.

The autonomic nervous system includes the following.

(1) Areas for visceral function located in the cerebral hemispheres

These are the structures in the limbic region which have been considered in Chapter 16. The hypothalamus, parts of the thalamus, and the prefrontal cortex are also involved in autonomic functions.

(2) Autonomic centres in the brainstem

These are located in the reticular formation and in the general visceral nuclei of cranial nerves.

(3) Autonomic centres in the spinal cord

These are located in the intermediolateral grey column.

(4) Peripheral part of autonomic nervous system

This is made up of all autonomic nerves and ganglia throughout the body. Many of these are intimately related to cranial and spinal nerves.

For details of peripheral autonomic pathways see the author's TEXTBOOK OF HUMAN ANATOMY. The description that follows aims at providing a simple account of neuronal arrangements within the system and the autonomic innervation of important organs.

Before we can consider the arrangement of neurons it is necessary to take a brief look at some aspects of gross anatomy.

THE SYMPATHETIC TRUNKS

The sympathetic trunks (right and left) are the most easily seen parts of the autonomic nervous system. They are placed on either side of the vertebral column. Above, they extend to the base of the skull; and below, to the coccyx. Each trunk bears a number of enlargements placed along its length. These are the *sympathetic ganglia*. The number of ganglia is variable. Generally there are three (superior, middle and inferior) in the cervical region; eleven in the thoracic region; four in the

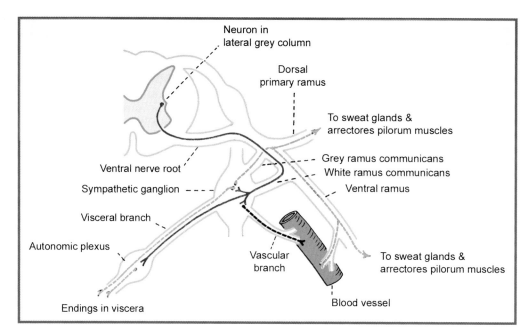

Fig. 19.1. Grey and white rami connecting a spinal nerve to the sympathetic trunk, and the fibres passing through them. Preganglionic fibres are shown in magenta.

lumbar region; and four in the sacral region, so that in all there are twenty two or twenty three ganglia on each trunk. The inferior cervical ganglion and the first thoracic are often fused to form a large **stellate ganglion**.

The sympathetic trunks are connected to the spinal nerves by a series of communicating branches or **rami communicantes**. These are of two types, white and grey. The white rami consist of myelinated fibres, while the grey rami are made up of unmyelinated fibres. The white rami carry fibres (originating in the spinal cord) from the spinal nerve to the sympathetic trunks. They are present only in the thoracic and upper lumbar regions. The grey rami carry fibres from the sympathetic trunk to spinal nerves. All spinal nerves receive grey rami. The fibres of the grey rami are distributed to peripheral tissues through the spinal nerves. The sympathetic trunks also establish communications with several cranial nerves through branches arising from the superior cervical ganglion.

In addition to communicating branches, the sympathetic trunks give off branches for supply of blood vessels and of viscera. The visceral branches are directed medially (Fig. 19.1) and take part in forming a series of autonomic plexuses in the thorax, abdomen and pelvis. Branches to peripheral parts of the body follow one of two routes. Some branches from the sympathetic trunks reach blood vessels directly and form perivascular plexuses on them. One such branch arises from the cranial end of the superior cervical ganglion and forms a plexus around the internal carotid artery. Other sympathetic fibres reach blood vessels (specially in the limbs) after running for part of their course through spinal nerves and their branches (Fig. 19.1).

Apart from supplying the blood vessels themselves, these sympathetic fibres innervate sweat glands and arrectores pilorum muscles of the skin.

AUTONOMIC PLEXUSES

It has been mentioned above that visceral branches of sympathetic trunks help to form various plexuses in the thorax, the abdomen and the pelvis. In addition to sympathetic fibres these plexuses contain parasympathetic fibres derived either from the vagus nerve, or from pelvic splanchnic nerves (see below). They also contain collections of neurons which are often referred to as ganglia. In the thorax there are the **superficial and deep cardiac plexuses** in relation to the heart, and the **pulmonary plexuses** in relation to the lungs (Fig. 19.2). In the abdomen there is a prominent **coeliac ganglion** on either side of the aorta. The two ganglia are interconnected by numerous fibres that form the **coeliac plexus**. This plexus is closely related to the coeliac trunk and sends ramifications along its branches. Other plexuses (or ganglia) are related to the abdominal aorta, to the superior mesenteric and inferior mesenteric arteries, and to other branches arising from the aorta. The pelvis has a **superior hypogastric plexus** (often called the **presacral nerve**) situated near the bifurcation of the aorta. When traced downwards, it divides into two **inferior hypogastric plexuses** (or **hypogastric nerves**) related to each internal iliac artery. Subsidiary plexuses run along branches of the internal iliac artery. Some plexuses are present in close relation to some viscera or even within their walls. The vesical plexus surrounds the urinary bladder. In the gut there is a **myenteric plexus** (of Auerbach) between the muscle coats; and a **submucosal plexus** (of Meissner).

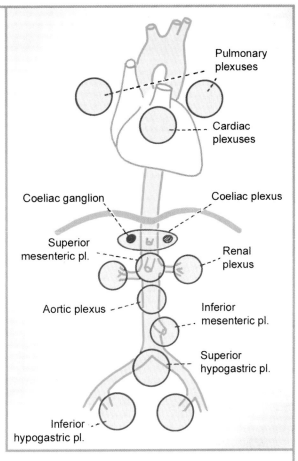

Fig. 19.2. Schematic representation of the location of important autonomic plexuses of the thorax and abdomen.

PREGANGLIONIC AND POSTGANGLIONIC NEURONS

The autonomic pathway, for innervation of smooth muscle or gland always consists of two neurons that synapse in a ganglion (Fig. 3.2). The first neuron carries the nerve impulse from the CNS to the ganglion and is called the **preganglionic neuron**. The second neuron carries impulses from the ganglion to smooth muscle or gland and is called the **postganglionic neuron**.

Sympathetic Preganglionic Neurons

The cell bodies of sympathetic preganglionic neurons are located in the intermediolateral grey column of the spinal cord in the thoracic and upper two (or three) lumbar segments (Fig. 19.3). Fibres arising from these neurons constitute the **thoracolumbar outflow**. Their axons leave the spinal cord through anterior nerve roots to reach the spinal nerves of the segments concerned. After a very short course in the ventral primary rami these fibres enter the white rami communicantes to reach the sympathetic trunk (Fig. 19.1).

On reaching the sympathetic trunk these fibres behave in one of the following ways (Figs. 19.1, 19.4).

(a) They may terminate in relation to cells of the sympathetic ganglion at the level concerned.

BASIC

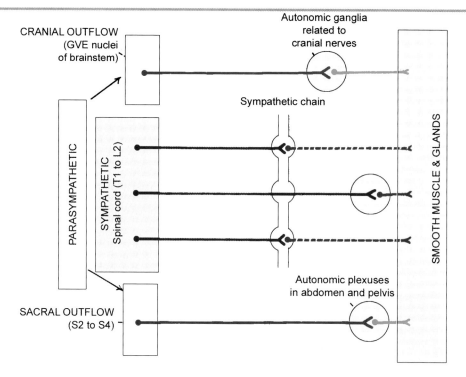

Fig. 19.3. Scheme to show the basic arrangement of sympathetic and parasympathetic neurons.

(b) They may travel up or down the sympathetic trunk to terminate in ganglia at a higher or lower level.

(c) They may leave the sympathetic trunk through one of its branches to terminate in a peripherally situated ganglion.

Sympathetic Postganglionic Neurons

These neurons are located primarily in ganglia on the sympathetic trunks. Some are located in peripheral autonomic plexuses (Figs 19.1, 19.5). Axons arising from sympathetic postganglionic neurons behave in one of the following ways.

(1) The axons may pass through a grey ramus communicans to reach a spinal nerve. They then pass through the spinal nerve and its branches to innervate sweat glands and arrectores pilorum muscles of the skin in the region to which the spinal nerve is distributed.

(2) The axons may reach a cranial nerve through a communicating branch and may be distributed through it as in the case of a spinal nerve.

(3) The axons may pass into a vascular branch and may be distributed to branches of the vessel. Some fibres from these plexuses may pass to other structures in the neighbourhood of the vessel.

(4) We have already seen that some axons, meant for innervation of blood vessels, travel for part of their course

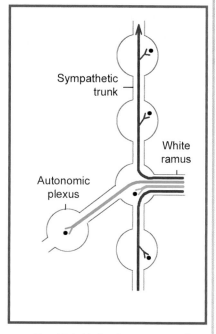

Fig. 19.4. Mode of termination of sympathetic preganglionic neurons.

in spinal nerves or their branches, and reach the vessels through vascular branches arising from these nerves. Many blood vessels in the peripheral parts of the limbs are innervated in this way.

(5) The axons of postganglionic neurons arising in sympathetic ganglia may travel through visceral branches and through autonomic plexuses to reach some viscera (e.g., the heart).

(6) The axons of postganglionic neurons located in peripheral autonomic plexuses innervate neighbouring viscera. These fibres often travel to the viscera in plexuses along blood vessels. For example, fibres for the gut travel along plexuses surrounding the branches of the coeliac, superior mesenteric and inferior mesenteric arteries.

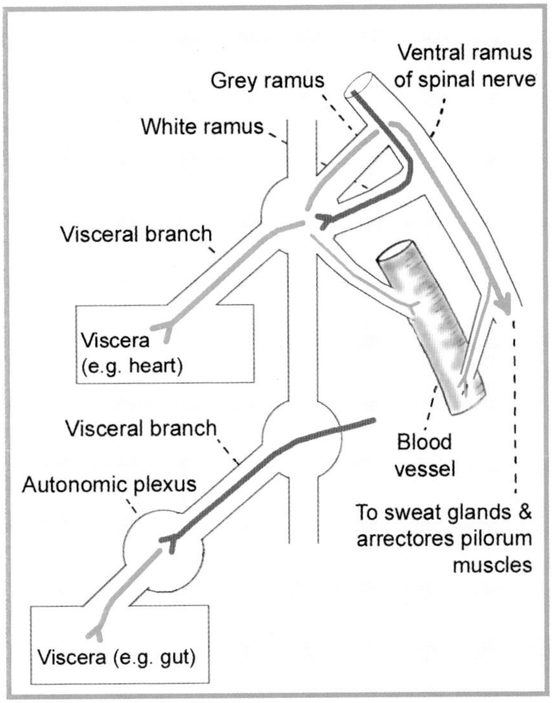

Parasympathetic Preganglionic Neurons

The parasympathetic preganglionic neurons are located in two distinct situations.

(1) The first group is located in the general visceral efferent nuclei of the brainstem. These are considered on page 109. Axons arising in these nuclei constitute the **cranial parasympathetic outflow** (Fig. 19.3). They pass through the third, seventh, ninth and tenth cranial nerves to terminate in peripheral ganglia. The largest part of this outflow is constituted by the vagus nerve. Its fibres terminate in relation to postganglionic neurons located in thoracic and abdominal autonomic plexuses.

(2) The second group of parasympathetic preganglionic neurons is located in the second, third and fourth sacral segments of the spinal cord (Fig. 19.3). Their axons constitute the **sacral parasympathetic outflow**. They emerge from the cord through the anterior nerve roots of the corresponding spinal nerves. The axons leave the spinal nerves to form the **pelvic splanchnic nerves** which end in pelvic autonomic plexuses (Fig. 19.6B).

Parasympathetic Postganglionic Neurons

(1) Postganglionic neurons related to the third, seventh and ninth cranial nerves are located in the ciliary, submandibular, pterygopalatine and otic ganglia. Some subsidiary ganglia may be located in the vicinity of these ganglia.

(2) Postganglionic neurons related to the vagus are located in thoracic and abdominal autonomic plexuses, close to, or within, the viscera supplied (Fig. 19.6). The axons arising from these postganglionic neurons innervate various thoracic and abdominal viscera including the greater part of the gut.

(3) Postganglionic neurons related to the sacral parasympathetic outflow are located in pelvic autonomic plexuses. They innervate the pelvic viscera. They also supply the rectum, the sigmoid colon, the descending colon, and the left one third of the transverse colon. Like the postganglionic neurons related to the vagus, these neurons are located close to, or within, the viscera supplied, their axons running a short course to supply the viscus concerned.

Fig. 19.5. Course and termination of sympathetic postganglionic neurons.

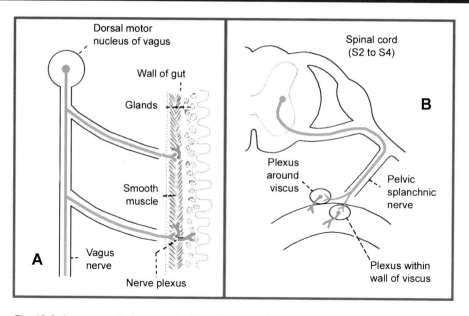

Fig. 19.6. Arrangement of preganglionic and postganglionic parasympathetic neurons related
(A) to the vagus, and (B) to pelvic splanchnic nerves.

SOME FURTHER DETAILS OF AUTONOMIC NEURONS

ADVANCED

Having considered the basic plan of the autonomic nervous system, we may now examine some further details of interest about autonomic neurons.

(1) The neurotransmitter acetylcholine is liberated at the terminals of preganglionic neurons, both sympathetic and parasympathetic. Acetylcholine is also liberated at the terminals of parasympathetic postganglionic neurons. However, the neurotransmitter liberated at the terminals of sympathetic postganglionic neurons is (as a rule) noradrenalin or adrenalin. Cells of the adrenal medulla which receive terminals of preganglionic sympathetic neurons, and produce noradrenalin and adrenalin, may be regarded as modified sympathetic postganglionic neurons. It may be noted that cells of the sympathetic ganglia and of the adrenal medulla have a common embryological origin from the neural crest.

Postganglionic sympathetic neurons innervating sweat glands are exceptional in that their terminals liberate acetylcholine.

(2) It is possible that some sympathetic preganglionic neurons may be located in spinal segments above T1 or below L3, and may leave the cord through corresponding spinal nerves.

(3) Some preganglionic sympathetic fibres may leave the spinal cord through dorsal nerve roots.

(4) Some sympathetic postganglionic neurons may be located in *intermediate ganglia* present on the trunks of spinal nerves, in the ventral rami or in rami communicantes.

(5) The number of postganglionic sympathetic neurons (or fibres) is much greater than that of preganglionic neurons, each preganglionic fibre synapsing with many postganglionic neurons. This results in considerable dispersal of the nerve impulse. A similar, but much lesser, dispersal of impulses also takes place in the parasympathetic nervous system. This is to be correlated with the fact that sympathetic stimulation produces widespread effects, whereas the effects of parasympathetic stimulation are much more localised.

(6) Some of the neurons in sympathetic ganglia are interneurons. Some of these are described as *small intensely fluorescent* (SIF) neurons. Some others are chromaffin.

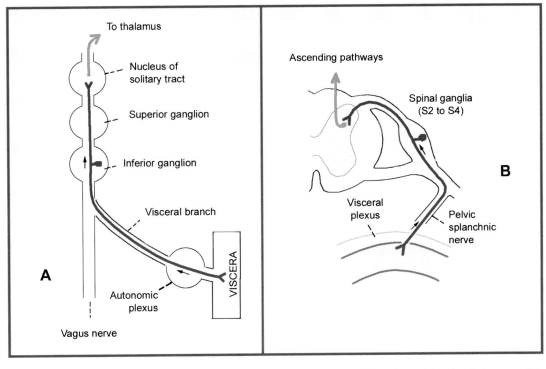

To thalamus

Nucleus of
solitary tract

Superior ganglion

Inferior ganglion

Visceral branch

A

Autonomic
plexus

VISCERA

Vagus nerve

Ascending pathways

Spinal ganglia
(S2 to S4)

B

Visceral
plexus

Pelvic
splanchnic
nerve

Fig. 19.7. Arrangement of afferent autonomic neurons related to the vagus (A), and to pelvic splanchnic nerves (B).

AFFERENT AUTONOMIC PATHWAYS

We have noted that sensory neurons related to the autonomic nervous system are general visceral afferent neurons; and that their arrangement is similar to that of afferent fibres in cerebrospinal nerves. The neurons concerned are located in spinal ganglia, or in sensory ganglia of cranial nerves. They carry impulses arising in viscera, and in blood vessels, to the central nervous system. They may be associated with the parasympathetic as well as the sympathetic systems. Accordingly, the cell bodies of the neurons in question may be located in one of the following situations.

Afferents Related to the Cranial part of the Parasympathetic System

These are general visceral afferent fibres related to the glossopharyngeal and vagus nerves. The cell bodies of the neurons concerned are located in sensory ganglia related to the cranial nerve in question. Their central processes terminate in the nucleus of the solitary tract (page 120). Some fibres may terminate in the dorsal vagal nucleus. The most important general visceral afferent fibres are those carried by the vagus nerve. Sensory fibres carried by the vagus innervate all organs to which its efferent fibres are distributed. The sensory fibres in the vagus are much more numerous than efferent fibres. Apart from carrying sensations afferent fibres are involved in various reflexes related to the organs concerned.

Glossopharyngeal afferents carry sensations from the pharynx and from the posterior part of the tongue. They also innervate the carotid sinus and the carotid body.

Afferents related to the Sacral part of the Parasympathetic System

These afferents are peripheral processes of unipolar neurons located in the dorsal nerve root ganglia of the second, third and fourth sacral nerves (Fig. 19.7B). These fibres run through the pelvic splanchnic nerves to innervate pelvic viscera. The central processes of these neurons enter

BASIC

the spinal cord. The spinal pathways carrying afferent impulses from the viscera are not fully established.

Afferents related to the Sympathetic Nervous System

Afferent fibres accompany almost all efferent sympathetic fibres. These afferent fibres are peripheral processes of unipolar neurons located in the spinal ganglia of spinal nerves T1 to L2 (or L3) (Fig. 19.8).

Some Further Comments on Autonomic Afferents

Some important points that may be noted about autonomic afferents are as follows.

(a) Autonomic afferents are necessary for various visceral reflexes. Most of these impulses are not consciously perceived.

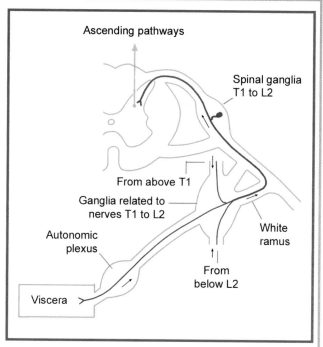

Fig. 19.8. Afferent autonomic pathways involving sympathetic nerves.

(b) Some normal visceral sensations that reach consciousness include those of hunger, nausea, distension of the urinary bladder or rectum, and sexual sensations. Sense of touch or pressure perceived by the tongue and pharynx, and the sensation of taste are also visceral sensations.

(c) Under pathological conditions visceral pain is perceived. This is produced by distension, by spasm of smooth muscle, or by anoxia.

(d) Sensory impulses from the same organ may travel both along sympathetic and parasympathetic nerves (see below).

Autonomic Nerve Supply of some Important Organs

The Eyeball

The **sphincter pupillae** is supplied by parasympathetic nerves. The preganglionic neurons concerned are located in the Edinger Westphal nucleus (page 118). Their axons travel through the oculomotor nerve and terminate in the ciliary ganglion. Postganglionic neurons are located in this ganglion. Their axons supply the sphincter pupillae and the ciliaris muscle (Fig. 19.9).

The **dilator pupillae** is supplied by sympathetic nerves. The preganglionic neurons concerned are located in the intermediolateral grey column of the first thoracic segment of the spinal cord. Their axons emerge through the anterior nerve root of the first thoracic nerve to reach the stellate ganglion. They, however, pass through this ganglion without relay, and ascend in the sympathetic trunk to reach the superior cervical sympathetic ganglion. Postganglionic neurons are located in this ganglion. Their axons pass through the internal carotid nerve. In the cavernous sinus they pass (through

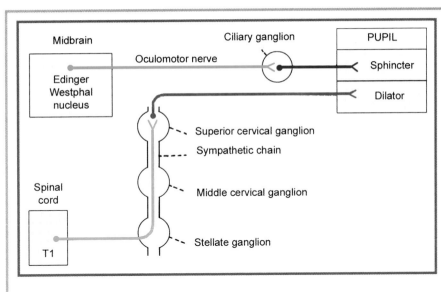

Fig. 19.9. Scheme to show the innervation of the pupil.

BASIC

communicating twigs) to the ophthalmic division of the trigeminal nerve. They travel through the nasociliary nerve and its long ciliary branches to the dilator pupillae.

Some sympathetic fibres reach the eyeball after passing through the ciliary ganglion. These fibres do not relay in this ganglion, but merely pass through it. They supply the blood vessels of the eyeball. Occasionally the fibres for the dilator pupillae may follow this route. Apart from the dilator pupillae and blood vessels, sympathetic fibres also supply the orbitalis muscle, smooth muscle in the eyelids, and probably also the ciliaris.

Horner's syndrome

Interruption of sympathetic supply to the head and neck results in Horner's syndrome. This consists of the following:
  (a)   Constriction of the pupil.
  (b)   Drooping of the upper eyelids (*ptosis*).
  (c)   Reduced prominence of the eyeball (*enophthalmos*).
  (d)   Absence of sweating on the face and neck.
  (e)   Flushing of the face.

CLINICAL

Salivary Glands

Submandibular and Sublingual glands

The secretomotor supply to the salivary glands is parasympathetic. Preganglionic neurons for the submandibular gland and for the sublingual gland are located in the superior salivary nucleus (page 119) (Fig. 19.10). Their axons pass through the facial nerve, its chorda tympani branch and then through the lingual nerve to reach the submandibular ganglion. The postganglionic neurons are located in this ganglion. Their axons reach the submandibular gland through branches from the ganglion to the gland. Some postganglionic neurons may be located in the hilum of the submandibular gland.

Fibres meant for the sublingual gland reenter the lingual nerve and pass through its distal part to reach the gland.

BASIC

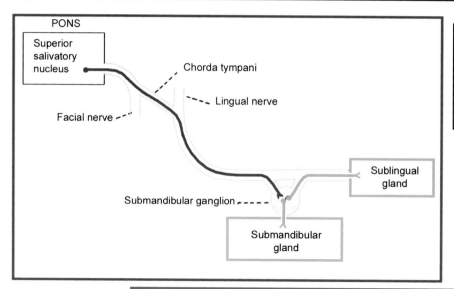

Fig. 19.10. Secretomotor pathways to the submandibular and sublingual salivary glands..

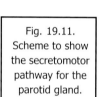

Fig. 19.11. Scheme to show the secretomotor pathway for the parotid gland.

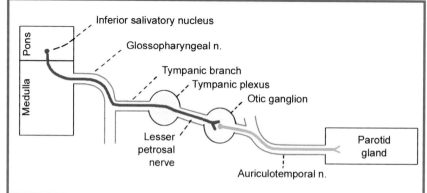

Parotid gland

The preganglionic neurons for the parotid gland are located in the inferior salivary nucleus (page 119). Their axons pass through the glossopharyngeal nerve and its tympanic branch, the tympanic plexus and the lesser petrosal nerve to terminate in the otic ganglion (Fig. 19.11). Postganglionic fibres arising in this ganglion reach the gland through the auriculotemporal nerve. (It has been reported that some parasympathetic fibres may reach the parotid gland through the facial nerve).

Sympathetic fibres travel to salivary glands along the blood vessels.

Lacrimal Gland

Preganglionic neurons for the lacrimal gland are located near the salivary nuclei. Their axons pass through the facial nerve, its greater petrosal branch, and through the nerve of the pterygoid canal to reach the pterygopalatine ganglion. Postganglionic fibres arising in this ganglion pass successively through the maxillary nerve, its zygomatic branch, the zygomaticotemporal nerve, a communicating branch from the zygomaticotemporal nerve to the lacrimal branch of the ophthalmic nerve, and finally through the lacrimal branch itself to reach the gland. However, some workers are of the opinion that postganglionic fibres reach the lacrimal gland through direct lacrimal rami from the pterygopalatine ganglion.

BASIC

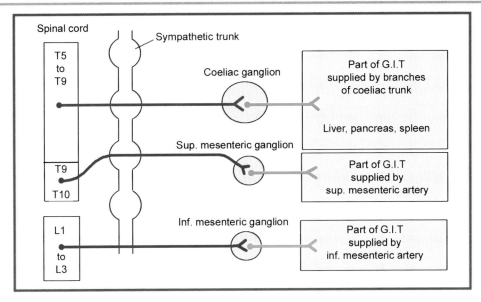

Fig. 19.12. Scheme to show the sympathetic innervation of the gut. The parasympathetic innervation is shown in Fig. 19.6.

Gastrointestinal Tract

1. The parasympathetic nerve supply of the greater part of the gastrointestinal tract (from the pharynx to the junction of the right two thirds of the transverse colon with the left one third) is through the vagus. The preganglionic neurons are situated in the dorsal nucleus of the vagus (Fig. 19.6A). (Some of them may lie in or near the nucleus ambiguus).

2. The left one third of the transverse colon, the descending colon, the sigmoid colon, the rectum and the upper part of the anal canal are supplied by the sacral part of the parasympathetic system. The preganglionic neurons concerned are located in the second, third and fourth sacral segments of the spinal cord (Fig. 19.6B). They emerge through the ventral nerve roots of the corresponding nerves, and pass into their pelvic splanchnic branches. The fibres to the rectum and the upper part of the anal canal pass through the inferior hypogastric plexus. The remaining fibres pass through the superior hypogastric plexus and are distributed along the inferior mesenteric artery.

3. The postganglionic parasympathetic neurons are located in the myenteric and submucosal plexus in the region to be supplied.

4. Preganglionic sympathetic neurons for the gut are located in the thoracolumbar region of the spinal cord (Fig. 19.12). Their axons pass through the sympathetic trunks without relay. They travel through the splanchnic nerves to terminate in plexuses (and ganglia) related to the coeliac artery, the superior mesenteric artery, the inferior mesenteric artery and the aorta itself. Postganglionic neurons are located in these plexuses. They travel along these blood vessels to reach the gut.

As a rule, parasympathetic nerves stimulate intestinal movement and inhibit the sphincters. They are secretomotor to the mucosal glands. Sympathetic fibres are distributed chiefly to blood vessels.

Afferent fibres travel both along sympathetic and parasympathetic pathways. Pain from most of the gastrointestinal tract travels along sympathetic nerves. However, pain from the pharynx and oesophagus is carried by the vagus, and that from the rectum and lower part of the pelvic colon by pelvic splanchnic nerves.

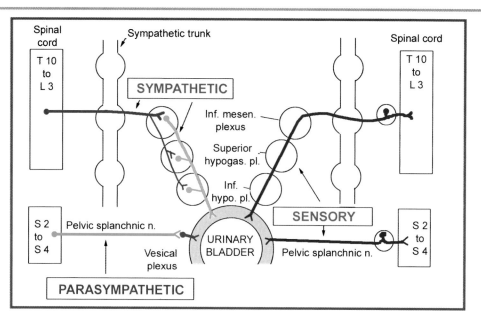

Fig. 19.13. Scheme to show the innervation of the urinary bladder.

Urinary Bladder

The parasympathetic nerves to the urinary bladder are derived from the sacral outflow. The preganglionic fibres pass through the pelvic splanchnic nerves and the inferior hypogastric plexuses to reach the vesical plexus. Parasympathetic postganglionic neurons are located in the vesical plexus. Parasympathetic stimulation is motor to the detrusor muscle and inhibitory to the sphincter.

Sympathetic preganglionic neurons are located in spinal segments T10 to L2. Their axons terminate in the inferior mesenteric, superior hypogastric, inferior hypogastric and vesical plexuses. Postganglionic neurons are located in these plexuses. According to classical teaching sympathetic stimulation has an effect opposite to that of the parasympathetic. However, some investigators believe that normal bladder function is controlled only by the parasympathetic nerves, and that sympathetic nerves are purely vasomotor in function.

Sensory fibres carry impulses of distension and of pain from the urinary bladder. They run through both sympathetic and parasympathetic pathways. In the spinal cord, fibres carrying the two types of sensation follow different routes. Fibres carrying pain are located in the anterior and lateral white columns while fibres carrying the sensation of bladder filling travel through the posterior column. As a result, intractable bladder pain (such as may occur because of carcinoma) can be relieved by cutting the anterior and lateral white columns of both sides (***bilateral anterolateral cordotomy***) without abolishing the sensation of bladder filling.

Severe lesions of the spinal cord above the sacral segments interfere with both afferent and efferent pathways. Normal micturition becomes impossible. However, the bladder empties reflexly when it is full (***automatic bladder***).

Ureter

Autonomic nerves to the ureter are predominantly sensory in function. They are derived mainly from segments T10 to L2 of the cord and also from segments S2 to S4. Distension by a stone causes severe pain (called ***renal colic***). This is referred to regions of skin innervated by segments T10 to L2. It, therefore, commences in the back over the lower ribs, and shoots downwards and forwards to the inguinal region, scrotum, and sometimes into the front of the thigh.

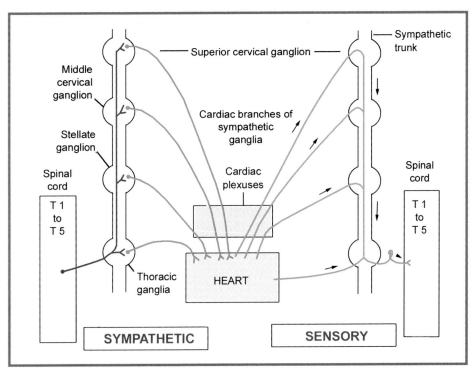

Fig. 19.14. Scheme to show the sympathetic innervation of the heart. Afferent fibres travelling along the sympathetic nerves are also shown.

Heart

Parasympathetic preganglionic neurons for the heart are located in the dorsal nucleus of the vagus. They reach the heart through cardiac branches of the vagus. The postganglionic neurons are located within the superficial and deep cardiac plexuses, and also in the walls of the atria. Their axons are distributed to the atria, the AV bundle, the SA node and the AV node.

Preganglionic sympathetic neurons are located in segments T1 to T5 of the spinal cord (Fig. 19.14). On reaching the sympathetic trunks their axons synapse with postganglionic neurons in the upper thoracic ganglia. Some fibres run upwards in the sympathetic trunk to end in cervical sympathetic ganglia. Postganglionic fibres leave these ganglia through their cardiac branches, and join the vagal fibres in forming the cardiac plexuses.

Contraction of cardiac muscle is not dependent on nerve supply. It can occur spontaneously. The nerves supplying the heart, however, influence heart rate.

Sympathetic stimulation increases heart rate and parasympathetic stimulation reduces it.

Sympathetic nerves supplying the coronary arteries cause vasodilatation increasing blood flow through them.

Afferent fibres from the heart travel through both sympathetic and parasympathetic pathways. Impulses of pain arising in the heart are carried mainly by the cardiac branches of the middle and inferior cervical sympathetic ganglia. Some fibres also pass through cardiac branches of thoracic sympathetic ganglia. These fibres pass through the sympathetic trunks and enter the spinal cord through spinal nerves T1 to T5. The cell bodies of the neurons concerned are located in the dorsal nerve root ganglia on these nerves. These pathways are important as they convey impulses of pain produced as a result of anoxia of heart muscle (*angina*). The pain is predominantly retrosternal, but it may be referred in various directions including the left shoulder and the inner side of the left arm. (Note that the inner side of the arm is supplied by segment T1). Afferent fibres running along the vagus are concerned with reflexes controlling the activity of the heart.

BASIC

CLINICAL

Bronchi

Parasympathetic preganglionic neurons, that supply the bronchi, are located in the dorsal vagal nucleus. The fibres travel through the vagus and its branches, to reach the anterior and posterior pulmonary plexuses. Postganglionic neurons are located near the roots of the lungs. Their axons run along the bronchi and supply them.

Preganglionic sympathetic neurons are located in the second to fifth thoracic segments of the spinal cord. Their axons terminate in the corresponding sympathetic ganglia. Postganglionic fibres arising in these ganglia reach the bronchi through branches from the sympathetic trunks to the pulmonary plexuses.

Parasympathetic stimulation causes bronchoconstriction, while sympathetic stimulation causes bronchodilatation. Parasympathetic stimulation also produces vasodilatation and has a secretomotor effect on glands in the bronchi. Sympathetic stimulation causes vasoconstriction.

Raynaud's disease (or phenomenon)

In all persons, exposure to cold can cause vasoconstriction. In some persons this response is abnormally high and vasoconstriction of arterioles in the distal part of the limb may seriously impair blood supply to the hands. In such cases a series of events may be observed. When the hand is cooled first there is a loss of colour (blanching) and the hand becomes pale. After an interval the arterioles dilate and blood starts flowing into the hand, but this blood is deoxygenated (because of stagnation in arteries). The hand becomes swollen and dark. As more blood flows into the hand the deoxygenated blood is washed off (with oxygenated blood) and the hand becomes red in colour.

Basically the condition is caused by abnormally active sympathetic nerves. It can be controlled with drugs. In more severe cases sympathetic denervation of blood vessels of the limb is necessary. This can be achieved by surgical removal of the upper thoracic sympathetic ganglia (preganglionic cervico-dorsal sympathectomy).

Thromboangitis obliterans (Buerger's disease)

In this condition arteries of the leg and foot are narrowed, and there is thrombophlebitis of veins. The condition is seen only in male smokers. Localized inflammatory changes are present in the walls of arteries and veins. Symptoms of arterial insufficiency are present. Gangrene of toes can occur. The condition can sometimes be controlled by complete abstinence from smoking, and may benefit from lumbar sympathectomy.

Some Recent Developments about the Autonomic Nervous System

In the preceding paragraphs the autonomic nervous system has been described in keeping with traditional teaching. Recent investigations have revealed many additional features of interest that are briefly considered below.

Enteric Nervous System

Although the presence of nerve plexuses in the wall of the gut, containing neuron somata in addition to nerve fibres, has been well known, their function has been obscure. Recent researches using immunochemical methods have revealed the presence of a large number of neuroactive substances in these plexuses. It has even been claimed that almost every neuroactive substance to be found in the CNS is also present in relation to the gut, suggesting much greater complexity of function of enteric plexuses than hitherto believed. The nerve plexuses of the gut are, therefore, now regarded as a third component of the autonomic nervous system (the other two components being sympathetic and parasympathetic) which is referred to as the enteric nervous system. Also see below.

Non-adrenergic, non-cholinergic neurons

The traditional concept of adrenergic (or noradrenergic) sympathetic postganglionic neurons, and cholinergic postganglionic parasympathetic neurons has been found to be simplistic for reasons discussed below.

Some autonomic neurons are neither adrenergic or cholinergic, and are described as "non-adrenergic, non-cholinergic" (NANC). The neuro-transmitter in these cells is probably ATP (adenosine triphosphate, which is a purine). Hence the neurons are sometimes referred to as purigenic.

Fig. 19.15. Classification of autonomic neurons of the basis of chemical coding

Neuron type	Neurotransmitters present	Neuromodulators present
Sympathetic	Naradrenalin ATP Neuropeptide Y	Enkephalin VIP Somatostatin Neuropeptide Y
Parasympathetic	Acetyl choline VIP ATP Nitrous oxide	Neuropeptide Y Dynorphins
Enteric NANC cells	ATP Nitrous oxide VIP	
Other enteric cells	Acetyl choline Substance P	
Sensory-motor cells	Substance P Chorionic gonadotropin releasing peptide ATP	VIP Dynorphins

Such fibres have been demonstrated in the gut wall, walls of blood vessels, urogenital tract, and also within the CNS. The neurons mainly terminate in relation to smooth muscle causing relaxation. They appear to be under control of sympathetic preganglionic neurons.

In addition to ATP numerous other neuroactive substances have been found in autonomic neurons. Some of them act as the main neurotransmitter, or as cotransmitters. (The concept of cotransmitters is based on the observation that one neuron may release more than one neurotransmitter at its endings.)

In addition to transmitters autonomic neurons may also contain neuromodulators. Autonomic neurons are classified into several types depending on their "chemical coding". Some examples are given in Fig. 19.15.

Sensorymotor neurons

It has been observed that many "afferent" autonomic neurons release neuroactive substances at their peripheral terminals. Such fibres are now referred to as sensory-motor neurons. The substances released are responsible for vasodilatation resulting from an axon reflex.

The neurotransmitters known to be released include substance P, ATP and chorionic gonadotropin releasing peptide (CGRP). Apart from vasodilatation the release of these substances can lead to alterations in contractility of smooth muscle. Effects on mast cells, leucocytes, and other cells are also described. Such nerves are believed to play an important role in the cardiovascular and gastrointestinal systems, and in the bronchial passages.

ADVANCED

BASIC

The interior of the brain contains a series of cavities (Fig. 20.1). The cerebrum contains a median cavity, the **third ventricle;** and two **lateral ventricles**, one in each hemisphere. Each lateral ventricle opens into the third ventricle through an **interventricular foramen**.

The third ventricle is continuous, caudally, with the **cerebral aqueduct** which traverses the midbrain and opens into the fourth ventricle.

The **fourth ventricle** is situated dorsal to the pons and medulla, and ventral to the cerebellum. It communicates, inferiorly, with the **central canal** which traverses the lower part of the medulla and the spinal cord. The entire ventricular system is lined by an epithelial layer called the **ependyma.**

The Lateral Ventricles

The lateral ventricles are two cavities, one situated within each cerebral hemisphere. Each ventricle consists of a central part which gives off three extensions called the anterior, posterior and inferior horns (Fig. 20.1).

The Central Part

The central part of the lateral ventricle is elongated anteroposteriorly. Anteriorly, it becomes continuous with the anterior horn, at the level of the interventricular foramen. Posteriorly, the central part reaches the splenium of the corpus callosum.

The central part is triangular in cross section (Fig. 20.2). It has a roof, a floor, and a medial wall. The roof and floor meet on the lateral side. The **roof** is formed by the trunk of the corpus callosum. The **medial wall** is formed by the septum pellucidum and by the body of the fornix. It is common to the two lateral ventricles. The **floor** is formed mainly by the superior surface of the thalamus (medially), and by the caudate nucleus (laterally). Between these two structures there are the stria terminalis (laterally) and the thalamostriate vein (medially). From Fig. 20.2 it will be seen that there is a space between the fornix and the upper surface of the thalamus. This is the **choroid fissure.**

A fold of pia mater, the **tela choroidea**, invaginates into the ventricle through the fissure and covers part of the thalamus. The tela choroidea is common to the two lateral ventricles, and to the third ventricle. Within each lateral edge of the tela choroidea there are plexuses of blood vessels that constitute the **choroid plexus** (Figs. 20.2, 20.7). The tela choroidea and other structures forming the walls of the ventricle are lined by ependyma.

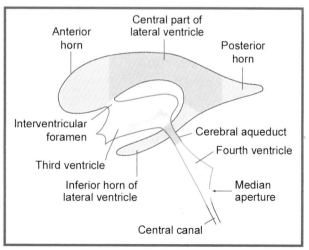

Fig. 20.1. The ventricular system of the brain seen from the lateral side.

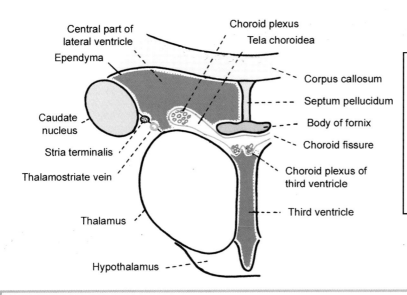

Fig. 20.2. Boundaries of the central part of the lateral ventricle and of the third ventricle. Note the relationship of the tela choroidea and the choroid plexuses to these ventricles.

The Anterior Horn

The anterior horn of the lateral ventricle, lies anterior to its central part, the two being separated by an imaginary vertical line drawn at the level of the interventricular foramen (Fig. 20.1). This horn is triangular in section. It has a roof, a floor and a medial wall (Fig. 20.3). It is closed, anteriorly, by the genu and rostrum of the corpus callosum.

The **roof** is formed by the most anterior part of the trunk of the corpus callosum. The floor is formed mainly by the head of the caudate nucleus. A small part of the floor, near the middle line, is formed by the upper surface of the rostrum of the corpus callosum. The **medial wall** (common to the two sides) is formed by the septum pellucidum. It may be noted that the tela choroidea and the choroid plexus **do not** extend into the anterior horn.

The Posterior Horn

The posterior horn of the lateral ventricle extends backwards into the occipital lobe. It has a roof, a lateral wall, and a medial wall (Fig. 20.4).

The **roof** and **lateral wall** are formed by the tapetum (page 93). The **medial wall** shows two elevations. The upper of these is the **bulb of the posterior horn**, which is produced by fibres of the

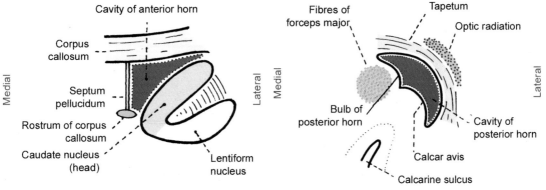

Fig. 20.3. Boundaries of the anterior horn of the lateral ventricle.

Fig. 20.4. Boundaries of the posterior horn of the lateral ventricle.

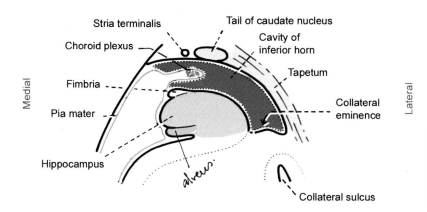

Stria terminalis
Tail of caudate nucleus
Choroid plexus
Cavity of inferior horn
Fimbria
Tapetum
Pia mater
Collateral eminence
Hippocampus
Medial
Lateral
alveus
Collateral sulcus

Fig. 20.5. Boundaries of the inferior horn of the lateral ventricle.

forceps major as they run backwards from the splenium of the corpus callosum. The lower elevation is called the ***calcar avis***. It represents white matter 'pushed in' by formation of the calcarine sulcus.

The Inferior Horn

The inferior horn of the lateral ventricle begins at the posterior end of the central part. It runs downwards and forwards into the temporal lobe, its anterior end reaching close to the uncus.

In considering the structures to be seen in the walls of the inferior horn it is useful to note that the anterior horn, the central part, and the inferior horn form one continuous C-shaped cavity. From Fig. 20.1 it will be obvious that the floor of the central part of the ventricle is continuous with the roof of

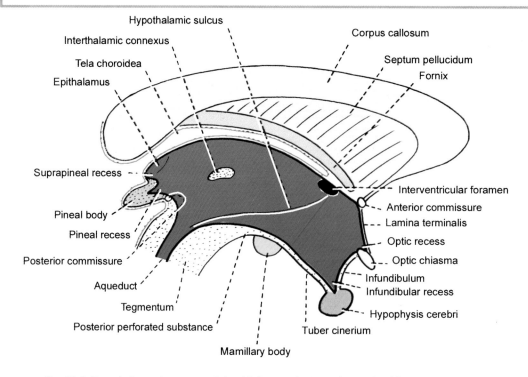

Hypothalamic sulcus
Interthalamic connexus
Corpus callosum
Tela choroidea
Septum pellucidum
Epithalamus
Fornix
Suprapineal recess
Interventricular foramen
Anterior commissure
Pineal body
Lamina terminalis
Pineal recess
Optic recess
Posterior commissure
Optic chiasma
Aqueduct
Infundibulum
Infundibular recess
Tegmentum
Hypophysis cerebri
Posterior perforated substance
Tuber cinerium
Mamillary body

Fig. 20.6. Boundaries and recesses of the third ventricle. Note the mode of formation of the tela choroidea that lies in the roof of the ventricle.

the inferior horn. It is also useful to recall that the body of the fornix divides, posteriorly, into two crura which become continuous with the fimbria and hippocampus.

In the central part of the ventricle, the choroid fissure lies below the fornix. When traced into the inferior horn, the fissure lies *above* the fimbria and hippocampus. The choroid plexus extends into the inferior horn through the choroid fissure.

In cross section, the inferior horn is seen to have a narrow cavity (Fig. 20.5). The cavity is bounded above, and laterally, by the *roof;* and below, and medially, by the *floor.* (Because of this orientation the lateral part of the roof is sometimes called the *lateral wall,* and the medial part of the floor is called the *medial wall.*)

The lateral part of the roof (or lateral wall) is formed by fibres of the tapetum. The medial part of the roof is formed by the tail of the caudate nucleus (laterally) and the stria terminalis (medially). These structures are continued into the roof of the inferior horn from the floor of the central part. Anteriorly, the tail of the caudate nucleus and the stria terminalis end in relation to the amygdaloid complex, which lies in the most anterior part of the roof.

The floor of the inferior horn is formed mainly by the hippocampus, along with the alveus and fimbria (page 236). In the lateral part of the floor there is an elevation, the *collateral eminence*, produced by inward bulging of the white matter which lies deep to the collateral sulcus.

The Third Ventricle

The third ventricle is the cavity of the diencephalon. It is a median cavity situated between the right and left thalami (Fig. 20.2). It communicates, on either side, with the lateral ventricle through the interventricular foramen (Figs. 20.1, 20.6). Posteriorly, it continues into the cerebral aqueduct which connects it to the fourth ventricle. The ventricle has two lateral walls, an anterior wall, a posterior wall, a floor and a roof.

Each *lateral wall* is marked by the *hypothalamic sulcus* (Fig. 20.6) which follows a curved course from the interventricular foramen to the aqueduct. Above the sulcus, the wall is formed by the medial surface of the thalamus. The two thalami are usually connected by a band of grey matter called the *interthalamic connexus,* which passes through the ventricle. The lateral wall, below the hypothalamic sulcus, is formed by the medial surface of the hypothalamus. A small part of the lateral wall, above and behind the thalamus, is formed by the epithalamus. The interventricular foramen is seen on the lateral wall, just behind the column of the fornix.

The *anterior wall* of the third ventricle is formed mainly by the lamina terminalis. Its upper part is formed by the anterior commissure, and by the columns of the fornix as they diverge from each other.

The *posterior wall* is formed by the pineal body and the posterior commissure.

The *floor* is formed by the optic chiasma, the tuber cinereum and the infundibulum, the mamillary bodies, the posterior perforated substance and the tegmentum of the midbrain.

The *roof* of the ventricle is formed by the ependyma that stretches across the two thalami (Fig. 20.2). Above the ependyma there is the tela choroidea. Within the tela choroidea there are two plexuses of blood vessels (one on either side of the middle line) which bulge downwards into the cavity of the third ventricle. These are the choroid plexuses of the third ventricle (See below) (Fig. 20.7).

The cavity of the third ventricle shows a number of prolongations or recesses (Fig. 20.6). The *infundibular recess* extends into the infundibulum. The *optic recess* lies just above the optic chiasma. The **pineal recess** lies between the superior and inferior laminae of the stalk of the pineal body. The **suprapineal recess** lies above the pineal body in relation to the epithalamus.

Tela Choroidea of the third and lateral ventricles

The tela choroidea is a double layered fold of pia mater that occupies the interval between the splenium of the corpus callosum and fornix, above, and the two thalami below. It is triangular in shape (Fig. 20.7). Its posterior end is broad and lies in the gap between the splenium (above) and the posterior part of the roof of the third ventricle (below) (Fig. 20.6). This gap is called the **transverse fissure**. The anterior end (representing the

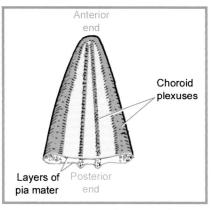

Fig. 20.7. Tela choroidea removed and viewed from above (schematic)

apex of the triangle) lies near the right and left interventricular foramina. The median part of the tela choroidea lies on the roof of the third ventricle. Its right and left lateral edges project into the central parts of the corresponding lateral ventricles (Fig. 20.2). When traced posteriorly, the two layers of pia mater forming the tela choroidea separate. The upper layer curves upwards over the posterior aspect of the splenium. The lower layer turns downwards over the pineal body and tectum (Fig. 20.6).

Choroid Plexuses

The choroid plexuses are highly vascular structures that are responsible for the formation of cerebrospinal fluid. The surface of each plexus is lined by a membrane formed by fusion of the ventricular ependyma with the pia mater of the tela choroidea. Deep to this membrane there is a plexus of blood vessels. Microscopic examination shows that the surface of the choroid plexus has numerous villous processes. Each process contains a plexus of capillaries that are connected to afferent and efferent vessels. Because of the presence of these processes the surface area of the

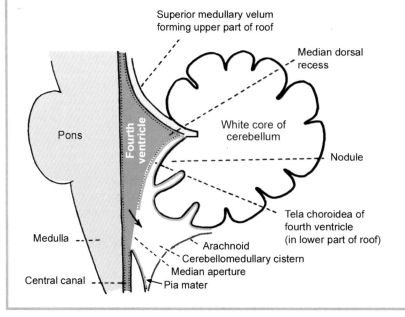

Fig. 20.8. Mid-sagittal section through the fourth ventricle and related structures. Note how the tela choroidea is formed.

choroid plexuses is considerable. It is further increased by the presence of microvilli (seen with the EM) present on the ependymal cells.

Four choroid plexuses are to be seen in relation to the tela choroidea of the third and lateral ventricles (Fig. 20.7). Two of these (one right and one left) lie along the corresponding lateral margins, and project into the central part of the corresponding lateral ventricle. Two other plexuses run parallel to each other, one on either side of the middle line. These are the choroid plexuses of the third ventricle. At each posterolateral angle of the tela choroidea the choroid plexus of the lateral ventricle continues into the inferior horn. The pial covering for this part of the plexus is provided by simple invagination of the pia, covering the medial aspect of the hemisphere, through the inferior part of the choroid fissure.

The tela choroidea and choroid plexuses of the fourth ventricle are considered on page 274.

The Fourth Ventricle

For a proper understanding of the anatomy of the fourth ventricle, it is necessary that some features of the gross anatomy of the cerebellum and of related structures be clearly understood. Reference to Fig. 20.8 will show that the cerebellum is intimately related to the ventricle. The upper part of the ventricle is related to the *superior (or anterior) medullary velum.* When traced inferiorly (and posteriorly) the velum merges into the white matter of the cerebellum. The lower part of the ventricle is related to the nodule (Figs. 20.8, 20.9A). It will be recalled that the nodule forms the anterior-most part of the inferior vermis. Immediately lateral to the nodule there is the tonsil of the cerebellum. If the tonsil is lifted away, we see that the nodule is continuous laterally with a membrane called the *inferior (or posterior) medullary velum* (Fig. 20.9B). Posteriorly, the inferior velum merges into the white matter of the cerebellum. This is seen in Fig. 20.10 which is a sagittal section along the axis XY shown in Fig. 20.9B. The inferior medullary velum has a thickened free edge which connects the nodule to the flocculus. This edge is the peduncle of the flocculus. In the intact brain, this peduncle is very near the posterior surface of the medulla, and is separated from the inferior cerebellar peduncle only by a narrow interval. With these facts clearly recorded we may now consider the anatomy of the fourth ventricle.

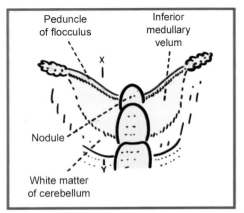

Fig. 20.9B. Similar view as in Fig. 20.9A after removal of the tonsil. This brings the inferior medullary velum into view. Note the peduncle of the flocculus connecting the nodule to the flocculus.

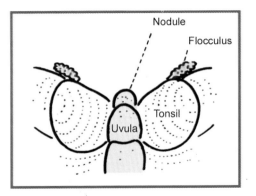

Fig. 20.9A. Part of the inferior aspect of the cerebellum showing the nodule and some related structures.

Fig. 20.10. Parasagittal section through the fourth ventricle a little lateral to the nodule (along axis XY of Fig. 20.9B) to show the relationship of the inferior medullary velum to the roof of the ventricle. Note that the lateral dorsal recess lies just superior to the velum.

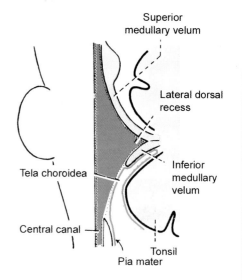

The fourth ventricle is a space situated dorsal to the pons and to the upper part of the medulla; and ventral to the cerebellum.

For descriptive purposes the ventricle may be considered as having a cavity, a floor, a roof and lateral walls.

The Cavity

The cavity of the ventricle is continuous, inferiorly, with the central canal; and, superiorly, with the cerebral aqueduct. It communicates with the subarachnoid space through three apertures, one median and two lateral (Figs 20.8, 20.13A). A number of extensions from the main cavity are described (Fig. 20.11). The largest of these are two *lateral recesses,* one on either side. Each ·lateral recess passes laterally in the interval between the inferior cerebellar peduncle (ventrally), and the peduncle of the flocculus (dorsally) (Fig. 20.13A). The lateral extremity of the recess reaches the flocculus. At this extremity, the recess opens into the subarachnoid space as the *lateral aperture.*

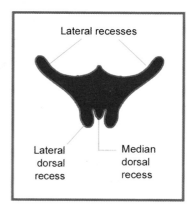

Fig. 20.11. Scheme of the cavity of the fourth ventricle to show the various recesses.

Another recess present in the middle line, is called the *median dorsal recess.* It extends into the white core of the cerebellum and lies just cranial to the nodule (Figs 20.8, 20.11). Immediately lateral to the nodule, another recess projects dorsally, on either side, above the inferior medullary velum. This is the *lateral dorsal recess* (Figs. 20.10, 20.11).

The Floor

Because of its shape, the floor of the fourth ventricle is often called the *rhomboid fossa* (Fig.20.12). It is divisible into an upper triangular part formed by the posterior surface of the pons; a lower triangular part formed by the upper part of the posterior surface of the medulla; and an intermediate part at the junction of the medulla and pons. The intermediate part is prolonged laterally over the inferior cerebellar peduncle as the floor of the lateral recess. Its surface is marked by the presence of delicate bundles of transversely running fibres. These bundles are the *striae medullares.*

The entire floor is divided into right and left halves by a *median sulcus.* Next to the middle line there is a longitudinal elevation called the *median eminence*. The eminence is bounded laterally by

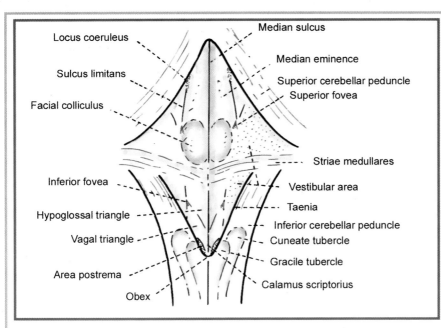

Fig. 20.12. Structures in the floor of the fourth ventricle.

BASIC

the **sulcus limitans.** The region lateral to the sulcus limitans is the **vestibular area** which overlies the vestibular nuclei. The vestibular area lies partly in the pons and partly in the medulla.

The pontine part of the floor shows some features of interest in close relation to the sulcus limitans and the median eminence. The upper-most part of the sulcus limitans overlies an area that is bluish in colour and is called the **locus coeruleus**. (Deep to the locus coeruleus there is the nucleus coeruleus which extends upwards into the tegmentum of the midbrain. It is regarded as part of the reticular formation).

Somewhat lower down, the sulcus limitans is marked by a depression, the **superior fovea.** At this level the median eminence shows a swelling, the **facial colliculus** (page 144).

The medullary part of the floor also shows some features of interest in relation to the median eminence and the sulcus limitans. The sulcus limitans is marked by a depression, the **inferior fovea.** Descending from the fovea, there is a sulcus that runs obliquely towards the middle line. This sulcus divides the median eminence into two triangles. These are the **hypoglossal triangle**, medially; and the **vagal triangle,** laterally. Between the vagal triangle (above) and the gracile tubercle (below), there is a small area called the **area postrema.** Finally, mention must be made of two terms often used in relation to the medulla. The lowest part of the floor of the fourth ventricle is called the **calamus scriptorius,** because of its resemblance to a nib. Each inferolateral margin of the ventricle is marked by a narrow white ridge or **taenia.** The right and left taeniae meet at the inferior angle of the floor to form a small fold called the **obex.** The term obex is often used to denote the inferior angle itself.

The Lateral Walls

The upper part of each lateral wall is formed by the superior cerebellar peduncle (Fig. 20.13B). The lower part is formed by the inferior cerebellar peduncle, and by the gracile and cuneate tubercles (Fig. 20.13C,D).

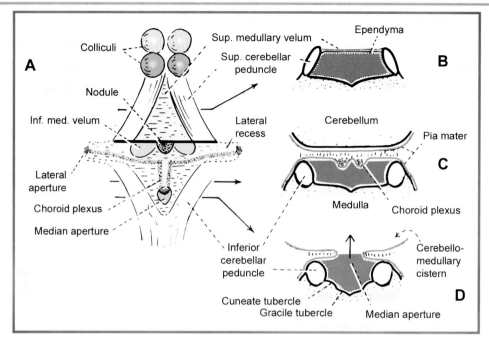

Fig. 20.13. Schemes to illustrate the formation of the roof of the fourth ventricle. The bold horizontal line in 'A' represents the white core of the cerebellum. The part above this line represents the upper part of the roof, and the part below the line represents the lower part of the roof. B, C and D represent transverse sections across the ventricle at the levels indicated.

The Roof

The roof of the fourth ventricle is tent-shaped and can be divided into upper and lower parts which meet at an apex (Figs. 20.8, 20.13A). The apex extends into the white core of the cerebellum. The upper part of the roof is formed by the superior cerebellar peduncles and the superior medullary velum (Figs. 20.13A,B). The inferior part of the roof is devoid of nervous tissue in most of its extent. It is formed by a membrane consisting of ependyma and a double fold of pia mater which constitutes the **tela choroidea of the fourth ventricle** (Fig. 20.13 A,C). Laterally, on each side, this membrane reaches and fuses with the inferior cerebellar peduncles. The lower part of the membrane has a large aperture in it. This is the **median aperture** of the fourth ventricle through which the ventricle communicates with the subarachnoid space in the region of the cerebellomedullary cistern. In the region of the lateral recess, the membrane is prolonged laterally and helps to form the wall of the recess. The inferior medullary velum forms a small part of the roof in the region of the lateral dorsal recess (Fig. 20.10). It may be noted that some authors describe the entire membranous structure, forming the lower part of the roof of the fourth ventricle, as the inferior medullary velum. The nodule is intimately related to the roof of the ventricle in the region of the median dorsal recess.

Tela Choroidea and Choroid Plexuses of the Fourth Ventricle

As stated above the **tela choroidea of the fourth ventricle** is made up of two layers of pia mater. The superior (or dorsal) layer lines the inferior vermis. On reaching the nodule (and more laterally, the inferior medullary velum), it is reflected on itself to form the inferior (or ventral) layer (Fig. 20.8). When traced laterally the dorsal layer is continuous with the pia mater covering the cerebellar hemispheres, while the ventral layer is continuous with the pia mater lining the medulla (Fig. 20.13C).

The **choroid plexuses of the fourth ventricle** are similar in structure to those of the lateral and third ventricles. They lie within the folds of pia mater that form the tela choroidea, and project into the cavity of the ventricle from the lower part of the roof (Fig. 20.13C). Each plexus (right or left) consists of a vertical limb lying next to the midline, and a horizontal limb extending into the lateral recess. The vertical limbs of the two plexuses lie side by side so that the whole structure is T-shaped. The lower ends of the vertical limbs reach the median aperture and project into the subarachnoid space through it. The lateral ends of the horizontal limbs reach the lateral apertures, and can be seen on the surface of the brain, near the flocculus.

BASIC

1. The **area postrema** is believed to be the site of the vomiting centre.
2. **Tumours** (medulloblastomas) are common near the roof of the fourth ventricle.
3. In **Arnold Chiari deformity** (mentioned on page 94) the medulla and the tonsils of the cerebellum come to lie in the vertebral canal. Apertures in the roof of the fourth ventricle are blocked leading to obstruction to flow of CSF and internal hydrocephalus. Cranial nerves arising from the medulla are stretched. This is a congenital anomaly. It is often associated with syringomyelia.

CLINICAL

The Cerebrospinal Fluid

The cerebrospinal fluid (CSF) fills the subarachnoid space. It also extends into the ventricles of the brain, and into the central canal of the spinal cord. It is formed by the choroid plexuses of the ventricles. The CSF formed in each lateral ventricle flows into the third ventricle through the interventricular foramen. From the third ventricle it passes through the aqueduct into the fourth ventricle. Here it passes through the median and lateral apertures in the roof of this ventricle to enter the part of the subarachnoid space which forms the cerebellomedullary cistern. From here the fluid enters other parts of the subarachnoid space. In passing from the posterior cranial fossa into the upper (supratentorial) part of the cranial cavity the CSF traverses the narrow interval between the free margin of the tentorium cerebelli and the brainstem. It leaves the subarachnoid space by entering the venous sinuses through arachnoid villi.

The CSF provides a fluid cushion which protects the brain from injury. It probably also helps to carry nutrition to the brain, and to remove waste products.

Samples of CSF are often required for help in clinical diagnosis. They are obtained most easily by **lumbar puncture** (page 276). In this procedure a needle is introduced into the subarachnoid space through the interval between the third and fourth lumbar vertebrae. Under exceptional circumstances CSF may be obtained by **cisternal puncture** in which a needle is passed into the cerebellomedullary cistern.

The total volume of CSF is about 140ml of which about 25ml is in the ventricles. The CSF is constantly replaced.

The CSF consists of water in which are present sodium chloride, potassium, glucose and proteins. The proportions of these substances differ considerably in blood and CSF and hence it is believed that CSF is formed by an active secretory process, and not by passive filtration. The epithelium and other tissues of the choroid plexuses form an effective barrier between the blood and the CSF. This blood - CSF barrier allows selective passage of substances from blood to CSF, but not in the reverse direction. The arachnoid villi provide a valvular mechanism for flow of CSF into blood without permitting back-flow of blood into the CSF.

ADVANCED

CLINICAL

Hydrocephalus

An abnormal increase in the quantity of CSF can lead to enlargement of the head in children. This condition is called **hydrocephalus.** Abnormal pressure of CSF leads to degeneration of brain tissue. Hydrocephalus may be caused by excessive production of CSF, by obstruction to its flow, or by impaired absorption through the arachnoid villi. It is classified as **obstructive** when there is obstruction to flow of CSF from the ventricular system to the subarachnoid space; or as **communicating** when such obstruction is not present. Obstruction is most likely to occur where CSF has to pass through narrow passages e.g., the interventricular foramina, the aqueduct, and the apertures of the fourth ventricle. In each of the above instances dilatation is confined to cavities proximal to the obstruction. Occasionally, meningitis may lead to obstruction of the narrow interval between the tentorium cerebelli and the brainstem. Meningitis may also lead to hydrocephalus by affecting the arachnoid villi, thus hampering the reabsorption of CSF. Also see Arnold Chiari malformation (page 275).

CSF and Injuries to the Skull

The skull is frequently injured by blows with a heavy object, and frequently in automobile accidents. Injury can be avoided by wearing a protective helmet.

1. Direct injury leading to fractures of the skull can damage any area of the brain. CSF can flow out and parts of brain can herniate out of the skull.

2. Even in the absence of a fracture direct injury can throw the brain against the opposite wall of the skull injuring it. This is contracoup injury.

In fractures of the base of the skull CSF may flow into the nose. Haemorrhage may take place into brain tissue, or into extradural space raising intracranial tension.

Lumbar Puncture

We have seen that a needle can be introduced into the subarachnoid space through the interval between the third and fourth lumbar vertebrae. This procedure, called lumbar puncture, is useful for several purposes.

(**a**) The pressure of CSF can be estimated, roughly, by counting the rate at which drops flow out of the needle; or more accurately, by connecting the needle to a manometer.

(**b**) Samples of CSF can be collected for examination. The important points to note about CSF are its colour, its cellular content, and its chemical composition (specially the protein and sugar content).

(**c**) Lumbar puncture may be used for introducing air or radio-opaque dyes into the subarachnoid space for certain investigative procedures. Drugs may also be injected for treatment.

(**d**) Mention may be made here of a use of lumbar puncture, not related to neurological diagnosis. Anaesthetic drugs injected into the subarachnoid space act on the lower spinal nerve roots and render the lower part of the body insensitive to pain. This procedure, called **spinal anaesthesia**, is frequently used for operations on the lower abdomen or on the lower extremities.

ADVANCED

Tanycytes & specialised areas of ependyma

At some isolated sites in the walls of the third and fourth ventricles, there are patches of ependyma where the ependymal cells are tall, columnar, and ciliated, and possess special histochemical properties. These cells are called **tanycytes**. Some areas where these patches are found (in the human brain) are as follows.

(**a**) The **subcommissural organ** is located over the dorsal wall of the aqueduct, just behind the posterior commissure.

(**b**) The **subfornical organ** is present in relation to the roof of the third ventricle, just below the body of the fornix.

(**c**) The **intercolumnar tubercle** or the **organ vasculosum** is present in relation to the anterior wall of the third ventricle (in the region where the columns of the fornix diverge).

ADVANCED

(**d**) In the floor of the fourth ventricle, the hypoglossal triangle is separated from the area postrema by a narrow ridge called the ***funiculus separans***. This ridge, and the area postrema, are lined by tanycytes.

Similar areas have been identified at various other sites in other species.

The functions attributed to tanycytes are:

(**a**) Secretion of neurochemical substances into CSF.

(**b**) Secretion of CSF itself.

(**c**) Transport of substances from CSF to underlying neurons or blood vessels.

(**d**) They may also act as chemoreceptors.

Ventriculography

CLINICAL

The ventricles of the brain can be studied in living subjects by taking radiographs after injecting a radio-opaque dye into the ventricular system. The procedure is called ventriculography. Parts of the ventricles can also be seen using CT scans and magnetic resonanace imaging.

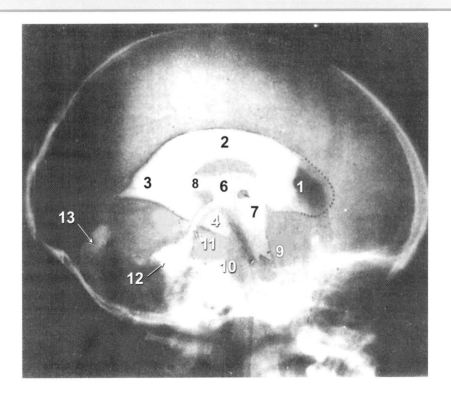

Fig. 20.14. Ventriculogram. Lateral view. A radiograph of the head was taken after injecting a radio-opaque dye into the ventricular system. The parts of the lateral ventricle seen are (1) anterior horn (part of which appears dark as air has entered it during injection); (2) central part; (3) posterior horn; (4) inferior horn. In relation to the third ventricle (6) we can identify the suprapineal recess (8), the optic recess (9) and the infundibular recess (10). The interthalamic connexus is seen as a dark area (7). Other structures seen are the aqueduct (11), and the fourth ventricle (12). Some dye that has reached the cisterna magna through the apertures of the fourth ventricle is also seen (13).

This figure is reproduced by kind courtesy of Prof. S.C. Srivastava

21 : Blood Supply of Central Nervous System

The nervous system is richly supplied with blood. Interruption of blood supply even for a short period can result in damage to nervous tissue. Traditionally it has been taught that lymphatics are not present in nervous tissue, but some workers have recently challenged this view.

Blood Supply of the Spinal Cord

The spinal cord receives its blood supply from three longitudinal arterial channels that extend along the length of the spinal cord (Fig. 21.1). The **anterior spinal artery** is present in relation to the anterior median fissure. Two **posterior spinal arteries** (one on each side) run along the posterolateral sulcus (i.e., along the line of attachment of the dorsal nerve roots). In addition to these channels the pia mater covering the spinal cord has an arterial plexus (called the **arterial vasocorona**) which also sends branches into the substance of the cord.

The main source of blood to the spinal arteries is from the vertebral arteries (from which the anterior and posterior spinal arteries take origin). However, the blood from the vertebral arteries reaches only up to the cervical segments of the cord. Lower down the spinal arteries receive blood through radicular arteries that reach the cord along the roots of spinal nerves. These radicular arteries arise from spinal branches of the vertebral, ascending cervical, deep cervical, intercostal, lumbar and sacral arteries (Fig. 21.2).

Many of these radicular arteries are small and end by supplying the nerve roots. A few of them, which are larger, join the spinal arteries and contribute blood to them. Frequently, one of the anterior radicular branches is very large and is called the **arteria radicularis magna**. Its position is variable. This artery may be responsible for supplying blood to as much as the lower two-thirds of the spinal cord.

The greater part of the cross sectional area of the spinal cord is supplied by branches of the anterior spinal artery (Fig. 21.1, left half). These branches enter the anterior median fissure (or sulcus) and are, therefore, called **sulcal branches.** Alternate sulcal branches pass to the right and left sides. They supply the anterior and lateral grey columns and the central grey matter. They also

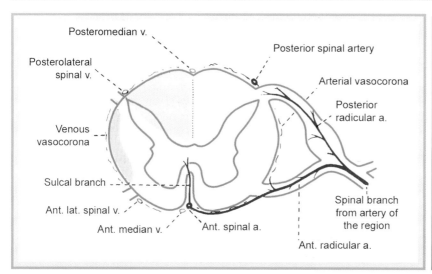

Posteromedian v.

Posterolateral spinal v.

Venous vasocorona

Sulcal branch

Ant. lat. spinal v.

Ant. median v.

Ant. spinal a.

Posterior spinal artery

Arterial vasocorona

Posterior radicular a.

Spinal branch from artery of the region

Ant. radicular a.

Fig. 21.1. Blood vessels supplying the spinal cord. In the left half of the figure the area showing green shading is supplied by the posterior spinal artery. The part showing pink shading is supplied by the arterial vasocorona, and the area with yellow shading is supplied by the anterior spinal artery.

supply the anterior and lateral funiculi. The rest of the spinal cord is supplied by the posterior spinal arteries. As already mentioned branches from the arterial vasocorona also supply the cord.

The veins draining the spinal cord are arranged in the form of six longitudinal channels. These are **anteromedian** and **posteromedian** channels that lie in the midline; and **anterolateral** and **posterolateral** channels that are paired (Fig. 21.1). These channels are interconnected by a plexus of veins that form a **venous vasocorona.** The blood from these veins is drained into radicular veins that open into a venous plexus lying between the dura mater and the bony vertebral canal (**epidural** or **internal vertebral venous plexus**) and through it into various segmental veins.

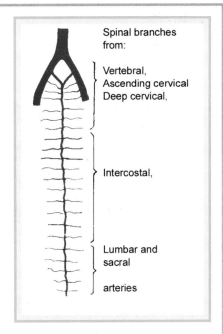

Fig. 21.2. Radicular arteries that contribute blood to the spinal arteries.

Thrombosis in the anterior spinal artery produces a characteristic syndrome. The territory of supply includes the corticospinal tracts. This leads to an upper motor neuron paralysis below the level of lesion. The spinothalamic tracts are also involved. This leads to loss of sensations of pain and temperature below the level of lesion. Touch and conscious proprioceptive sensations are not affected as the posterior column tracts are not involved. The extent of damage varies depending on the efficiency of anastomoses in the region.

Arteries Supplying the Brain

The brain is supplied by branches of the **internal carotid** and the **vertebral** arteries (Figs. 21.3, 21.4). Each internal carotid artery gives off two major branches to the brain. These are the **anterior cerebral** and **middle cerebral** arteries.

The two vertebral arteries ascend on the anterolateral aspect of the medulla. At the lower border of the pons they unite to form the **basilar** artery.

The basilar artery lies in the midline, ventral to the pons. At the upper border of the pons it bifurcates into two **posterior cerebral** arteries. The internal carotid and vertebro-basilar systems are connected by the **posterior communicating** arteries. The two anterior cerebral arteries are connected by the **anterior communicating** artery. As a result of these anastomoses an arterial ring, the **circulus**

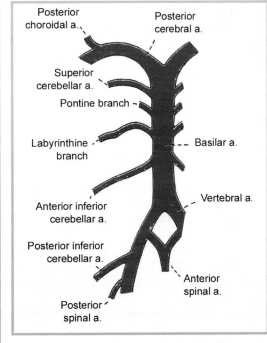

Fig. 21.3. Branches of the vertebral and basilar arteries.

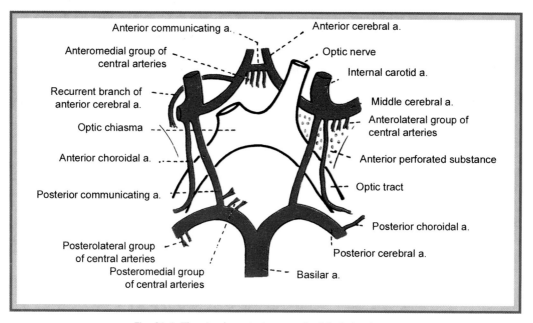

Fig. 21.4. The circulus arteriosus and related structures.

arteriosus (or circle of Willis) is formed in relation to the base of the brain (Fig. 21.4).

In addition to the larger arteries mentioned above, two smaller branches of the internal carotid system must be noted. One of these is the ***anterior choroidal*** artery which arises directly from the internal carotid, runs backwards in relation to the optic tract, and enters the inferior horn of the lateral ventricle through the choroid fissure. The other is the ***recurrent branch*** of the anterior cerebral artery (also called the ***artery of Heubner***). This artery runs backwards and laterally to enter the anterior perforated substance.

Thrombosis in the artery of Heubner results in contralateral paralysis of the face and upper extremity.

The anterior, middle and posterior cerebral arteries give rise to two sets of branches, cortical and central. The ***cortical branches*** ramify on the surface of the cerebral hemispheres and supply the cortex. The ***central*** (or ***perforating***) ***branches*** pass deep into the substance of the cerebral hemisphere to supply structures within it. They consist of six main groups: anteromedial and posteromedial (which are median and unpaired); right and left anterolateral; and right and left posterolateral (Fig. 21.4). The arteries of the ***anteromedial group*** arise from the anterior cerebral and anterior communicating arteries. They enter the most medial part of the anterior perforated substance. The arteries of the ***anterolateral group*** are the so-called ***striate arteries***. They arise mainly from the middle cerebral artery. Some of them arise from the anterior cerebral artery. The anterolateral group of perforating arteries enter the anterior perforated substance and divide into two sets, medial and lateral. The ***medial striate arteries*** ascend through the lentiform nucleus. They supply this nucleus and also the caudate nucleus and the internal capsule. The ***lateral striate arteries*** ascend lateral to the lower part of the lentiform nucleus; they then turn medially and pass through the substance of the lentiform nucleus to reach the internal capsule and the caudate nucleus. One of these lateral striate arteries is usually larger than the others. It is called ***Charcot's artery***, or ***artery of cerebral haemorrhage***. The ***posteromedial group*** of central arteries arise from the posterior cerebral and posterior communicating arteries. They enter the interpeduncular region. The central branches of the ***posterolateral group*** arise from the posterior cerebral artery, as it winds around the cerebral peduncle.

Each vertebral artery gives off *anterior* and *posterior spinal* arteries (that supply the medulla in addition to the spinal cord), and the *posterior inferior cerebellar* artery which supplies the medulla in addition to the cerebellum. The basilar artery gives off the *anterior inferior cerebellar* arteries, and the *superior cerebellar* arteries to the cerebellum, and numerous branches to the pons. We have already noted that the posterior cerebral arteries are the terminal branches of the basilar artery. In addition to central and cortical branches, the posterior cerebral artery gives off the *posterior choroidal* artery.

At this stage it may be noted that because of anastomoses between the major arteries supplying the brain, blood supply of the area supplied by one artery can be taken over by another artery in the event of it becoming blocked. This remark applies, however, only to the main arteries, and *not* to their smaller branches (see below).

Arterial Supply of the Cerebral Cortex

The cerebral cortex is supplied by cortical branches of the anterior, middle and posterior cerebral arteries.

Superolateral surface

The greater part of the superolateral surface is supplied by the middle cerebral artery (Fig. 21.5). The areas *not* supplied by this artery are as follows.

(**a**) A strip half to one inch wide along the superomedial border extending from the frontal pole to the parieto-occipital sulcus is supplied by the anterior cerebral artery.

(**b**) The area belonging to the occipital lobe is supplied by the posterior cerebral artery.

(**c**) The inferior temporal gyrus (excluding the part adjoining the temporal pole) is also supplied by the posterior cerebral artery.

Medial surface

The main artery supplying the medial surface is the anterior cerebral (Fig. 21.6). The area of this surface belonging to the occipital lobe is supplied by the posterior cerebral artery.

Inferior Surface

The lateral part of the *orbital surface* is supplied by the middle

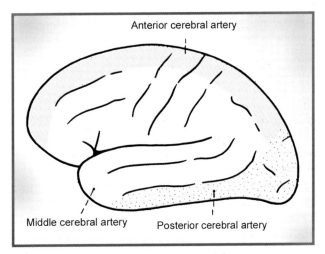

Fig. 21.5. Distribution of the anterior, posterior and middle cerebral arteries on the superolateral surface of the cerebral hemisphere.

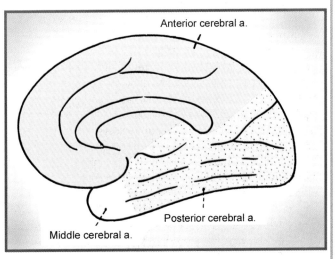

Fig. 21.6. Arteries supplying the medial surface of the cerebral hemisphere.

cerebral artery, and the medial part by the anterior cerebral artery (Fig. 21.7).

The **tentorial surface** is supplied by the posterior cerebral artery. The temporal pole is, however, supplied by the middle cerebral artery (Fig. 21.7).

Additional points of interest

From the description given above it will be clear that the main somatic motor and sensory areas are supplied by the middle cerebral artery except in their uppermost parts (leg areas) which are supplied by the anterior cerebral. The acoustic area is supplied by the middle cerebral artery, and the visual area by the posterior cerebral.

The part of the visual area responsible for macular vision lies in the region where the territories of supply of the middle and posterior cerebral arteries meet. It may receive a supply from the middle cerebral artery, either directly, or through anastomoses with branches of the posterior cerebral artery. This is one explanation for the observation that macular vision is often spared in cases of thrombosis of the posterior cerebral artery. The phenomenon can also be explained by the observation that dye injected into the carotid system (for angiographic studies) often passes into the posterior cerebral artery through the posterior communicating artery.

The cortical arteries give off branches that run perpendicularly into the substance of the cerebral hemisphere. Some of these are short and end within the grey matter of the cortex. Others are longer and penetrate into the subjacent white matter. While cortical branches may anastomose with each other on the surface of the brain, the perpendicular branches (both long and short) behave as terminal or end arteries. Each branch supplies a limited area of brain tissue, and does not anastomose with neighbouring arteries. As a result, blockage of such a branch leads to death (necrosis) of brain tissue in the region of supply.

Having studied the blood supply of the cerebral hemispheres we can now understand the effects of interruption of blood flow through major arteries.

1. **Thrombosis in the main stem of the anterior cerebral artery** (beyond the anterior communicating artery) leads to the following.

(a) Paralysis (or weakness) of muscles of the leg and foot of the opposite side (by involvement of the upper part of the motor area).

(b) Loss (or dulling) of sensations from the leg and foot of the opposite side (by involvement of the upper part of the sensory area).

(c) Sense of stereognosis is impaired (by involvement of parietal lobe).

(d) Personality changes (by involvement of frontal lobe).

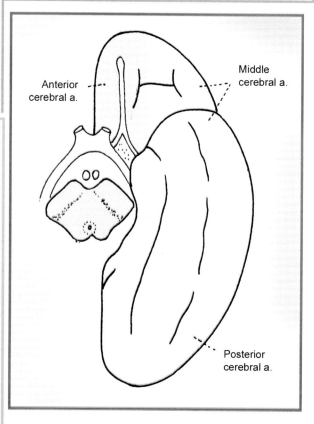

Fig. 21.7. Arteries supplying the orbital and tentorial surfaces of the cerebral hemisphere.

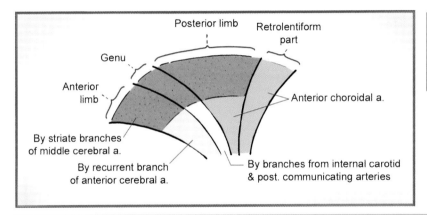

Fig. 21.8. Scheme to show the arterial supply of the internal capsule.

2. **Thrombosis in the main stem of the middle cerebral artery** leads to the following.

(a) Hemiplegia and loss of sensations on the opposite half of the body. The face and arms are most affected. Foot and leg are spared.

(b) Aphasia (by involvement of Broca's and Wernicke's areas), specially if the thrombosis is in the left hemisphere in a right handed person.

(c) Homonymous hemianopia on opposite side (by involvement of optic radiation).

(d) Hearing may be affected but this may be compensated by the opposite hemisphere.

3. **Thrombosis in the main stem of the posterior cerebral artery** leads mainly to visual effects. There is homonymous hemianopia on the opposite side. For reasons explained above, above the macular area is often spared.

Arteries Supplying the Interior of the Cerebral Hemisphere

Internal capsule

The main arteries supplying the internal capsule are the medial and lateral striate branches of the middle cerebral artery, the recurrent branch of the anterior cerebral, and the anterior choroidal artery. The internal capsule may also receive direct branches from the internal carotid artery, and branches from the posterior communicating artery (Fig. 21.8).

The **upper parts** of the anterior limb, the genu, and the posterior limb are supplied by striate branches of the middle cerebral artery. The **lower parts** of these regions are supplied as follows.

(**a**) The lower part of the anterior limb is supplied by the recurrent branch of the anterior cerebral artery.

(**b**) The lower part of the genu is supplied by direct branches from the internal carotid, and from the posterior communicating artery.

(**c**) The lower part of the posterior limb is supplied by the anterior choroidal artery.

The **retrolentiform part** of the internal capsule is supplied by the anterior choroidal artery. The **sublentiform part** is probably supplied by the anterior choroidal artery.

For some clinical correlations see pages 104 and 243.

Thalamus

The thalamus is supplied mainly by perforating branches of the posterior cerebral artery (Fig. 21.9). The posteromedial group of branches (also called **thalamo-perforating** arteries) supply the medial and anterior part. The posterolateral group (also called **thalamo-geniculate** branches) supply the posterior and lateral parts of the thalamus. The thalamus also receives some branches from the posterior communicating, anterior choroidal, posterior choroidal, and middle cerebral arteries.

Hypothalamus

The anterior part of the hypothalamus is supplied by central branches of the anteromedial group (arising from the anterior cerebral artery). The posterior part is supplied by central branches of the posteromedial group (arising from the posterior cerebral and posterior communicating arteries).

Corpus Striatum

The main arterial supply of the *caudate nucleus* and *putamen* is derived from the medial and lateral striate branches of the middle cerebral artery (Fig. 21.10). In addition, their anteriormost parts (including the head of the caudate nucleus) receive their blood supply through the recurrent branch of the anterior cerebral artery, and their posterior parts (including the tail of the caudate nucleus) through the anterior choroidal artery.

The main supply of the *globus pallidus* is from the anterior choroidal artery. Its lateral segment also receives blood through the striate arteries. The medialmost part of the globus pallidus receives branches from the posterior communicating artery.

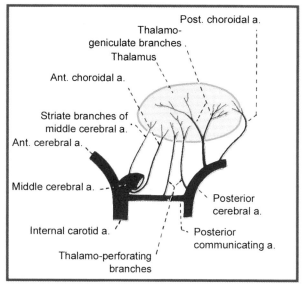

Fig. 21.9. Scheme to show the arteries supplying the thalamus.

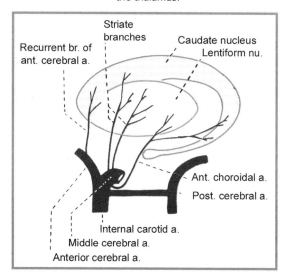

Fig. 21.10. Scheme to show the arteries supplying the corpus striatum.

Arterial Supply of the Brainstem

Medulla

The medulla is supplied by various branches of the vertebral arteries. These are the anterior and posterior spinal arteries, the posterior inferior cerebellar artery, and small direct branches (Fig. 21.11). The anterior spinal artery supplies a triangular area next to the midline. This area includes the pyramid, the medial lemniscus, and the hypoglossal nucleus. The posterior spinal artery supplies a small area including the gracile and cuneate nuclei. The posterior inferior cerebellar artery supplies the retro-olivary region. This region contains several important structures including the spinothalamic tracts, the rubrospinal tract, the nucleus ambiguus, the dorsal vagal nucleus, and descending autonomic

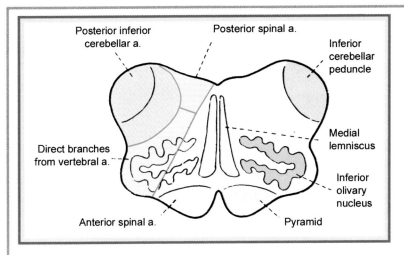

Posterior inferior cerebellar a.

Posterior spinal a.

Inferior cerebellar peduncle

Medial lemniscus

Direct branches from vertebral a.

Inferior olivary nucleus

Anterior spinal a.

Pyramid

Fig. 21.11. Cross section through the medulla to show the regions supplied by different arteries.

fibres. The posterior inferior cerebellar artery also supplies part of the inferior cerebellar peduncle. The rest of the medulla is supplied by direct bulbar branches of the vertebral arteries.

Thrombosis in an artery supplying the medulla produces symptoms depending upon the structures involved. Two characteristic syndromes are the *medial medullary syndrome* produced by thrombosis in the anterior spinal artery, and the *lateral medullary syndrome* produced by thrombosis in the posterior inferior cerebellar artery.

In the medial medullary syndrome the ventral and medial part of the medulla is damaged. Involvement of corticospinal fibres (pyramids) leads to contralateral hemiplegia. Damage to the hypoglossal nucleus leads to ipsilateral (lower motor neuron type of) paralysis of muscles of the tongue. Involvement of the medial lemniscus leads to loss of the sensation of fine touch, sense of movement and sense of position.

In the lateral medullary syndrome the structures damaged include the following.

(**1**) Damage to the lateral spinothalamic tract leads to contralateral loss of sensations of pain and temperature.

(**2**) Damage to the spinal nucleus and tract of the trigeminal nerve leads to loss of sensations of pain and temperature over the region supplied by the trigeminal nerve.

(**3**) Damage to the nucleus ambiguus leads to difficulty in swallowing (dysphagia) and in speech (dysarthria).

(**4**) Damage to the cerebellum and to the inferior cerebellar peduncle causes loss of equilibrium (ataxia) and giddiness.

(**4**) Involvement of descending autonomic fibres leads to Horner's syndrome (page 259).

Pons

The pons is supplied by branches from the basilar artery. The medial portion of the ventral part of the pons is supplied by *paramedian branches.* The lateral portion of the ventral part is supplied by *short circumferential branches.* The dorsal part of the pons is supplied by *long circumferential branches.* The dorsal part also receives branches from the anterior inferior cerebellar and superior cerebellar arteries. The paramedian branches of the basilar artery may extend into this region from the ventral part of the pons.

Pontine haemorrhage

Haemorrhage into the pons leads to coma (and is often fatal). The reticular formation, autonomic nervous system and the hypothalamus are affected. Apart from coma the condition is marked by pin point pupils and hyperpyrexia Bilateral facial paralysis and paralysis of all four limbs can occur if the haemorrhage is extensive.

Midbrain

The midbrain is supplied mainly by branches of the basilar artery. These are the posterior cerebral and superior cerebellar arteries and direct branches from the basilar artery. Branches are also received from the posterior communicating and anterior choroidal arteries. Branches arising from these vessels may either be ***paramedian,*** which supply parts near the midline; or ***circumferential*** which wind round the midbrain to supply lateral and dorsal parts. One of the latter arteries is called the ***quadrigeminal artery.*** It is the main source of blood to the colliculi.

Arteries Supplying the Cerebellum

The superior surface of the cerebellum is supplied by the ***superior cerebellar*** branches of the basilar artery. The anterior part of the inferior surface is supplied by the ***anterior inferior cerebellar*** branches of the same artery. The posterior part of the inferior surface is supplied by the ***posterior inferior cerebellar*** branch of the vertebral artery.

Venous Drainage of the Brain

The veins draining the brain open into the dural venous sinuses (Fig. 21.12). These are the superior sagittal, inferior sagittal, straight, transverse, sigmoid, cavernous, sphenoparietal, petrosal and occipital sinuses. Ultimately, the blood from all these sinuses reaches the sigmoid sinus which becomes continuous with the internal jugular vein. The intracranial venous sinuses communicate with veins outside the skull through emissary veins. For details about intracranial venous sinuses see the author's Textbook of Anatomy.

The venous drainage of individual parts of the brain is described below.

Veins of the Cerebral Hemisphere

The veins of the cerebral hemisphere consist of two sets, superficial and deep.

The superficial veins drain into neighbouring venous sinuses. The ***superior cerebral veins*** drain the upper parts of the superolateral and medial surfaces, and end in the superior sagittal sinus. Some veins from the medial surface join the inferior sagittal sinus. ***Inferior cerebral veins*** drain the lower part of the hemisphere. On the superolateral surface, they drain into the ***superficial middle cerebral vein*** which lies superficially along the lateral sulcus and its posterior ramus. The posterior end of this vein is connected to the superior sagittal sinus by the ***superior anastomotic vein***; and to the transverse sinus by the ***inferior anastomotic vein.*** The superficial middle cerebral vein terminates in the cavernous sinus. Veins from the inferior surface of the cerebral hemisphere drain into the transverse, superior petrosal, cavernous and sphenoparietal sinuses. Some may ascend to join the inferior sagittal sinus.

The deep veins of the cerebral hemisphere are the two ***internal cerebral veins***, that join to form the ***great cerebral vein*** (Fig. 21.13); and the two ***basal veins,*** that wind round the midbrain to end in the great cerebral vein. Each internal cerebral vein begins at the interventricular foramen, and

BASIC

runs backwards in the tela choroidea, in the roof of the third ventricle. It has numerous tributaries. One of these is the **thalamostriate vein** which lies in the floor of the lateral ventricle (between the thalamus, medially; and the caudate nucleus, laterally). Each basal vein begins near the anterior perforated substance. It is formed by union of the following.

(**a**) The anterior cerebral vein, which accompanies the anterior cerebral artery.

(**b**) The deep middle cerebral vein, which lies deep in the stem and posterior ramus of the lateral sulcus.

(**c**) Some **inferior striate veins** that emerge from the anterior perforated substance.

The great cerebral vein, formed by union of the two internal cerebral veins, passes posteriorly beneath the splenium of the corpus callosum, to end in the straight sinus. It receives the basal veins, some veins from the occipital lobes, and some from the corpus callosum.

The deep cerebral veins described above are responsible for draining the thalamus, the hypothalamus, the corpus striatum, the internal capsule, the corpus callosum, the septum pellucidum, and the choroid plexuses. Many tributaries of the internal cerebral veins extend beyond the corpus striatum into the white matter of the hemispheres. Here they establish communications with superficial veins. They can thus serve as alternative channels for draining parts of the cerebral cortex.

The upper part of the **thalamus** is drained by the tributaries of the internal cerebral vein (including the thalamostriate vein). The lower part of the thalamus, and the hypothalamus, are drained by veins that run downwards to end in a plexus of veins present in the interpeduncular fossa. This plexus drains into the cavernous and sphenoparietal sinuses, and into the basal veins.

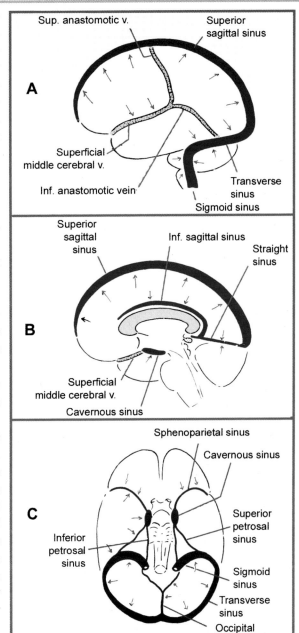

Fig. 21.12. Diagrams to show the position of the intracranial venous sinuses in relation to (A) the lateral, (B) medial, and (C) inferior aspects of the brain.

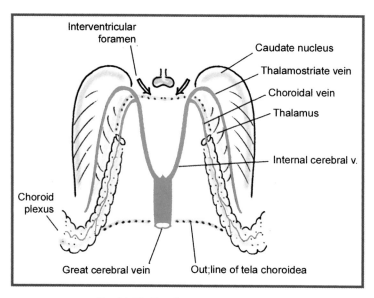

Fig. 21.13. The deep cerebral veins.

The **corpus striatum** and **internal capsule** are drained by two sets of striate veins. The **superior striate veins** run dorsally and drain into tributaries of the internal cerebral vein. The **inferior striate veins** run vertically downwards and emerge on the base of the brain through the anterior perforated substance. Here they end in the basal vein.

Veins of the cerebellum and brainstem

The veins from the upper surface of the **cerebellum** drain into the straight, transverse, and superior petrosal venous sinuses. Veins from the inferior surface drain into the right and left sigmoid, and inferior petrosal, sinuses; the occipital sinus and the straight sinus.

The veins of the **midbrain** drain into the great cerebral vein or into the basal vein. The **pons** and **medulla** drain into the superior and inferior petrosal sinuses, the transverse sinus and the occipital sinus. Inferiorly, the veins of the medulla are continuous with the veins of the spinal cord.

BLOOD-BRAIN BARRIER

It has been observed that while some substances can pass from the blood into the brain with ease, others are prevented from doing so. This has given rise to the concept of a selective barrier between blood and the brain. Anatomically, the structures that could constitute the barrier are as follows.

(**a**) Capillary endothelium.

(**b**) Basement membrane of the endothelium.

(**c**) Closely applied to the vessels there are numerous processes of astrocytes. It has been estimated that these processes cover about eighty five percent of the capillary surface.

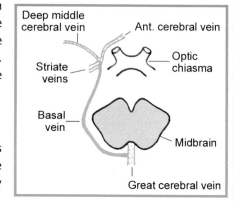

Fig. 21.14. Formation of the basal vein.

Some areas of the brain (and related structures) appear to be devoid of a blood-brain barrier. These include the pineal body, the hypophysis cerebri, the choroid plexus, the median eminence (hypothalamus) and some specialised areas of ependyma in the walls of the third and fourth ventricles.

The blood brain barrier can break down following ischaemia or infection in the brain. The barrier can also break down in trauma and through the action of toxins. Some drugs, including some antibiotics, pass through the barrier but some others cannot.

In infants bilirubin can pass through the barrier. There is danger of encephalitis if bilirubin levels are high (seen as jaundice in the newborn or **kernicterus**).

(**d**) Traditionally it has been taught that the subarachnoid space is continuous with perivascular spaces (present around blood vessels passing into the brain). However, it has now been shown that the perivascular spaces, and the subpial space, are completely cut off from the subarachnoid space by pia mater (which is reflected onto arteries as a sleeve). The pia mater, therefore, contributes to the establishment of the blood brain barrier.

CONTROL OF CEREBRAL BLOOD FLOW

Cerebral blood flow is influenced by sympathetic nerves. (which are present around arteries as they pass through the subarachnoid space). Adrenergic nerve fibres within the brain also end on blood vessels.

Blood flow through the brain does not markedly vary with alterations in blood pressure. Blood flow through a part of the brain increases when that part is "active". Such areas can be visualised by using the technique of **positron emission tomography** (PET). Studies using the technique are throwing much light on functions of various areas. PET can be combined with **magnetic resonance imaging** (see Chapter 22) to provide accurate localisation of the areas showing altered blood flow.

BASIC

Intracranial haemorrhage

An intracranial haemorrhage may be of the following types.

1. **Extradural haemorrhage** (between dura mater and overlying bone) is usually a result of fracture of the skull. In factures of the base of the skull blood may leak into the nose, the pharynx or the ear. An extradural haematoma may form. One important cause of this is bleeding from the middle meningeal artery in fractures of the squamous temporal bone.

2. **Subdural haemorrhage** (between dura mater and arachnoid mater) is usually caused by rupture of cerebral veins as they pass through this space to reach venous sinuses. This can happen in head injuries. Such bleeding can be extensive and can act as a space occupying lesion.

3. **Subarachnoid haemorrhage** (between arachnoid mater and pia mater) often occurs by rupture of aneurysms on the base of the skull.

4. **Haemorrhage into brain tissue** (e.g. cerebral haemorrhage) is usually a result of rupture of an artery supplying the region.

CLINICAL

22 : Some Investigative Procedures

In many of the preceding chapters we have briefly mentioned some of the manifestations of neurological disorders. Diagnosis of the site, and nature, of disease depends on an analysis of the total picture presented by the patient. It is here that knowledge of neuroanatomy becomes important. It is this knowledge that enables the physician to pinpoint the region, involvement of which could explain the various manifestations observed.

In some cases considerable help in localisation of lesions and in diagnosis of their nature, may be obtained by the use of certain investigative procedures that are briefly mentioned below.

Lumbar Puncture

See Chapter 20, page 276.

Traditional Radiological Procedures

(**1**) Plain radiographs of the skull may give evidence of disease when the skull bones are affected, or when there are areas of calcification.

(**2**) Air injected into the subarachnoid space through lumbar puncture ascends in the spinal subarachnoid space to the cranial cavity. The air can be seen in radiographs. This procedure is called **pneumoencephalography.** The air injected may enter the ventricles. Their outlines can then be seen. (This procedure is no longer used and is of historical interest only).

(**3**) See ventriculography, Chapter 20, page 277.

(**4**) The vascular system of the brain can be visualised by injecting radio-opaque material into the common carotid or vertebral arteries (**Cerebral angiography**). Radiographs taken immediately after the injection reveal the arterial pattern. The capillary and venous patterns can be seen after brief intervals.

(**5**) The spinal subarachnoid space can be visualised by injecting radio-opaque material (**myelography**).

Abnormal appearances seen with the procedures mentioned above help in determining the nature and location of tumours or other masses present in relation to the brain or spinal cord.

Computed Tomography

The term **tomography** has been applied to radiological methods in which tissues lying in a particular plane are visualised.

In recent years a technique has been developed in which a series of levels studied in this way are analysed using computers. Such analysis provides images giving a remarkable degree of detail (Fig. 22.1). The procedure is called **computed tomography** or CT scan.

The technique has revolutionised neurological diagnosis, and has rendered many older techniques obsolete. Tumours, areas of haemorrhage, and various other lesions can be identified with confidence.

In Fig. 22.1 note that the overall appearance is similar to that of a radiograph, as the most radio-opaque structures (eg., bones) appear white; the most radio-lucent structures (e.g., air filled cavities) appear black; and other tissues show shades of grey. Also note the distinctive granular appearance of normal brain tissue. Large masses of grey matter (e.g., the thalamus) appear somewhat lighter in colour than surrounding matter and can, therefore, be distinguished. The appearances that are characteristic of normal tissue are altered by disease.

Magnetic Resonance Imaging (MRI)

This is a complex technique in which radio-active materials, strong magnetic fields, and radio pulses are used to create images of outstanding clarity (Figs 22.2 to 22.4)). The images are distinctly superior

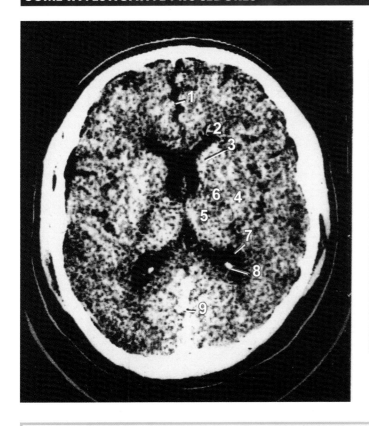

Fig. 22.1. Transverse sectional view of the cerebral hemisphere obtained in a living person by CT scan. The cut passes through the internal capsule.

1. Median longitudinal fissure.
2. Anterior horn of lateral ventricle. 3. Caudate nucleus.
4. Lentiform nucleus.
5. Thalamus. 6. Internal capsule (posterior limb). 7. Lateral ventricle at junction of central part and posterior horn.
8. Choroid plexus.
9. Falx cerebri.

This fugure is reproduced by courtesy of Prof. S.C. Srivastava

to those of CT scans. The technique is specially useful for demonstrating normal and abnormal tissues, particularly in the posterior cranial fossa and in the vertebral canal.

MRI images are of two standard types. In T1 images (also called T1 weighted images) the areas occupied by CSF are black while other tissues are seen in shades of grey (Fig. 22.2). In T2 images (also called T2 weighted images) areas occupied by CSF are white. Images intermediate between T1 and T2 (called **proton density images**) can also be obtained. Such images show grey and white matter of the brain in very good contrast.

Using MRI, sectional appearances in sagittal, coronal and transverse planes can be obtained. The ability to image structures in multiple planes makes spatial localisation and differentiation of lesions more accurate. Sagittal sections (Fig. 22.3) are particularly useful in demonstrating the brainstem and spinal cord, without overlying bone artefacts. Coronal sections provide a good display of the cerebral and cerebellar hemispheres; and brainstem displacement can be seen when present.

In additional to sectional images in different planes three dimensional pictures can also be produced (by combining information from a series of sectional views).

The main advantages of MRI are high contrast, good soft tissue discrimination, absence of bone and metal artefacts, and the use of non-ionizing radiation. MRI is a powerful diagnostic tool, and it can detect the majority of intracranial lesions.

However, like all other techniques, MRI has its limitations. These are high cost, long time required for collecting data, and the fact that the patient being investigated has to be confined within a tube for a prolonged period (during which there can be difficulty in monitoring a critically ill patient). The machine is very noisy. Very fat persons or those with metallic implants or pacemakers cannot be subjected to this technique.

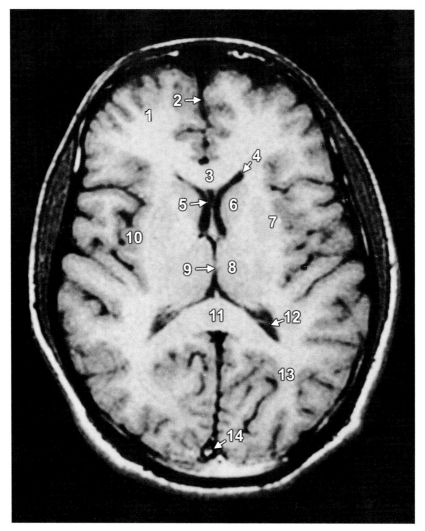

Fig. 22.2. Sectional view of cerebral hemisphere obtained in a living person by the technique of magnetic resonance imaging (MRI).

1. Frontal lobe. 2. Median longitudinal fissure. 3. Genu of corpus callosum.
4. Anterior horn of lateral ventricle. 5. Septum pellucidum (double layered).
6. Caudate nucleus. 7. Lentiform nucleus. 8. Thalamus. 9. Third ventricle.
10. Insula. 11. Splenium of corpus callosum. 12. Posterior horn of lateral ventricle.
13. Occipital lobe. 14. Superior sagittal sinus.
Figures 22.2 to 22.4 are reproduced by kind courtesy of Dr. R.K. Yadav.

MR Angiography

Modifications of the standard MRI techniques can used to obtain images of selected tissues only. Large blood vessels can be demonstrated without injecting contrast media into them. Blood flow through vessels can also be measured. Three dimensional images of intracranial arteries can also be obtained. However, MR angiography is not an acceptable substitute for conventional angiography for imaging of small blood vessels; and in patients with suspected subarachnoid haemorrhage, or aneurysms.

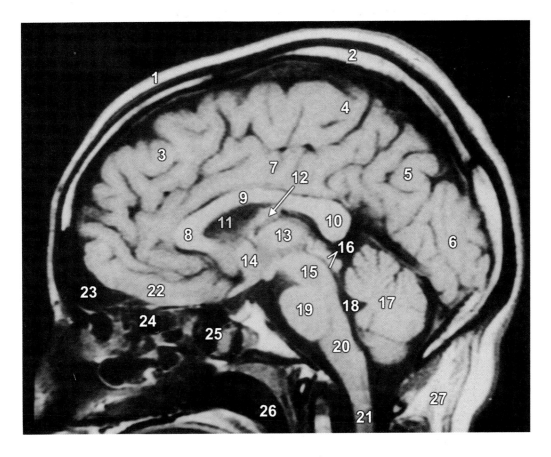

Fig. 22.3. Sagittal sectional view. Magnetic resonance imaging (T1).
Note the vast amount of detail that can be seen.
1. Scalp. 2. Skull. 3. Medial frontal gyrus. 4. Paracentral lobule. 5. Precuneus. 6. Cuneus.
7. Gyrus cinguli. 8, 9, 10. Genu, trunk and splenium of corpus callosum. 11. Lateral ventricle.
12. Fornix. 13. Thalamus. 14. Hypothalamus. 15. Midbrain. 16. Colliculi and aqueduct.
17. Cerebellum (Vermis). 18. Fourth ventricle. 19. Pons. 20. Medulla, 21. Spinal cord.
22. Gyrus rectus. 23. Frontal air sinus. 24. Ethmoidal air sinuses. 25. Sphenoidal sinus.
26. Nasopharynx. 27. Fat in suboccipital region.

Digital Subtraction Angiography (DSA)

This is a computerised technique in which blood vessels can be imaged using very low concentrations of contrast media (thus reducing chances of adverse effects that sometimes occur in conventional angiography). Bones and other tissues are removed from the image (by the computer through a technique called digital substraction) revealing blood vessels clearly (Fig. 22.4).

There are two variations of DSA, one using intravenous injection of contrast medium, and the other in which the medium is injected directly into arteries.

Intravenous DSA is easy to perform, there being no need for anaesthesia. Discomfort to the patient is minimal. However, resolution of the images obtained is not very good. As dye reaches all intracranial arteries simultaneously, there is overlapping of vessels of the right and left sides resulting in confusion.

In arterial DSA a small quantity of much diluted contrast medium is injected directly into the selected artery. Images of excellent quality are obtained (Fig. 22.4). The recording and playback facilities provided by DSA equipment considerably shorten the time required for the procedure.

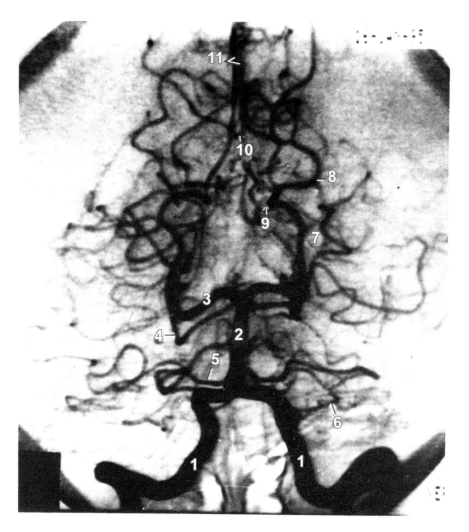

Fig. 22.4. Digital subtraction angiography (DSA). Diluted contrast medium was injected into the left vertebral artery (1). The dye has filled the vertebral artery of the opposite side, the basilar artery (2), and the posterior cerebral artery (3). The posterior inferior cerebellar branch of the vertebral artery (6), the anterior inferior cerebellar (5) and superior cerebellar branches (4) of the basilar artery are seen. Dye has flowed through the posterior communicating artery (7) into the carotid system. The terminal part of the internal carotid artery (9), the middle cerebral artery (8), and the anterior cerebral arteries (11) are outlined. The anterior communicating artery can also be identified (10). Numerous small branches of various arteries are also seen.

Ultrasound methods

Ultrasound waves applied to any part of the body are reflected back by various structures. The reflected waves (or echo) can be picked up and visualised on a screen. Images of internal organs can be obtained in this way. In the field of neurology ultrasound waves can be used to detect a shift of midline structures e.g., the falx cerebri.

The technique is called *echoencephalography.*

Xenon Scan

Various other scanning methods using radioactive isotopes are being introduced. If solutions containing a radioactive isotope of xenon are injected into the common carotid artery, radiations can be picked up using a gamma camera. Using this method it is possible to determine the blood flow through different parts of the brain; and to see the changes that take place during various kinds of activity. For example, if a hand is moved while such pictures are being taken the 'hand area' of the motor cortex shows increased blood flow.

Positron Emission Tomography (PET)

In this technique positron emitting isotopes (radionucleides including ^{15}O, ^{11}C and ^{18}F) are used. The technique allows measurement of blood flow through specific areas of brain tissue. Using this method it is possible to determine areas of brain that are 'active' when performing a particular action. PET is a technique for functional rather than structural imaging. It can be combined with MRI for accurate localisation of areas involved. PET can also be used to measure oxygen uptake, or glucose utilisation. Regions containing specific neuropeptides can be recognised.

Electrophysiological Methods

(1) Information about the functioning of the brain can be obtained by a study of the patterns of electrical activity within it. Electrodes are applied over the scalp at various points. These are connected to a machine which records the electrical potentials. The procedure is called **electroencephalography** or EEG).

(2) Electrical activity precedes or accompanies muscle contraction. This can be recorded by suitable machines. The procedure is called **electromyography** or EMG. It is employed for the study of various disorders of skeletal muscle. It is also a valuable tool for investigating the normal actions of muscles.

(3) The rate of conduction in nerve fibres can also be measured by electrical methods.

(4) One of the standard methods of neurophysiological investigation has been to stimulate a particular part of the nervous system and to record **evoked potentials** from other regions. Most such experiments have been done on animals after exposing the regions concerned. Sophisticated instruments are now available that enable similar studies to be done in human subjects through surface electrodes. Using such methods it is possible to determine the integrity (or otherwise) of various pathways.

The brief review of techniques given above will show that the study of neurology is a rapidly advancing science. With advances in instrumentation it is inevitable that our concepts of structure, function, and disease in the nervous system will undergo many modifications. Any student would be well advised, therefore, to keep a very open mind receptive to new ideas and concepts.

RELATED TOPICS IN OTHER CHAPTERS

Index

Gyrus (continued)
  semilunaris, 225
  splenial, 233
  supramarginal, 82
  temporal, inferior, 82
  temporal, middle, 82
  temporal, superior, 82
  temporal, transverse, 82, 91
  uncinate, 225
Haemorrhage, 2
  extradural, 289
  into brain tissue, 289
  pontine, 286
  subarachnoid, 289
  subdural, 289
Heart, innervation, 263
Hemianopia, 249
  heteronymous, 249
  heteronymous, bitemporal, 249
  homonymous, 249
  nasal, 249
Hemibalism, 213
Hemiplegia, 103
Herpes zoster, 33
Hippocampus, 233, 237
Hydrocephalus, 276
  congenital, 94
Hydromyelia, 94
Hyperaesthesia, 111
Hypoaesthesia, 111
Hypoalgesia, 111
Hypophysis, 198
  neuro-, 199
Hypothalamus, 83, 87, 88, 193
  connections of, 196
  control of adenohypophysis, 200
  control of hypophysis cerebri, 198
  functions of, 201
  regions of, 195
  zones of, 193
Incisure, preoccipital, 80
Indusium griseum, 233
Insula, 81
Internal capsule, 87, 91, 104, 240
  anterior limb of, 92
  fibres passing through, 240
  genu of, 92
  posterior limb of, 92
  retrolentiform part, 92
  sublentiform part, 92

Internode, 14
Ischaemic neuritis, 20
Isthmus, 84
Joint, flail, 181
Junction,neuromuscular, 42
Kernicterus, 289

Lamina
  alar, 62
  basal, 62
  cribrosa, 248
  terminalis, 84
Lemniscus, 7
  lateral, 123
  medial, 67, 70, 107, 138
  spinal, 109, 123
Leptomeninges, 30
Lesion, space occupying, 3
Limen insulae, 85

Lobe
  frontal, 80, 81
  limbic, 228
  occipital, 80
  parietal, 80
  piriform, 225
  temporal, 80, 82
Lobule
  paracentral, 84
  parcentral, 80
  parietal, inferior, 82
  parietal, superior, 82
Locus coeruleus, 157, 273
Lumbar puncture, 34, 275, 276
Macrocephaly, 27, 94
Macula lutea, 245
Magnetic resonance imaging, 290
Medulla
  central canal of, 66
  development of, 160
  gross anatomy, 63
  internal structure, 137
  internal structure, preliminary, 66
Melatonin, 202
Meningocoele, 94
Meningoencephalocoele, 94
Meningomyelocoele, 94
Mesaxon, 5
Meta-thalamus, 191
Microcephaly, 27, 94